OCULAR HISTOLOGY

BEN S. FINE, M.D.

**Research Associate, Department of Ophthalmic
Pathology, Armed Forces Institute of Pathology;
Associate Research Professor of Ophthalmology,
The George Washington University;
Senior Attending Ophthalmologist, The Washington
Hospital Center, Washington, D.C.;
Clinical Professor of Pathology,
Uniformed Services University of the Health Sciences,
Bethesda, Maryland**

MYRON YANOFF, M.D., F.A.C.S.

**Chairman and William F. Norris and George E. deSchweinitz
Professor of Ophthalmology, Department of Ophthalmology,
University of Pennsylvania School of Medicine and
Presbyterian-University of Pennsylvania Medical Center;
Director, Scheie Eye Institute, Philadelphia, Pennsylvania**

with a contribution by

FREDERICK A. JAKOBIEC, M.D., D.Sc.,
TAKEO IWAMOTO, M.D.

OCULAR HISTOLOGY

A TEXT AND ATLAS

SECOND EDITION

WITH 18 COLOR ILLUSTRATIONS

MEDICAL DEPARTMENT
Harper & Row, Publishers
Hagerstown, Maryland
New York, San Francisco, London

79 80 81 82 83 84   10 9 8 7 6 5 4 3 2 1

For information address Medical Department, Harper & Row, Publishers, Inc.,
2350 Virginia Avenue, Hagerstown, Maryland 21740

Library of Congress Cataloging in Publication Data

Fine, Ben S
  Ocular histology.

  Includes bibliographies and index.
  1. Eye—Anatomy. I. Yanoff, Myron, joint author.
II. Title.
QM511.F55 1979   611'.0189'84   78–18686
ISBN 0–06–140819–0

To our wives and children

CONTENTS

Contributors   ix

Forewords to the First Edition   xi

Preface to the Second Edition   xiii

Preface to the First Edition   xv

1 Electron Microscopy: Techniques and Interpretation   1

2 The Cell and Its Contents   17

3 Cell Interrelations   31

4 Extracellular Materials   37

5 Arrangement of Tissues and Cells   51

6 The Retina   59

7 The Vitreous Body   129

8 The Lens   147

9 The Cornea and Sclera   161

10 The Uveal Tract 195

11 The Anterior Chamber Angle 249

12 The Optic Nerve 271

13 The Ocular Adnexa: Lids, Conjunctiva, and Orbit 289
Frederick A. Jakobiec, Takeo Iwamoto

Index 343

CONTRIBUTORS

TAKEO IWAMOTO, M.D.

Associate Professor of Clinical Ophthalmology, College of Physicians and Surgeons, Columbia University, New York, New York

FREDERICK A. JAKOBIEC, M.D., D.Sc.

Assistant Professor of Clinical Ophthalmology and Surgical Pathology, College of Physicians and Surgeons, Columbia University; Director, Algernon B. Reese Laboratory of Ophthalmic Pathology, Edward S. Harkness Eye Institute, New York, New York

BRUCE H. SMITH

Captain, MC, USN; Director, Armed Forces Institute of Pathology, Washington, D.C.

LORENZ E. ZIMMERMAN, M.D.

Chief, Ophthalmic Pathology Branch, Armed Forces Institute of Pathology, Washington, D.C.

FOREWORDS TO THE FIRST EDITION

This text and atlas of ocular histology is published as a part of the observances of the golden anniversary of the American Registry of Pathology, which had its origins in the Registry of Ophthalmic Pathology in 1921. Fifty years ago, when American ophthalmic pathology was in its infancy, the members of the American Academy of Ophthalmology and Otolaryngology had the foresight to create a histopathology laboratory for the study of ocular tissues at the old Army Medical Museum, which was then under the guidance of Major George Callender, the curator. Since then, the Registry of Ophthalmic Pathology has grown to include over 90,000 specimens, and the Registry itself has expanded to encompass 27 separate registries under the overall name of the American Registry of Pathology, itself one of four departments in the Armed Forces Institute of Pathology. The Registry of Ophthalmic Pathology, now under the guidance of Dr. Lorenz E. Zimmerman, has become a major force in ophthalmic pathology today, and is responsible for a very heavy program in consultation, education, and research in this specialty.

The years of experience and the careful and dedicated work of the authors are clearly demonstrated in this volume. The staff of the Armed Forces Institute of Pathology takes pride in having been able to assist the authors in the preparation and completion of this excellent book.

BRUCE H. SMITH
Captain, MC, USN
Director, Armed Forces
Institute of Pathology
1971

As this new book by two former Fellows at the Armed Forces Institute of Pathology (AFIP) goes to press, we are celebrating the fiftieth anniversary of the establishment of our Ophthalmic Pathology Laboratory. The necessary organizational agreements for this laboratory were concluded in 1921, and the facility became operational in 1922. Under the guidance of such dedicated pioneers as Callender, Ash, DeCoursey, and Wilder, this laboratory produced many prize-winning exhibits, a number of important research papers based on cases contributed to the Registry of Ophthalmic Pathology, and a series of atlases published by the American Registry of Pathology.

During the period between its founding in 1921 and 1955, the laboratory was housed in the old Army Medical Museum building on the Mall near the Capitol. Space was extremely limited, facilities outmoded, and modern research impossible. By the end of World War II a backlog of several thousand cases had accumulated, and this situation continued during the hectic period of the Korean conflict. Needless to say, the staff in its cramped quarters was nearly overwhelmed.

In 1955, the AFIP moved into its new home on the grounds of the Walter Reed Army Medical Center, a modern research building where more space for a larger staff and excellent facilities for experimental pathology and electron microscopy became available for the first time. It was shortly after we moved into the new building that Ben Fine—still in residency at the District of Columbia General Hospital—began to visit the AFIP to study ophthalmic pathology at every opportunity. Upon completion of his clinical training, he was awarded a full-time NIH fellowship in ophthalmic pathology at the AFIP, and rapidly became one of our most active investigators. Soon after the arrival of the first electron microscope at the AFIP in 1958, Ben Fine teamed with A.J. Tousimis, then a graduate student in biophysics working at the AFIP, and began his electron microscopic studies of ocular tissues.

Thus began not only Ben Fine's career as one of the world's foremost authorities on electron microscopy of the eye, but also the modern training program in ophthalmic histology and pathology at the AFIP. Before our move into the new building, training and research programs were necessarily limited to descriptive pathology, clinicopathologic investigations, and a very limited amount of histochemistry. In our new quarters it gradually became possible to broaden the training and research opportunities, and Ben Fine was the first and certainly one of the most outstanding of a group of about 50 Fellows who have profited by the opportunities made possible through this expanding program.

Myron Yanoff, another former Fellow in Ophthalmic Pathology at the AFIP, is also a pioneer. As the scope of ophthalmic pathology and ophthalmic research is rapidly enlarging, a number of those who have embarked on careers in ocular pathology during the past few years have found it desirable to avail themselves of more than the ordinary formal training, with the expanded objectives of Board certification in both pathologic anatomy and ophthalmology. Myron Yanoff was one of the first to obtain such dual certification.

Together, Drs. Fine and Yanoff are a most interesting team. While both have maintained an active practice of clinical ophthalmology, they are nevertheless completely dedicated to their half-time laboratory work. Both are stimulating teachers who are playing important roles in the formal education of residents and Fellows under their tutelage. The need for a suitable textbook on ocular histology to assist them in their teaching activities provided the incentive for the preparation of this volume. Needless to say, I encouraged them to proceed with their plans, as have the various administrative officers who have been at the AFIP since their work was started. The result is this book—one of the very first to incorporate electron microscopic observations into a detailed presentation of the normal structure of ocular tissues.

I am very proud that the authors of this new book are among my former Fellows, and that the environment of our laboratory, now observing its golden anniversary, was so conducive for their work. I trust that those who use it will find this book a fitting gem to set off this golden crown.

LORENZ E. ZIMMERMAN, M.D.
Chief, Ophthalmic Pathology Branch
Armed Forces Institute of Pathology
1972

PREFACE TO THE SECOND EDITION

It is more than six years since the first edition of Ocular Histology was published. Since that time anatomic studies of ocular tissues both normal and abnormal have continued to expand. Additional methods of inquiry, such as the use of the scanning electron microscope, electron dense tracers, and freeze fracture etching, have been widely applied. This second edition incorporates some examples of the new techniques and brings to the reader the new findings as well as interpretations in ocular histology.

Although our intent is to present normal ocular structure, it is difficult (and in fact undesirable) to divorce this presentation completely from changes that occur in pathologic ocular tissues or from clinical observations. For this reason a number of normal clinical observations (e.g., fundus photographs or fluorescein angiograms), which also represent one aspect of gross anatomy, are included in the text.

The presentation on ocular basement membranes has been expanded to include some changes associated with aging, as well as some basement membrane alterations present in pathologic tissues. An examination of basement membranes produced by abnormal cells often can provide us with a better understanding of cell function or malfunction, even though the cell structures themselves may appear normal. Our classification of basement membranes, therefore, has been improved and expanded to include both normal and abnormal structures that cells may produce.

We have also considerably revised the description of the foveomacular region of the retina. Descriptive terminology in this area differs widely in usage between anatomist and clinician and this has lead to confusion. We point out the different usages of terms and offer a method of equating the anatomic terms with the clinical ones. Anatomic terms are used here preferentially with the widely used clinical equivalents in parentheses.

Although every attempt was made to limit the size of the new edition and to present our material concisely, we found it necessary to add text and figures to existing chapters. A number of line drawings have been improved, and a few have been added. An entirely new chapter by Drs. Jakobiec and Iwamoto on the ocular adnexa, including lids, conjunctiva, and orbit, will make this book more useful than before to students of ophthalmology and ocular pathology.

Although cytologic terminology has become more uniform since our first edition, there still remains a number of alternate terms used widely by different investigators. Some of the alternate terms are included in parentheses or footnotes. Above all, we have tried to present as consistent a terminology as possible to best meet the needs of the student, the researcher, and the clinician.

We are grateful to Efrain Perez-Rosario for his continued assistance in all aspects of tissue preparation for both scanning and transmission electron microscopy, to James Stripling for technical assistance, to Phyllis Stripling for retyping the manuscript, and to Elizabeth McDonnell for preparing additional line drawings.

B.S.F.
M.Y.

PREFACE TO THE FIRST EDITION

This book is an outgrowth of a series of lectures presented to postgraduate students attending the biannual course in ophthalmic pathology at the Armed Forces Institute of Pathology and to those attending the postgraduate course in ophthalmology at the University of Pennsylvania in Philadelphia.

Although a number of references currently are available for ophthalmic histology, the observations that can be made by electron microscopy remain rather widely scattered throughout the literature and therefore are not readily available to the student. We have endeavored to assemble a text that would bridge the gap between conventional light microscopy and electron microscopy. We also have attempted to provide a short introduction to contemporary cytology which may serve as a background for the more extensive presentations that are currently available.

Our aim is to present, in as systematic and simplified a manner as possible, a cytologic *method* or approach for examining the way in which ocular tissues are assembled and arranged, and to point out, wherever possible, any clinical relevance that the anatomic observations may have. We hope that this dual approach will be of value to ophthalmologists, to those who require a contemporary histologic basis from which to investigate a variety of problems in ocular pathology, as well as to others interested in the visual sciences.

It is in this sense of contemporary cytology that the eye, despite its content of tissues with high degrees of specialization, may be considered a sequestered microcosm of the tissues of the body. The eye not only contains examples of most other tissues, but frequently, because of their high degree of functional specialization, may dramatically illustrate a high degree of morphologic exaggeration. For example, the photoreceptor outer segments provide striking illustrations of the degree to which a cilium of a sensory cell may be altered; the pigmented or light-absorbing cells produce melanin granules not in one but in at least two characteristic and rather large sizes; the vitreous body is not only highly transparent, but also one of the most delicate collagenous tissues to be found in man; and the anterior lens capsule is by far the thickest basement membrane in the body. On the other hand, this high degree of specialization does not completely obscure the close relationship of ocular tissues to others: the retina is still part of the central nervous system, the cornea and lens are derivatives of the skin, and the ciliary epithelium is a neuroepithelial gland. From the characteristic and highly specialized morphologic features, therefore, we can, in turn, often infer something about function.

The cytologic examples used are all taken from ocular tissues, primarily human. Most of the preparations are original, as are some of the concepts; for the latter we accept responsibility. In instances where there is a difference of opinion, either in definition or in terminology, or where additional clarification seems warranted, explanatory footnotes are included. The point of view preferred by the authors is presented as the "accepted opinion." No doubt in time some of the concepts and even some of the terminology presented will be further modified.

The authors wish to thank all who have helped in the preparation of this text. In particular, we also wish to dedicate this book in part to Dr. Maximilian Salzmann, who, by 1912, had already stated most of what we have come to say here, and to Dr. Lorenz E. Zimmerman, for creating the environment in which this work was possible.

Our special thanks to Margaret J. Patton for her invaluable and patient assistance in the preparation of the manuscript; to Genevieve C. Overmyer, for all of the related typing of the manuscript; and to Drs. David Barsky, Joseph W. Berkow, Jay L. Helfgott, David M. Kozart, Michael Ramsey, Benjamin Rones, Harold G. Scheie, Mark O. M. Ts'o, Roderick Willis, and Lorenz E. Zimmerman, for encouragement and editorial comments. In addition, we are grateful to John C. Barber, Elizabeth McDonnell, and Frances Schulz, of the Armed Forces Institute of Pathology, for their help with many of the line drawings; and to Drs. Mark O. M. Ts'o, Michael Mund, Merlyn Rodrigues, Peter Wobmann, and Max Helfgott, for their kindness in contributing illustrations. John M. Wehrung, Director of the Sperry Rand Microanalysis Laboratory in Rockville, Maryland, gave us invaluable assistance with the scanning electron microscopy.

Finally, we extend our sincere appreciation to Efrain Perez-Rosario, who for more than a decade has assisted in all of the preparation and sectioning techniques required for our various publications and for this book.

Acknowledgment is given for the support received for much of this work from contract No. DA–49–193–MD–2680, from the Medical Research and Development Command, United States Army, Washington, D.C., and from research grants Nos. EY–00289, EY–00397, and EY–00133 and training grant No. EY–00032 from the National Eye Institute (formerly part of the National Institute for Neurological Diseases and Blindness), National Institutes of Health, Bethesda, Maryland.

B.S.F.
M.Y.

OCULAR HISTOLOGY

chapter 1

ELECTRON MICROSCOPY: TECHNIQUES AND INTERPRETATION

THE TRANSMISSION ELECTRON MICROSCOPE   3

TISSUE PREPARATION   3

  SECTIONING, MOUNTING, AND

      EMBEDDING   3

  FIXATION   4

SPECIAL METHODS OF EXAMINATION   4

  SHADOW-CASTING   5

  SURFACE REPLICATION   5

  FREEZE-FRACTURE–ETCH   6

  SCANNING ELECTRON MICROSCOPY   7

  "STAINING" AND HISTOCHEMICAL

      METHODS   9

  TRACERS FOR TRANSPORT MECHANISMS   10

  AUTORADIOGRAPHY   11

PHOTOGRAPHY   12

  TECHNIQUE   12

  INTERPRETATION   12

THE TRANSMISSION ELECTRON MICROSCOPE

The transmission electron microscope (TEM) is the electronic counterpart of the inverted compound light microscope (15) (Fig. 1–1). The source of light is replaced by a source of electrons, usually a heated tungsten filament from which the electrons are boiled off. The electrons (at a potential of 50–60 kV generally) are fired down an evacuated column (*i.e.*, a vacuum approximately that of a good television tube) through the central apertures of a series of circular electromagnets. Control of current flow through these circular electromagnets collimates, spreads, or contracts this beam, which, like the electromagnetic spectrum, travels in waves. As with the light microscope, the first lens, the one near the illuminating source, is called the condenser lens; the next, near the specimen, is called the objective lens; the last, which is not a lens into which the observer looks but rather one that projects the image onto a fluorescent screen, is called a projector lens. The screen fluoresces generally in some shade of green, and the image is viewed as a shadow on this green background. A permanent record is obtained by moving the screen aside temporarily and allowing the imaged beam to fall directly on a photographic emulsion (glass plate or cut film).

A latent image is produced in silver halide crystals and is brought out subsequently by conventional photographic development techniques. Because the various wavelengths within the electron beam cannot be separated out, all the photographs are in shades of black and white. The vacuum of the column generally precludes the examination of living tissue. With the transmission electron microscope direct magnifications of from ~500 × to ~150,000 × can be obtained with resolutions that may exceed 5 A. Greater enlargement can be secured by conventional photographic methods, but the usefulness of this procedure is limited.

TISSUE PREPARATION

SECTIONING, MOUNTING, AND EMBEDDING

Because an electron beam of 50–60 kV cannot penetrate conventional tissue slices or sections,

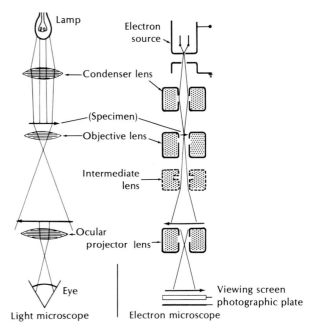

FIG. 1–1. Schematic drawing illustrating analogy between compound light microscope and transmission electron microscope. (Fine BS *et al.*: Arch Ophthalmol 62:931, 1959)

methods were developed to cut sections thin enough to allow *some* of the electrons to be *transmitted* through them (18, 26). The sections necessarily range from 200–600 A in thickness.* Because specimens are difficult to hold rigidly for thin sectioning, plastic embedding materials were introduced (methacrylates at first, now almost universally replaced by epoxy [21] or other resins). The tissue embedded in plastic and mounted in a special microtome is cut with either a glass or a diamond knife. The diamond knife is most useful for cutting hard or dense

* A conventional section of ocular tissue measures 8–10μ in thickness; a tissue section for electron microscopy measures 200–600 Angstroms (A) or 20–60 nm. This difference can better be appreciated when the following relations are considered:

1 millimeter (mm) = 1000 microns (μ) or micrometers (μm)
1 micron (μ) = 1000 millimicrons (mμ) or nanometers (nm)
1 millimicron (mμ) = 10 Angstroms (A)
1 Angstrom (A) = 0.1 nanometer (0.1 nm)

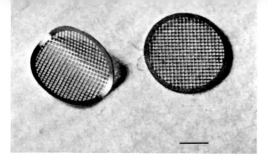

FIG. 1–2. Copper screens, or grids, commonly used to support tissue sections in electron microscope. Marker indicates 1 mm.

tissue (e.g., melanin-bearing cells or dense collagen, as in the cornea and sclera).

Microtomes of special design move the tissue forward in exceedingly small increments using either mechanical or thermal advancing mechanisms. More specialized microtomes automatically advance and section the tissue so that, with care, it can be sectioned serially.

The plastic-embedded tissue sections are then mounted on copper screens (or when necessary for special techniques, nickel or gold screens) called **grids** (Fig. 1–2), which are placed into the microscope column for examination. Only that tissue lying within an aperture in the grid can, of course, be observed. When a small area is to be examined, a number of sections usually are prepared in the event the area of interest is obscured by the metallic supporting gridwork. To minimize such occurrences or to permit proper sequencing when serial sections are examined, a variety of specially designed grids are available.

FIXATION

It has long been known that autolytic changes (especially vacuolation of the cytoplasm and chromatin aggregation of the nucleus) can occur in tissues prepared for light microscopy and are caused either by delay in fixation or improper fixation. Proper fixation is even more critical when the higher resolving power of the electron microscope is used for examination. Tissues, therefore, are usually fixed promptly on separation from their blood supply (immersion fixation) or *in situ* by intraarterial injection of the fixative (perfusion fixation). Because the fixative used most often (buffered osmium tetroxide) penetrates poorly, the tissue usually is cut into small blocks (~1–2 cu mm), so that the layer of interest lies within 1–2 mm of the fixative. A surface layer, such as retina, which is less than 1 mm thick, can be suitably fixed by

immersion alone while it is still adherent to its backing of adjacent tissues (choroid and sclera). Those tissues that are of no particular interest may be subsequently discarded.

The osmium tetroxide* fixative blackens all the tissue it touches so that topographic orientation may be difficult after fixation and small lesions may be hard to find. A more suitable, all-around fixative, cold 2% glutaraldehyde,† can, if used with care, penetrate larger blocks of tissue without blackening them and produce results roughly equivalent to initial fixation with buffered osmium. The osmium tetroxide, however, enhances the contrast of all cell membranes and most of their cytoplasmic particles. For adequate contrast enhancement in tissue sections, therefore, initial fixation in glutaraldehyde must be followed by treatment with osmium tetroxide unless, of course, there is special reason, as in a conflict of densities, to delete this additional step.

SPECIAL METHODS OF EXAMINATION

Various special examination techniques are available in electron microscopic studies. The topography, or three-dimensional appearance, of material to be examined can be obtained by the use of shadow-casting, surface replication,

---

* We have found Dalton's chrome-osmium fixative (10) very useful. Fixation times vary from a short exposure of 35 min for a tissue as delicate as the retina to as long as 1 hour for a tissue as dense as cornea.

† Cold (~5° C) glutaraldehyde as a 2% solution in phosphate buffer is a useful general fixative. This fixative also permits certain histochemical reactions to be carried out (e.g., as for horseradish peroxidase) prior to examination of the tissue by TEM. More recently, a mixture of Formalin (40% formaldehyde) and glutaraldehyde, either five parts Formalin and 0.5 part glutaraldehyde (31) or four parts Formalin and and one part glutaraldehyde (23) in the cold (~5° C) has been found to be a useful general fixative for ocular and other tissues.

or scanning electron microscopy (SEM). The contrast among cell components can be enhanced by "staining" or other histochemical methods, transport mechanisms can be followed by use of tracers such as ferritin, saccharated iron oxide, or horseradish peroxidase or by methods of autoradiography using radioactive tracers.

SHADOW-CASTING

This old method, used in transmission electron microscopy to enhance the three-dimensional appearance of particles or particulate matter, entails "spraying" them with a thin molecular layer of metal from an elevated, angled point source (15) (Fig. 1–3). Since the spray comes in from an angle, a zone behind the object (shadow) does not become coated. When the shadow-cast preparation is subsequently examined in the electron microscope, the region of the shadow allows the electron beam of the microscope to pass through more easily, producing greater exposure to the photographic plate. On the usual positive print (Fig. 1–4 A) the shadow is white, but the final illustration is deliberately reversed to show the shadow as dark (Fig. 1–4B).

The metallic coating is produced by vaporizing a small amount of metal (e.g., uranium,* palladium, chromium) on a heated tungsten filament in a vacuum chamber (Fig. 1–3). Since the filament is placed at a predetermined distance and height from the object to be coated, the three dimensions of the object can be determined by simple measurements. Tissue sections can also be studied by shadow-casting. For this purpose, they must be embedded in a plastic (e.g., methacrylate) that can be removed to produce some exposed three-dimensional material. The technique is nicely illustrated in the examination of the vitreous body (see Ch. 7) where the structural filaments and ground substances are seen almost *in situ*.

SURFACE REPLICATION

In a surface replication, either a thin or a thick plastic coat is applied to a surface, allowed to harden, and peeled away (11) The thin coat may be examined directly in the electron microscope or may be shadow-cast for enhancement of the surface detail. The thick coat may be

* Designated "U-shad" in this text.

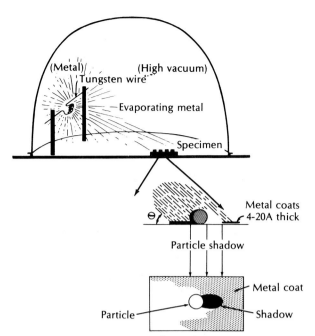

FIG. 1–3. Schematic drawing illustrating technique of shadow-casting. (Fine BS *et al.*: Arch Ophthalmol 62:931, 1959)

FIG. 1–4. Effect of shadow-casting. A. Melanin granules with light shadows. B. Reversal of photographic process produces dark shadows but white melanin granules. (× 10,000)

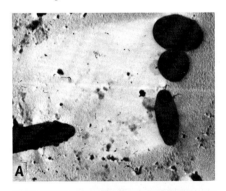

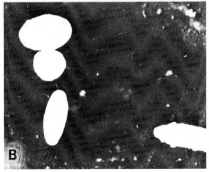

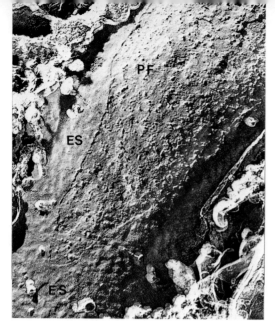

FIG. 1–5. Freeze-fracture-etch of plasmalemmal unit membrane of a protozoan. Unit membrane is split. **ES,** extracellular surface; **PF,** protoplasmic face of membrane. Note granularity characteristic of a fracture face. (× 25,000) (Courtesy of Dr. Russell Steere)

FIG. 1–6. Schematic drawing of scanning electron microscope. Transmission electron microscope is modified to scan or play a narrow beam of electrons over surface of specimen. The series of lines ultimately produced on display screen by secondary electrons is photographed with camera attachment.

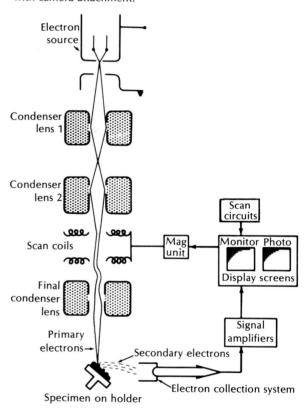

used to obtain a positive replica or it may be examined directly, in the manner of the thin coat.

FREEZE-FRACTURE-ETCH

A small piece of tissue, either fresh or fixed with or without cryoprotective agent, is frozen rapidly in liquid nitrogen. The tissue is attached to a cold specimen holder (−98 to −50° C), and then mechanically broken. The specimen fracture faces can then be shadowed directly (see section on shadow-casting earlier in this chapter) with metal, or the temperature is raised (to −98° C) to allow some of the surface ice to sublime off. The latter additional procedure exposes the free surface of the tissue which is said to be "etched." The fracturing process generally passes through the middle plane of unit membranes so that two inner surfaces or *faces* can be examined. The etching allows examination of the exposed *surface* of the specimen lying beneath the fracture plane. The exposed surfaces and/or faces are then shadow-cast with a metallic coating (e.g., platinum) producing a replica. Additional support for the nonuniform replica is provided by applying an overall film of carbon. The tissue is subsequently digested away, the replica floating free in the solution. After suitable washing, the replica is mounted on a grid for direct examination with the TEM, where it can be photographed.

The cell membrane has two hydrophilic *surfaces,* one facing the cell cytoplasm or protoplasm, and the other, the extracellular space. When exposed (Fig. 1–5), the two surfaces of the membrane are called **PS** (protoplasmic surface) and **ES** (extracellular surface) respectively (4). When split along the hydrophobic portion of the membrane by freeze fracture the two new *faces* so exposed are called **PF** (protoplasmic face) and **EF** (extracellular face). An older terminology used the terms **A face** (protoplasmic face) and **B face** (extracellular face) for the newly exposed surface of the split cell membrane.

SCANNING ELECTRON MICROSCOPY

The scanning electron microscope (SEM) is the electronic counterpart of the stereoscopic (dissecting) light microscope.

In scanning electron microscopy (Fig. 1–6) the electron beam is focused to an exceedingly small spot. The electron beam (or "probe") plays over (or "scans") the surface of a metal-coated, dried specimen. The beam or scan, controlled by deflecting magnetic fields, traverses the specimen in a series of sequential lines. Bombardment of the metal-coated ("shadowed") specimen produces *secondary* electrons, which are collected, translated into light, and subsequently converted into a series of corresponding sequential lines on an oscilloscope, much as is done on a television screen. The picture produced on the screen may be photographed, the photography being generally carried out on a second screen that duplicates the one used for viewing.

Preparation of specimens for scanning electron microscopy is essentially similar to their preparation for transmission electron microscopy except that upon reaching the stage of final dehydration in 100% propylene oxide, the tissue is not embedded in plastic but dried out by a method that prevents shrinkage or distortion of the tissue, a method called **critical point** drying (2, 9). The method involves drying the tissue without creating surface tension problems. Carbon dioxide was the gas used originally; while others have added the use of various fluorocarbons.

Slow air drying may be used on occasion if the tissues normally are resistant to distortion and rapid or preliminary observations are desired. The fixed, dried specimen is then mounted whole on a specimen mount ("pedestal" or "stub," Fig. 1–7) by means of an electrically conducting cement or tape. The mounted specimen is then lightly coated (shadowed) in a vacuum chamber with a thin film of metal (e.g., aluminum, gold, gold-palladium) to enhance the production of secondary electrons as well as to carry away charges that may be generated at the point of impact by the electron probe.

By this technique, striking three-dimensional enlargement of surfaces can be readily obtained (Fig. 1–8). Because of the great depth of field, direct magnification of from $\sim$20 $\times$ $\sim$50,000 $\times$ can be obtained, and resolutions to $\sim$150 Å or better. Information deep to the surface cannot be obtained unless the surface layer is removed by either chemical or physical means (Fig. 1–9).

For direct correlation of the surface view with internal structure, the dried specimen can be removed from the mount, reinfiltrated with propylene oxide, and subsequently embedded in Epon as for transmission electron microscopic examination. Thin (1.5μ) sections of this material can be made for correlative light microscopic study (Fig. 1–10) and thinner sections for correlative electron microscopic (*i.e.*, TEM) study (Fig. 1–11, see also Ch. 7).

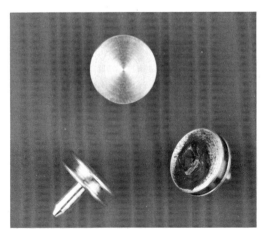

FIG. 1–7. Aluminum specimen mount (stub) for scanning electron microscope, without specimen, showing surface area for mounting (**above**), side view of stub (**left**), and stub with fixed, dried specimen mounted and prepared for examination (**right**). Diameter of mounting area here is 12 mm. Specimen mount illustrated here is aluminum pin-type variety designed for Cambridge scanning electron microscope, manufactured by Cambridge Instruments, England. Mounts for other makes of scanning electron microscopes differ in configuration and may be much larger in diameter.

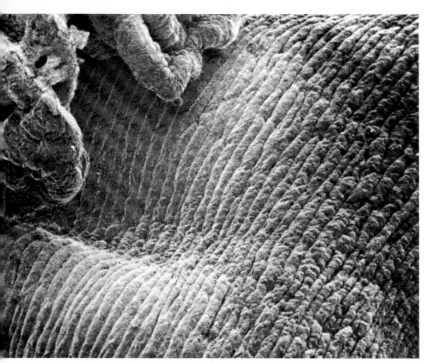

FIG. 1–8. Scanning electron micrograph of posterior surface of rhesus monkey iris. Circumferential furrows and ridges are clearly displayed. At left, overlying ciliary crests (processes) are seen. (× 165)

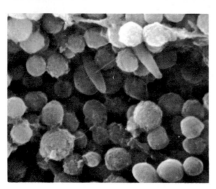

FIG. 1–9. Scanning electron micrograph of melanin granules within cells of iris pigment epithelium. Granules were exposed by tearing away enveloping cytoplasm. (× 7300)

FIG. 1–10. Epon-embedded section of iris stained with toluidine blue, made by embedding dried specimen in Figure 1–8 in Epon. (× 210) (AFIP Neg. 70-4570)

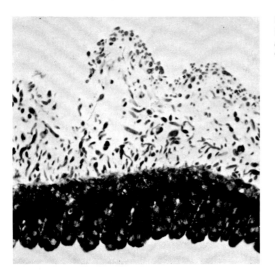

FIG. 1–11. A. Scanning electron micrograph of posterior surface of iris pigment epithelial layer. (× 1500) B. Transmission electron micrograph of same material after reinfiltration and embedding, showing that cell cytoplasm between granules is moderately well preserved except for many cytoplasmic holes. Thin basement membrane (**BM**) is poorly outlined. (× 16,500) C. Electron micrograph of iris stromal melanocyte. Myriad pinholes are present in cytoplasm between melanin granules and within substance of nucleus (**N**). (× 16,500)

"STAINING" AND HISTOCHEMICAL METHODS

Various compounds are used to enhance the contrast of membranes and particles in a cell or of various extracellular materials. Uranyl acetate, lead citrate, and lead hydroxide are used to treat tissue sections already improved from the native state by fixation with osmium tetroxide. In addition, lead citrate and lead hydroxide enhance the contrast of glycogen particles. Seligman *et al.* (27) have introduced a histochemical procedure, the thiosemicarbazide (TSC) method, for the demonstration of glycogen. This method is the electron miscropic equivalent of the periodic acid-Schiff (PAS) treatment so widely used in light microscopy (see Ch. 4). Thiosemicarbazide-positive particles can be even more accurately identified as glycogen when digested with diastase (3, 14) (Fig. 1–12).

The contrast of extracellular materials such as collagen and elastin can often be enhanced by treatment of the tissue section with either phosphotungstic acid or with the TSC method. More recently, another method (silver tetraphenylporphine sulfonate—Ag-TPPS) has been introduced (1), which stains the elastin of elastic tissue exceedingly densely and with considerable specificity (see Ch. 10).

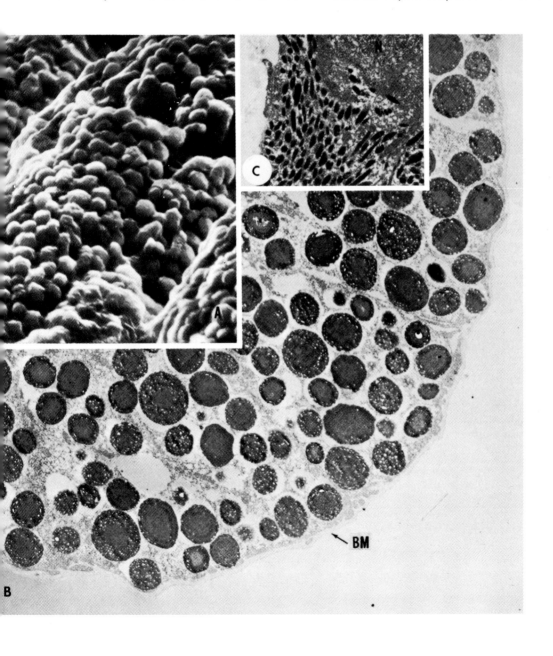

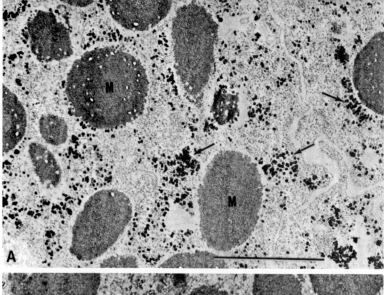

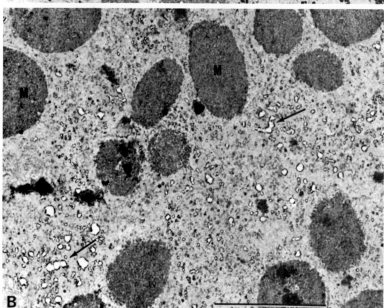

FIG. 1–12. Thiosemicarbazide method for glycogen detection. A. In TSC-treated section of iris pigment epithelium, glycogen particles (**arrows**) are exceedingly dense. (× 33,000) B. Pretreatment of tissue section with diastase digests out particles (**arrows**), identifying them as glycogen. (× 33,000) **M,** melanin granules. (Berkow JW, Fine BS: Am J Ophthalmol 69:994, 1970)

FIG. 1–13. Ferritin particles placed outside the vessel cross endothelial lining of an iris vessel. Note particles in large (macro) pinocytotic vesicles (**arrows**) as well as in lumen (**L**) and outside the vesicle (× 65,260) (Fine BS: Invest Ophthalmol 3:609, 1964)

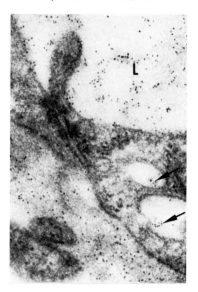

TRACERS FOR TRANSPORT MECHANISMS

A tracer useful for studying normal inter- or intracellular transport by electron microscopy should, of course, be one that has inherent electron density (e.g., ferritin [13], Fig. 1–13) or one that, by suitable treatment, can be made electron-dense (e.g., peroxidase or horseradish peroxidase [16], see Fig. 1–14) in the tissue prior to examination.

The tracer should follow as closely as possible normal pathways and should not stimulate or induce a new or abnormal activity on the part of the cells (e.g., pinocytosis or phagocytosis). For small passageways a small molecule is used (e.g., horseradish peroxidase, mol. wt 40,000; mol. diam, ~50 A). For larger passageways, a larger molecule may be used (e.g., ferritin—mol. wt ~60,000; mol. diam, ~100 A). For extremely large avenues, such as those that may be seen by light microscopy, much larger molecules can be used (e.g., dextrans [28] requiring subsequent color staining—i.e., PAS treatment for recognition) or carbon particles (e.g., India ink) (Fig. 1–15), which possess native density to visible light. Fluorescein, an extremely small molecule, may also be used for light microscopy by examining sections of frozen tissue under ultraviolet light (24).

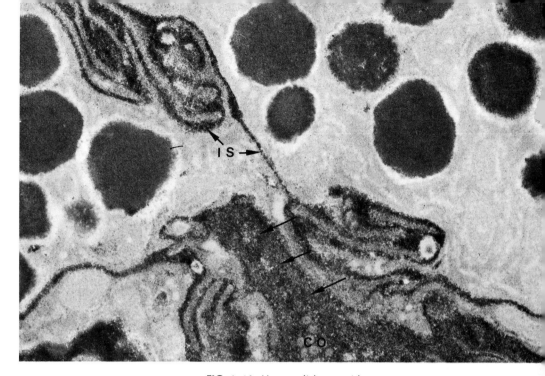

FIG. 1–14. Horseradish peroxidase can be seen passing between collagen fibrils (**CO**), through the thick basement membrane of ciliary pigment epithelium (**arrows**) and along the intercellular spaces (**IS**) between adjacent pigment epithelial cells. (Rhesus monkey × 26,000)

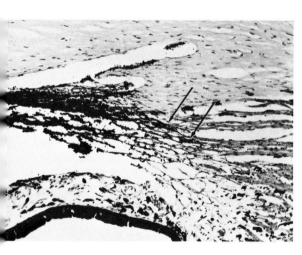

FIG. 1–15. India ink passing along trabecular meshwork. Ink (**arrows**) is present in anterior ciliary muscle. (Alcian blue stain, × 115) (Fine BS: Invest Ophthalmol 3:609, 1964)

AUTORADIOGRAPHY

The pathway of various components being synthesized in a tissue can be traced by injecting radioactive precursor chemicals into living animals (5, 7, 17, 19, 21, 22, 32–34). The tissues from each animal are fixed and sectioned sequentially in time. The sections are applied to a photographic emulsion to record the site or sites of activity at the light microscopic level. Adequate intracellular localization by these methods necessarily is poor. It is almost two decades since the technique was applied and refined for use at the electron microscopic level. The modification allowed more accurate localization of the injected radioisotopes to the various intracellular organelles. Although the procedure is highly technical and time-consuming, the principle remains the same. The thin section for electron microscopy is placed on a grid and coated directly with a thin film of photographic emulsion, a preparation selected for its extra fine grain size and the high density of the crystals, which have greatest sensitivity to the radiation. The coated sections are stored in the dark for periods of days to months depending upon intensity of the radiation and the sensitivity of the emulsion. The film is developed and the exposed silver halide crystals can be seen overlying the tissue section. For improved resolution, the gelatin film is removed, a procedure which does not significantly alter the disposition of the developed crystals.

Unfortunately, at the TEM level the developed silver halide crystals are present as "filaments" with length and tortuosity. Interpretation becomes difficult because it is unclear whether the point of initial exposure lies at one end of the filament, the other end, or at its middle. An error of localization of up to 100–200 A can be made. Numerous samples and a statistical analysis tend to reduce these limitation, but some uncertainty will remain (6).

PHOTOGRAPHY

TECHNIQUE

The photographic techniques used in electron microscopy are generally those of conventional black-and-white photography.

INTERPRETATION

The photograph contains the information. Unlike the light micrograph, in which the observed detail is *less* than can be seen by the examiner, the detail in the electron micrograph is *greater* than can be seen by the unaided eye of the examiner on the fluorescent screen. This higher information content in the micrograph is due to the combination of the extreme thinness of the tissue sections and the high resolution and depth of field of the electron microscope.

The information in the photograph is in shades of black and white, which indicate relative tissue densities to the electron beam. Structures are therefore described as electron-dense or electron-lucent, or simply as dense or lucent. In experiments *not* employing contrast enhancements, the relative tissue densities remain quite constant and therefore are believed to reflect the *in-vivo* situation. Thus, a very lucent tissue or cytoplasm (within limits) might be interpreted as "watery." Intracellular particles may vary from being extremely electron-dense to being invisible ("negative staining").

Note in Figure 1–16 the ganglion cell cytoplasm present on the lower left, and a number of bipolar cells on the right that are surrounded by the lucent cytoplasm of the Müller cells. Above are the complex interdigitating neurites of the inner plexiform layer. Diagonal scratches in the tissue section were produced by defects in the sharp cutting edge of the knife. These microscratches are analogous to the larger ones of light microscopy. Note also that the nuclei are dense. A nucleus, however, is less dense than its nucleolus. The other nuclei in the photograph do not necessarily lack nucleoli; these may lie in another plane of section in such thin slices. The small dense bodies in the ganglion cell cytoplasm are more dense than

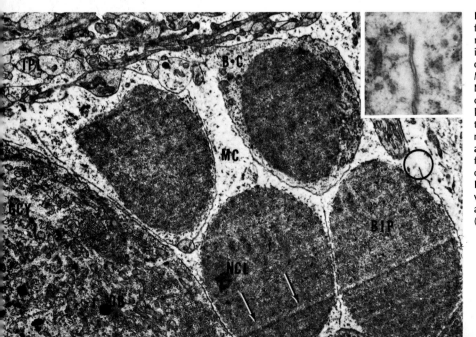

FIG. 1–16. Sample electron micrograph from innermost bipolar cell layer of retina, illustrating some problems in interpretation. **GCY,** ganglion cell cytoplasm; **BIP,** bipolar cell; **MC,** Müller cell; **IPL,** inner plexiform layer; **NCL,** nucleolus; **B•C,** bipolar cell cytoplasm; **DB,** dense body. **Arrows,** knife marks, or microscratches, across tissue section. Note break in plasma membrane of adjacent cells (**encircled area** and **enlarged inset**). Such sharp fractures of surface membranes occur during fixation and/or tissue processing. Lucency of cytoplasm in immediate vicinity of plasma membrane fracture also indicates artifact of preparation. (× 5500; **inset,** × 25,000)

the bipolar cell nucleolus. The cytoplasm of the bipolar cell is more dense than the lucent cytoplasm of the adjacent Müller cells. That there are in reality two separate but adjacent cells can only be appreciated at higher magnification, which shows the two adjacent cell plasma membranes together with a uniform ("typical") intercellular space.

Misinterpretation of electron micrographs can be easily avoided if the basic principles of cells, cell membranes, intercellular spaces, and planes and thinness of sectioning are constantly kept in mind. For example, in Figure 1–17 continuity of the extracellular collagen with the cytoplasm of the cell is apparent. Closer examination, however, reveals that 1) the plasma membranes of the cell have been sectioned obliquely in some areas (Fig. 1–17, **free arrows**), whereas they have been sectioned normally in other areas (Fig. 1–17, **N, arrows**); 2) the spaces around the collagen fibrils are much less dense than the cytoplasm of the cell, which is quite homogeneous, clearly indicating that these fibrils lie in a different matrix or milieu (in this case extracellular); 3) although it is possible that the extracellular fibrils are being produced by adjacent cells, the evidence must, of necessity, be indirect, since no filament or fibril can be found traversing a *normally* sectioned plasma membrane.

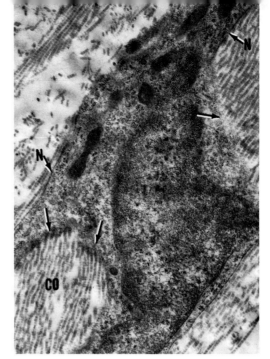

FIG. 1–17. Electron micrograph illustrating problems in interpretation. Oblique sectioning (**free arrows**) of cell lying in matrix of collagen fibrils (**CO**) gives false impression that collagen is either within cell or being directly extruded from it. Appearance of correctly sectioned plasma membrane (**N arrows**) refutes this interpretation. ($\times$ 10,800)

G. 1–18. Iris stroma cells. Effect of ative on cell appearance. A. Initial ation with glutaraldehyde produces aracteristic clumping of nuclear romatin. ($\times$ 14,000) B. Initial fixation osmium tetroxide produces a more mogeneous-appearing nucleus. 12,000)

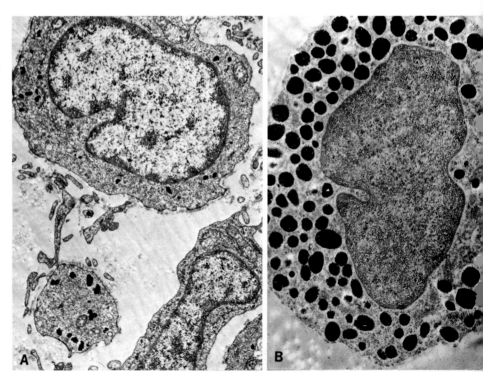

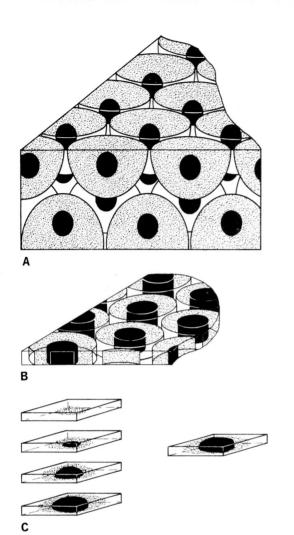

FIG. 1–19. Schematic representation of relative volumes of tissues. A. Conventional light microscopic section (~8–10μ in thickness). B. Epon-embedded sections for light microscopy (~1–2μ in thickness). C. Epon-embedded sections for electron microscopy (~200–600 A in thickness).

initially to an osmium tetroxide fixative (see Ch. 6 and 12).

What can be observed at any one time is limited by the volume of tissue examined (Fig. 1–19). Conventional light microscopic sections with a thickness of 8–10μ have a surface area limited only by the size of the original specimen or the size of the supporting slide. Thin sections* of plastic-embedded material for light microscopy with a thickness of 1–1.5μ have a surface area generally limited to the size of the small fragment of embedded tissue. The much thinner sections for electron microscopy, 200–600 A in thickness, have a surface area limited to a few square millimeters at most.

The tissue sections embedded in plastic for light microscopic examination may be stained by such dyes as paraphenylenediamine (12), toluidine blue (32), methylene blue (25), hematoxylin-phloxin (25), or hematoxylin-eosin (8). These sections are useful for preliminary evaluation of the tissue prior to electron microscopic examination and also provide two-dimensional detail better than can be seen in conventional sections for light microscopy.

Further examples of correct interpretation, or of misinterpretation, of electron micrographs are noted throughout the text.

The appearance of the cell varies with the type of fixative used (29). For example, nuclear chromatin aggregation is characteristic of initial exposure to Formalin or glutaraldehyde (Fig. 1–18, A) while a more homogeneous appearance is produced by initial exposure to Dalton's chrome-osmium fixative (Fig. 1–18B). Another example is the appearance of cytoplasmic tubules in some cells treated initially with glutaraldehyde (Fig. 6–61) compared with cytoplasmic filaments in the same cells exposed

* Electron microscopists who deal mainly with very thin plastic-embedded tissue sections for TEM study, generally describe them as "thin" or "semi-thin" sections. Plastic-embedded sections cut at 1.5μ in thickness for light microscopic comparison, therefore, are referred to as "thick" sections. This terminology, of course, neglects the much thicker 8–10μ "conventional" sections used for light microscopy. To avoid this potential conflict in terminology of "thick" and "thin" sections, all photographs of Epon-embedded light microscopic sections (i.e., ~1.5μ thick) are designated throughout this text as "Epon sections," and when stained with paraphenylenediamine, are also designated as "PD." Plastic embedments other than Epon (e.g., methacrylate) are noted. All other light microscopic sections are of the 8–10μ thick conventional type, with the staining technique specified: H&E, hematoxylin and eosin; PAS, periodic acid-Schiff; Masson, Masson trichrome. All illustrations are from human material unless otherwise noted.

REFERENCES

1. Albert EN, Fleischer E: A new electron-dense stain for elastic tissue. J Histochem Cytochem 18:697, 1970
2. Anderson TF: Techniques for the perservation of three dimensional structure in preparing specimens for the electron microscope. Trans NY Acad Sci 13:130, 1951
3. Berkow JW, Fine BS: Glycogen in normal human iris pigment epithelium. Am J Ophthalmol 69:994, 1970
4. Branton S, Bullivant S, Gilula NB, et al.: Freeze-etching nomenclature. Science 190:54, 1975
5. Caro LG: Electron microscopic radioautography of thin sections: The Golgi zone as a site of protein concentration in pancreatic acinar cells. J Biophys Biochem Cytol 10:37, 1961
6. Caro LG: High resolution autoradiography. II. The problem of resolution. J Cell Biol 15:189, 1962
7. Caro LG, Van Tubergen RP, Kolb JA: High resolution autoradiography. I. Methods. J Cell Biol 15: 173, 1962
8. Chang SC: Hematoxylin-eosin staining of plastic embedded tissue sections. Arch Pathol Lab Med 93:344, 1972
9. Cohen AL, Marlow DP, Garner GE: A rapid critical point method of using fluorocarbons ("freons") as intermediate and transitional fluids. J Microscopie 7:331, 1968
10. Dalton AJ: A chrome osmium fixative for electron microscopy. Anat Rec 121:281, 1955
11. Dawes CJ: Biological Techniques in Electron Microscopy. New York, Barnes & Noble, 1971
12. Estable-Puig JF, Bauer WC, Blumberg JM: Para-phenylenediamine staining of osmium-fixed, plastic-embedded tissue for light and phase microscopy. J Neuropathol Exp Neurol 24:531, 1965
13. Fine BS: Observations on the drainage angle in man and rhesus monkey. A concept of the pathogenesis of chronic simple glaucoma. A light and electron microscopic study. Invest Ophthalmol 3: 609, 1964
14. Fine BS: Free-floating pigmented cyst in the anterior chamber. Am J Ophthalmol 67:494, 1969
15. Fine BS, Tousimis AJ, Zimmerman LE: Some general principles of electron microscopy. Arch Ophthalmol 62:931, 1001, 1959
16. Graham RC, Karnovsky MJ: The early stages of absorption of injected horseradish peroxidase in the proximal tubules of mouse kidney: ultrastructure cytochemistry by a new technique. J Histochem Cytochem 14:291, 1966
17. Hay ED, Revel JP: The fine structure of the DNP component of the nucleus. An electron microscopic study utilizing autoradiography to localize DNA synthesis. J Cell Biol 16:29, 1963
18. Hayat MA: Principles and Techniques of Electron Microscopy—Biological Applications, Vol I. New York, Van Nostrand Reinhold, 1970
19. Herron WL, Riegel BW, Myers OE, Rubin ML: Retinal dystrophy in the rat: a pigment epithelial disease. Invest Ophthalmol 8:595, 1969
20. LeBlond C, Warren KB (eds): The Use of Radio-autography in Investigating Protein Synthesis. New York, Academic Press, 1966
21. Luft JH: Improvements in epoxy resin embedding methods. J Biophys Biochem Cytol 9:409, 1961
22. Magalhaes MM, Coimbra A: Electron microscope radioautographic study of glycogen synthesis in the rabbit retina. J Cell Biol 47:263, 1970
23. McDowell EM, Trump BF: Histologic fixatives suitable for diagnostic light and electron microscopy. Arch Pathol Lab Med 100:405, 1976
24. McMahon RT, Tso MOM, McLean IW: Histologic localization of sodium fluorescein in human ocular tissues. Am J Ophthalmol 80:1058, 1975
25. Munger BL: Staining methods applicable to sections of osmium-fixed tissue for light microscopy. J Biophys Biochem Cytol 11:502, 1961
26. Pease DC: Histological Techniques for Electron Microscopy, 2nd ed. New York, Academic Press, 1964
27. Seligman AM, Hanker JS, Wasserkrug H, Dmochowski H, Katzoff L: Histochemical demonstration of some oxidized macromolecules with thiocarbohydrazide (TCH) or thiosemicarbazide (TSC) and osmium tetroxide. J Histochem Cytochem 13:629, 1965
28. Simionescu N, Simionescu M, Palade GE: Permeability of intestinal capillaries. Pathway followed by dextrans and glycogen. J Cell Biol 53:365, 1972
29. Trump BF, Ericsson JLE: The effect of the fixative solution on the ultrastructure of cells and tissues. Lab Invest 14:1245, 1965
30. Trump BF, Smuckler EA, Benditt EP: A method for staining epoxy sections for light microscopy. J Ultrastruct Res 5:343, 1961
31. Yanoff M: Formaldehyde-glutaraldehyde fixation. Am J Ophthalmol 76:303, 1973
32. Young RW: Visual cells and the concept of renewal. Invest Ophthalmol 15:700, 1976
33. Young RW, Bok D: Participation of the retinal pigment epithelium in the rod outer segment renewal process. J Cell Biol 42:392, 1969
34. Young RW, Bok D: Autoradiographic studies on the metabolism of the retinal pigment epithelium. Invest Ophthalmol 9:524, 1970

chapter 2

THE CELL AND ITS CONTENTS

NUCLEUS, CYTOPLASM, AND PLASMA
    MEMBRANE   19
  CELL MEMBRANE (PLASMALEMMA)   19
CYTOPLASMIC ORGANELLES   20
  ENDOPLASMIC RETICULUM   20
  MITOCHONDRIA   23
  THE GOLGI COMPLEX   23
  CENTRIOLES AND CILIA   24
  FILAMENTS, MICROTUBULES, AND GROUND
    SUBSTANCE   25
CYTOPLASMIC INCLUSIONS   26
  RIBOSOMES   26
  GLYCOGEN   26
  PIGMENT GRANULES   26
  LIPOIDAL BODIES   27
  LYSOSOMES (CYTOSOMES)   27
  SECRETION GRANULES OR VACUOLES   29

Electron microscopy is a method of studying histology at the cytologic level (4, 13). In applying this technique to ocular tissues, therefore, we are concerned not only with histologic terminology but also with cytologic terminology. Where applicable, light microscopic cytologic terminology has been carried over without modification into electron microscopic cytology. On occasion some newer cytologic terms dictated by electron microscopic observations have been added.

NUCLEUS, CYTOPLASM, AND PLASMA MEMBRANE

When a cell is fixed and stained for light microscopy with such dyes as hematoxylin and eosin (H&E) (15, 22), it is clearly shown to contain a nucleus, the dense blue-staining (basophilic or hematoxylinophilic), rather centrally located structure, and a pink-staining (acidophilic or eosinophilic) cytoplasm. The cytoplasmic portion of the living cell appears delicately structured expect for a rather narrow uniform zone around the periphery. The nonstructured periphery is called the **ectoplasm** (Fig. 2–1). The greater volume of apparently structured cytoplasmic protoplasm is called the **endoplasm.** The entire cell is bounded by the plasma membrane (also called **cell membrane, cell-limiting membrane,** or **plasmalemma**), which cannot be visualized with the light microscope.

With proper fixation and sectioning at right angles to the cell surface, the sharp profile of the plasmalemma appears in an electron micrograph (Fig. 2–2) as a continuous dense line ~75 A in thickness. At higher magnification, however, three further subdivisions of this single membrane are recognizable: a central lucent zone lying between two denser zones, each ~25 A in thickness. Each of the three parts is called a **leaflet.** The composite trilaminar membrane is known as a **unit membrane** (26). With few exceptions, the micrographs presented in this monograph demonstrate these membranes

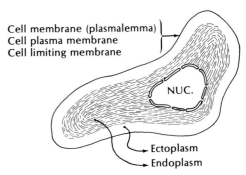

Cell membrane (plasmalemma)
Cell plasma membrane
Cell limiting membrane

NUC.

Ectoplasm
Endoplasm

FIG. 2–1. The cell.

at *low* magnification, and therefore the unit membrane is seen only as a single line (see Ch. 3).

CELL MEMBRANE (PLASMALEMMA)

The classic concept considered cell membrane structure to be composed of two layers of phospholipid in which the hydrophilic polar ends were directed away from each other toward layers of protein. By high-resolution electron microscopy the cell membrane, sectioned normal to the surface, as mentioned in the foregoing section, is seen as a three-layered structure, two outer dense layers separated by a middle lucent layer. The dense layers, however, are somewhat asymmetric, the outer being thicker than the inner. All of the carbohydrate portions of the membrane glycoprotein and/or glycolipid lie in the outermost layer and project into the cell *coat* or *glycocalyx** (2, 9). Because some regulated passage of nonlipid soluble materials is known to traverse the cell membrane, the classic concept has been modified to include structural proteins that traverse the membrane and so provide "pores" or passage-

* The cell coat of glycocalyx is considered to be mostly a secretory product of the cell consisting of glycoproteins, glycolipids, and polysaccharides. The plasmalemmal structural components may project into this surface layer.

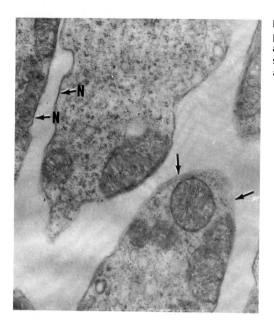

FIG. 2–2. Plasma membrane, sectioned perpendicularly (**N arrows**), appears as a single dense line. Membrane, sectioned obliquely (**free arrows**), appears blurred or indistinct. (× 14,000).

FIG. 2–3. Transmission electron micrograph, showing interconnected beadlike structures (reticulum) within attenuated cytoplasm of a monolayer of cultured cells. **Arrow,** free surface of cell; **M,** mitochondrion. (Porter KR et al.: J Exp Med 81:233, 1945)

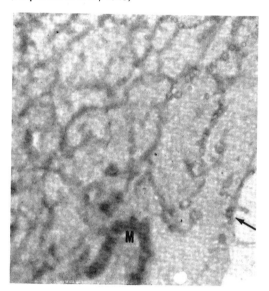

ways for them. The observation of numerous small trypsin-digestible bodies lying exposed to view in a membrane cloven through its middle layer by freeze-fracture-etching supports the concept of the presence of protein molecules intercalated as integral components of the unit membrane (see Fig. 3–7).

Additionally, a number of special mechanisms are considered to reside within the cell membrane, a *sodium pump* to maintain proper ionic concentrations within the cell, and *active transport mechanisms* requiring expenditure of energy to transport such materials as amino acids, glucose, and lipids into the cell.

Currently, the overall view of plasmalemmal structure is that of the *fluid mosaic* model (28), in which the structural lipids and proteins are arranged in a kind of mosaic arrangement. The membranes are considered quasi-fluid structures in which the structural materials are free to rotate while remaining within the layers.

Oblique sectioning of a unit membrane produces a blurred zone of moderate density. If the membrane undulates as it passes in and out of the plane of the thin section, it may seem to appear and disappear (Fig. 2–2). Superimposition of two cells whose plasmalemmas are cut obliquely at the overlap may give a false impression of cell continuity and be misinterpreted as a single continuous cell. Careful tracing of the cell boundaries is essential to proper interpretation.

CYTOPLASMIC ORGANELLES

ENDOPLASMIC RETICULUM

Before the development of thin-sectioning techniques, a method had to be found that would permit an electron beam to pass through cells. In 1945, Porter et al. (23) examined the attenuated periphery of a monolayer of cultured cells in the electron microscope (Fig. 2–3). They noted that in addition to the already well-recognized discrete, threadlike structures —the mitochondria—the peripheral cytoplasm contained a system of interconnecting lines and irregular enlargements forming a cytoplasmic network or reticulum. The network, therefore, was called the **endoplasmic reticulum.**

Subsequent development of suitable thin-sectioning techniques revealed that the network was not limited to the endoplasm, that it

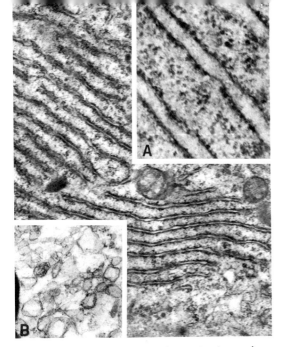

FIG. 2–4. Stacks of organized granular endoplasmic reticulum in cell from nonpigmented ciliary epithelium. This highly organized appearance indicates high degree of synthetic activity by cell. (× 15,000) A. Ribosomes aligned along one surface of parallel cytoplasmic membranes (Nissl substance of ganglion cell). (× 45,000) B. Portion of endoplasmic reticulum that is free of granules (agranular or smooth-surfaced) and less well arranged. (× 30,000)

was not connected to the surface plasma membrane except in unusual circumstances, and that its membrane-bound tubules and cisterns permeated much of the cytoplasm of most cells. In cells engaged actively in the synthesis of certain proteins (e.g., acinar cells of the pancreas [27]), this system appeared "highly organized" or layered, and the membranes were coated on one side with small, dark particles ~150 A in diameter (17, 18) (Fig. 2–4). The particles (once known as "Palade granules" but now termed **ribosomes**) were demonstrated to contain ribonucleoprotein, the material that accounts for cytoplasmic basophilia. Where the particles occur bound to the cytoplasmic membranes of the endoplasmic reticulum, the reticulum is known as **granular** (rough-surfaced) endoplasmic reticulum (e.g., ganglion cells of the retina, discussed in Ch. 6, and nonpigmented epithelial cells of the ciliary body pars plana, discussed in Ch. 10). The remaining reticulum is known as the **agranular** (smooth-surfaced) reticulum (e.g., retinal pigment epithelium and Müller cells discussed in Ch. 6).

The system of endoplasmic reticulum ends blindly at the nucleus as several double-membraned arcuate expansions encircling the nucleus (Fig. 2–17) to form the nuclear double membrane (Fig. 2–5). Apertures or *pores* lying between these expansions maintain continuity between the nuclear and cytoplasmic compartments. The resting nucleus (within the nuclear membrane) is easily separable into two parts,

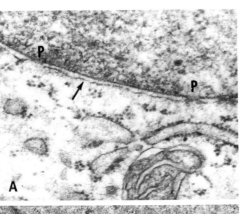

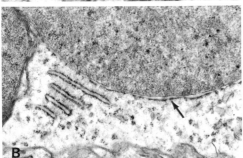

FIG. 2–5. Nuclear double membrane formed by endoplasmic reticulum. In A double membrane is agranular (**arrow**). Note condensation of nuclear chromatin on inner side of nuclear pores (**P**), as well as appearance of a thin membrane across pore at right. (× 42,000) In B outer membrane is studded with ribosomes (**arrow**). (× 16,000) C. The nuclear pores are sectioned obliquely— light apertures representing pores sectioned closer to cytoplasmic side, and darker apertures representing pores sectioned closer to nuclear chromatin. (× 21,000)

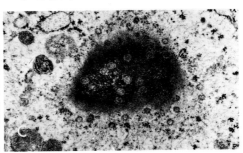

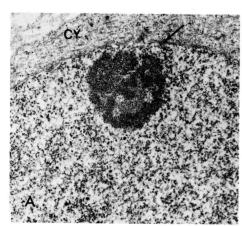 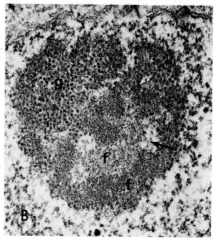

FIG. 2–6. Nucleoli. A. Nucleolus of cone cell body. **Arrow,** double membrane of nucleus; **CY,** perikaryonal cytoplasm. (× 16,000) B. Nucleolus showing dense strands composed of granules (**g**) and fine filaments (**f**); **arrow,** a lucent area. (× 30,000)

the nuclear chromatin and the nucleolus. The division is most obvious in cells that are initially fixed in osmium tetroxide where the chromatin appears homogeneously distributed in the nuclear sap or ground substance (Fig. 1–18). With initial fixation in an aldehyde (formaldehyde or glutaraldehyde), the chromatin forms dense clumps, most noticeable along the nuclear membrane (condensed chromatin). The aggregation along the nuclear membrane makes it stand out well on hematoxylin and eosin stained sections. Clumps of chromatin also appear scattered throughout the clear nuclear sap and may even be associated with the periphery of the nucleolus.

The chromatin (*i.e.,* basophilic material on H&E stained sections) contains the deoxyribonucleic acid (DNA) as well as other materials, including a small amount of ribonucleoprotein (RNA). The nucleolus (Fig. 2–6) (or nucleoli if there are more than one) lies freely (*i.e.,* without membrane) within the nucleus. The nucleolus is composed of a dense, filamentous network containing granules of ribonucleoprotein (ribosomal RNA or rRNA) which are being formed there. The nucleolar strands are frequently separated by patches of more lucent material generally considered to represent enclosed areas of nuclear sap.

Ribonucleoprotein derived from the nuclear DNA is in the form of delicate threads that are termed the messenger RNA (mRNA). These reach the cytoplasmic ribosomes (granular endoplasmic reticulum) presumably by passage through the nuclear pores. At the ribosomal site the mRNA, with the assistance of a transfer RNA

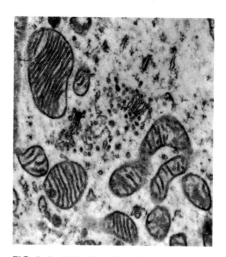

FIG. 2–7. Mitochondria with their characteristic internal double-membraned cristae. (× 22,000)

FIG. 2–8. Schematic drawing of sectioned mitochondria. **Arrows,** Double membrane of outer wall.

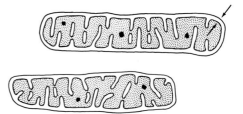

(tRNA) directs the production of appropriate proteins by the cytoplasmic RNA.

MITOCHONDRIA

In addition to the widely distributed endoplasmic reticulum, the cytoplasm contains a number of discrete organelles (Fig. 2–3) previously described by light microscopists as slender thread-like granules—mitochondria. These organelles move about freely in the living cell and can be stained supravitally with Janus green. By electron microscopy (4, 13, 16), in tissue sections they generally appear (Fig. 2–7) as elongated, spherical and sometimes branching structures bounded by a double membrane, each of which is a unit membrane (Fig 2–8, 3–7; e.g., retinal photoreceptors, Ch. 6). The inner membrane is thrown into folds (Fig. 2–9), forming the cristae mitochondriales or simply **cristae.** The rather uniform intermembrane space between the outer membranes is continued into the cristal folds as the **intracristal space.** The homogeneous mitochondrial ground substance or **matrix** occupies all the space between the double-walled cristae and lies therefore in the intercristal spaces. A number of discrete, very dense granules (300–500 A in diameter) are frequently present within the mitochondrial matrix. They are called **mitochondrial** or **matrix** granules. The composition and function of the mitochondrial granules is controversial. Occasionally intra-mitochondrial granules considered to be glycogen have been reported in such tissues as rat retina (14). Crystalline formations have also been reported.

Mitochondria may differ considerably in appearance from tissue to tissue (compare corneal endothelium with neural retina), varying in both cristal arrangement and length, to density of the intercristal matrix.

The mitochondria function as the main source of cell energy by converting adenosine diphosphate (ADP) to adenosine triphosphate (ATP) by oxidative phosphorylation. The ATP then provides the necessary energy for various parts of the cells by giving up its energy rich terminal phosphate groups to another molecule and, in so doing, is itself reduced to adenosine diphosphate (ADP), ready to be recycled again by oxidative phosphorylation. Biochemical assay of isolated mitochondrial fragments (21) indicates that the phosphorylating and respiratory enzymes are in general bound to the membranes, while the enzymes of the Krebs citric acid cycle are within the matrix. The mitochondria are therefore sometimes called the "powerhouses" of the cell.

There is evidence that the membrane-bound enzymes are not haphazardly arranged but are properly (morphologically as well as biochemically) sequenced along the membranes. "Elementary particles" (21) (with globular heads 80–100 A in diameter), which can be observed by rapid freezing and high-resolution electron microscopy to be attached exclusively to the matrix side of the inner mitochondrial membrane, are also considered possible foci in which enzymes are arranged to perform specific functions.

Mitochondria readily swell or contract with osmotic changes, and therefore their variable morphologic appearance in this regard is sometimes physiologic, sometimes artifactitious.

THE GOLGI COMPLEX

Without direct connection to the endoplasmic reticulum, the Golgi apparatus or complex is a second, smaller system of agranular, membrane-bound, flattened vesicles or saccules (7) (Fig. 2–10). Since the apparatus lacks granules, it does not stain with the usual methods for light microscopy and in H&E-stained sections occasionally may be seen as a "negatively stained" area (an unstained area in a region otherwise well stained, e.g., the juxtanuclear "halo" in a plasma cell). In highly oriented or polarized cells such as those in various epithe-

FIG. 2–9. Continuity (**at arrow**) of mitochondrial inner wall and a crista. (× 100,000)

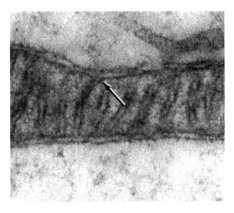

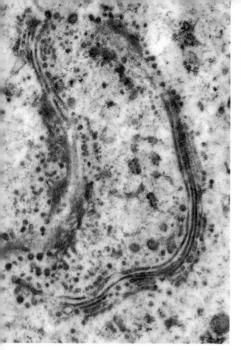

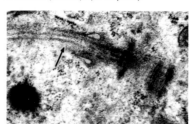

FIG. 2–10. Golgi complex, showing several stacks of agranular membranes and associated free vesicles of varying sizes. (× 24,000)

FIG. 2–11. Two centrioles. Centriole at right is unmodified. Centriole at left has become modified into a basal body for a cilium (**arrow**). (× 27,000)

lia, the Golgi apparatus generally is found on the apical side of the nucleus and forms a "crown" to the apical pole of the nucleus. It is recognized in sections as several layers of agranular, flattened vesicles surrounded by clusters of large and small rounded vesicles (e.g., nonpigmented epithelial cells of the ciliary body pars plana, Ch. 10).

The Golgi saccules act as a form of temporary way station for secretory materials passing from the rough endoplasmic reticulum (RER) toward the cell surface. The synthesized materials leave the RER contained in small transfer vesicles, which arrive at the Golgi at its forming or *immature* face. The materials undergo condensation and modification (especially their carbohydrate content) within the Golgi. The altered secretory materials then leave the Golgi from its appropriate surface (the *mature* face) as larger mature secretory vacuoles or granules to be extruded at the apical surface of the cell.

Union of the mature granules with the cell surface membrane also provides the cell surface with its glycoprotein coating, a phenomenon enormously exaggerated around the retinal rods and cones as the interreceptor mucoid (Ch. 6; see also the unicellular mucous glands of the conjunctival epithelium, Ch. 9).

The vesicles should not be confused with *coated* vesicles, which carry a fuzzy coating on their cytoplasmic surface. Coated vesicles bud off from the cell surface in a variety of absorptive epithelia and also are believed to bud off from the endoplasmic reticulum.

CENTRIOLES AND CILIA

Within each cell are two short, cylindrical structures (centrioles) usually located in the vicinity of the Golgi apparatus. The region they occupy is known in light microscopy as the centrosome. The centrioles are best observed as two small blue dots when stained with iron hematoxylin. They generally are composed of nine short microtubules ("filaments") arranged as a short cylinder.

More detailed investigation has shown that the microtubules are arranged in twos or threes (doublets or triplets). In many epithelia one centriole comes to lie near the apical cytoplasm of the cell (Fig. 2–11), and its tubules become enormously elongated, protruding from the apical end and pushing the apical plasma membrane outward. From the basal end of the centriole one or two rootlets project deep into the apical cytoplasm. These rootlets consist of exceedingly delicate filaments with cross-striations of ~600 A. This composite structure is known as a **cilium** (Fig. 2–12). and the *fixed centriole* is known as a **basal body.** The second

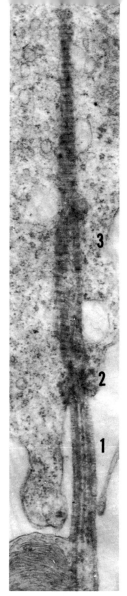

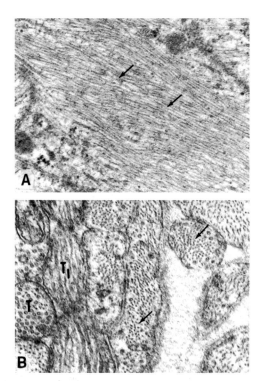

FIG. 2–12. Rabbit retina, showing typical cilium with ciliary extension (**1**), fixed basal body (**2**), and cross-striated rootlets (**3**). (× 25,000)

FIG. 2–13. Optic nerve, intracellular filaments and tubules. A. Longitudinal appearance of filaments (**arrows**). (Glutaraldehyde fixation × 30,000). B. Cross-sectional appearance of filaments (**arrows**). Cells containing microtubules are axons. **T**, Tubules cut in cross-section. **T$_l$**, Tubules cut longitudinally. (Glutaraldehyde fixation, × 36,000)

centriole is not modified and remains as a *free* centriole. Cross-sections of the shafts of cilia generally show nine peripheral bundles of tubules (doublets or triplets). In "motile" cilia two additional microtubules are present axially, to produce what is called a 9 + 2 pattern. A few special "nonmotile" cilia (*e.g.*, photoreceptors) lack central or axial microtubules and have the 9 + 0 pattern when viewed in cross section.

A few ciliated cells can be found in almost every ocular tissue when examination is made by electron microscopy, even when the tissue being examined is not generally noted for its content of cilia (*e.g.*, uveal tract).

FILAMENTS, MICROTUBULES, AND GROUND SUBSTANCE

Many delicate filaments may be found intracellularly. They range from 50–80 A in diameter and vary in concentration from one cell type to another (Fig. 2–13). Epithelial cells, especially those of epidermis or its ocular counterpart, the corneal epithelium (Fig. 3–3, 9–5), contain large numbers of such delicate intracellular filaments. The filaments are sometimes considered to be a type of "endoskeleton" of the cell, and their relation to other structural configurations (*terminal web, terminal bar,* and *desmosomes*) is noted later. Smooth and striated muscle cells contain special varieties of intracytoplasmic filaments which are so characteristic that the cells can be identified from small fragments (30).

Some microfilaments appear to play a part in ameboid movement. *Some* of these filaments are sensitive to cytochalasin B, an alkaloid that impairs a variety of cell activities. It generally is assumed that the cytochalasin-B-sensitive microfilaments are the contractile machinery of nonmuscle cells (e.g., fibroblasts, glial cells).

Actin is present in its globular form (G-actin) in a wide variety of cells (e.g., retinal pigment epithelium) (5). It may quickly polymerize into its fibrous form (F-actin). Such transformation appears to account for the well known sol-gel transitions that occur in the cytoplasm of moving cells.

In addition to filaments that may be present under all conditions of fixation, **microtubules** (~200–500 A in diameter) often may be found, especially in certain cells that have been *initially* fixed in an aldehyde (e.g., glutaraldehyde or formaldehyde; Fig. 2–13). The "tubular" structures may therefore be present in either filament form (~50–80 A in material initially fixed in osmium tetroxide) or microtubule form (~200–250 A in material initially fixed in glutaraldehyde), depending upon the fixative initially used. In certain ocular tissues (e.g., the retina) such variations can be produced readily.

Excluding the free ribonucleoprotein particles (mRNA, ribosomal rosettes, or polysomes) and the glycogen particles (~300 A in diameter), the remainder of the cytoplasmic substance generally appears as a watery (i.e., lucent) material containing a very diffuse grayish substance. This "leftover" watery region is referred to as the cytoplasmic **ground substance.**

CYTOPLASMIC INCLUSIONS

RIBOSOMES

Free clusters of ribonucleoprotein particles (ribosomes, RNP), measuring ~150 A, may be present in the ground substance of the cytoplasm, sometimes in the form of small rosettes (polysomes). Cytoplasmic basophilia is due to the presence of the ribosomes.

Although striking in appearance in cells highly specialized to produce secretory granules (e.g., pancreatic acinar cells, mucus-producing cells, etc.), rough endoplasmic reticulum is present in all nucleated cells to synthesize the materials required for a cell's needs, internal as well as external.

GLYCOGEN

The appearance of glycogen, a polymer of glucose, in an electron micrograph varies with the cell type and with the method of fixation

(3, 20, 24). With good fixation, the irregularly shaped particles average 200–300 A in diameter (thus generally larger than ribosomes) and are sometimes called **beta particles.** The beta particles are distinguished from clusters of such particles, which are called **alpha particles** or rosettes.

If unstained, aggregates or clusters of the particles may be recognized by their "negative" appearance. Treatment of a tissue section with a lead stain (e.g., lead hydroxide) accentuates the density of these particles and facilitates their identification. They can also be demonstrated by the thiosemicarbazide (TSC) method (Fig. 1–12A). Diastase digestion may be necessary at the electron microscopic level to identify individual or widely scattered particles of glycogen (Fig. 1–12B).

PIGMENT GRANULES

In normal ocular tissue, two varieties of pigment granules can be seen by light microscopy. The most obvious granule is melanin, which is extremely dense to both light and electron microscopy. The less obvious granule is lipofuscin. Melanin granules are found within many of the cells of the neuroepithelial layers and within the pigment-bearing cells of the uveal tract. The melanin granules of these two different ocular coats are easily distinguished from each other when viewed by light microscopy because those of the neuroepithelium are larger and therefore appear darker than those of the uveal tract (Fig. 2–14). In fact, the neuroepithelial granules are large enough (~1μ) to be observed as discrete by oil-immersion light microscopy. Those of the uveal tract lie close to the limits of resolution (~0.3–0.5μ) of the light microscope. Melanin granules are also easily recognized by electron microscopy (Fig. 2–15) because of their exceedingly dense appearance, their regular contours, and, with glass-knife sectioning, their often "fractured" appearance. Diamond knives generally cut the melanin granules more smoothly. The second variety of granule (lipofuscin) may be confused with the melanin granule because of its slightly yellow-orange to brownish color by light microscopy and its proximity to the melanin granule. By electron microscopy the lipofuscin granules are more easily sectioned and are less dense (Fig. 6–16). They appear more numerous in certain cells as the organism ages (i.e., few are found

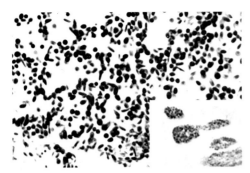

FIG. 2–14. Light micrographs of melanin granules of neuroepithelium, and of uveal tract (**inset**). Note that neuro-epithelial granules are larger and appear more dense. (Epon, × 1000) (AFIP Neg. 68-9944).

in infant eyes, more in young adult eyes, and most in aged eyes). Lipofuscin can be identified in normal or abnormal (e.g., as over a malignant melanoma) pigment epithelial cells by their positive acid-fast staining or by their auto-fluorescence with ultraviolet light (Fig. 2–16).

The visual pigments in the photoreceptor outer segments or the yellow material within the neurosensory retina producing the macula lutea cannot be identified as such by electron microscopy. They, therefore, lie dispersed at the molecular level.

Other pigments may be present, such as hemoglobin in red blood cells (Fig. 6–76). Products of hemoglobin (hemosiderin, ferritin) or iron, silver, or copper deposits of foreign origin, found in pathologic tissue (30), are not considered here.

LIPOIDAL BODIES

Normal cells may contain fat droplets (lipoidal bodies), which appear by electron microscopy to be greatly varied. Some are homogeneous while others show lamellar configurations. Some have less density; others have greater density; some may even appear to lose their central substance in the process of fixation and staining. Sick, degenerating, or altered cells may accumulate lipids by imbibition from the exterior or simply by accumulating lipids released from the cells' own cytoplasm. These are described elsewhere.

LYSOSOMES (CYTOSOMES)

A heterogeneous group of "dense bodies" (actually variable in appearance and density) is found in many cells throughout the body. Attempts have been made to characterize these bodies according to their function. One variety,

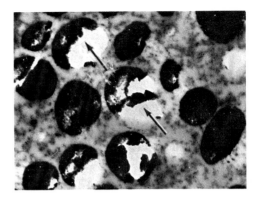

FIG. 2–15. Electron micrograph of neuroepithelial melanin granules. Note extreme density of granules, their circular and oval profiles, and their often "fractured" appearance (**arrows**). (× 10,000)

FIG. 2–16. Pigment epithelial cells overlying a malignant melanoma. Their large content of autofluorescent lipofuscin is evident when examined by ultraviolet light. (AFIP Neg. 75-9358)

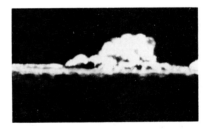

originally fractionated from rat liver cells, was found on biochemical assay to contain acid hydrolases or "lytic" enzymes; hence the term **lysosome**. Although originally proposed as the place where cell autolysis (8) (e.g., "suicide bags") begins, the dense bodies are now thought, on morphologic grounds, to be a heterogeneous group, unlikely to function in all cells in the same way; hence the nonspecific term, cytosome (10, 29). A lysosome can be identified in a tissue section only by histochemi-

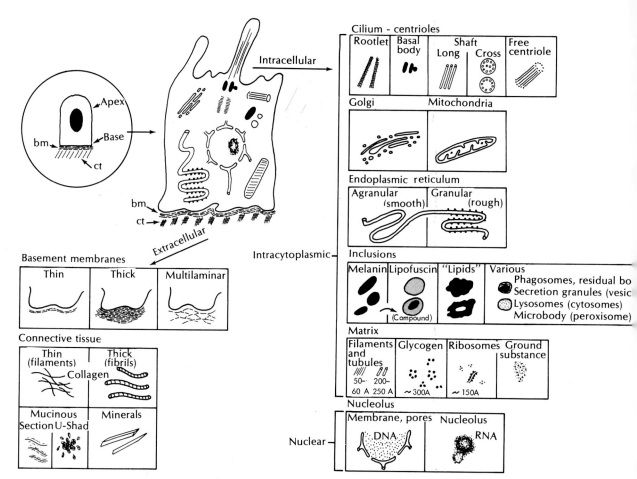

FIG. 2–17. Schematic drawing of cell, its components (organelles), its contents (inclusions) and relationship to extracellular materials.

cal means (12). Morphologic identification *in situ*, therefore, is generally limited to the histochemical demonstration of preferably two or more hydrolases in the same location (12). Biochemical assay is generally carried out on relatively homogeneous preparations of the bodies collected by either differential or zonal centrifugation.

The dense bodies or "primary" lysosomes generally have a single limiting membrane and are usually PAS-positive, exhibit metachromasia, and often stain for acid mucopolysaccharides.

"Secondary" lysosomes is a term generally applied to *digestive* vacuoles that may be present in a cell. Such vacuoles contain material that may be recognized as having been taken in

from outside the cell (phagocytosis or heterophagocytosis) or as material actually derived from parts of its own cytoplasm, *e.g.*, mitochondria (autophagocytosis). The cell may be unable to extrude some of the dense end products of intracytoplasmic digestion, and such bodies are often termed **residual bodies** (see Ch. 6).

In many ocular tissues (especially ganglion cells of the retina) dense cytoplasmic bodies of unknown composition appear more dense with age and are neither PAS-positive by light microscopy nor the equivalent TSC-positive by electron microscopy. The dense bodies in the ganglion cells may possibly function as "waste-baskets" for materials that cannot be removed in any other way. Some of the increase in density with age may therefore be due to increasing polymerization of these sequestered materials.

The granules of such cells as blood neutrophils contain a variety of enzymes and therefore are generally considered good examples of "true," *i.e.*, primary, lysosomes.

Other dense cytoplasmic bodies, differing in appearance, can be observed in various tissues and are sometimes named "microbodies" (1, 11, 25). They have been observed in kidney tubules and liver. The former are single membrane-bound structures, ~0.5μ in diameter, with a finely granular matrix of moderate density. A dense core or **nucleoid** is sometimes observed as in rat liver. Microbodies have been found to contain a variety of oxidases, hence the proposed alternate name of **peroxisome.** Their functions are not known.

SECRETION GRANULES OR VACUOLES

Secretory cells (19) synthesize a "useful" material to be extruded to the exterior via a lumen, as in exocrine cells, or directly into the tissue fluids or bloodstream, as in endocrine cells. The cells produce materials that range from mucous vesicles of the salivary glands to the denser, enzyme-packed granules of the pancreas. The secretory materials are thought to be synthesized at least partially within the highly organized forms of granular endoplasmic reticulum (6). They are transferred to the Golgi apparatus, presumably by isolated vesicles, where they are either concentrated or chemically altered or both. Subsequently, they are extruded to the exterior, generally through the plasmalemma of the cell via the apical cytoplasm.

Figure 2–17 summarizes schematically the structure of a cell and its relation to various extracellular materials (Ch. 4).

REFERENCES

1. Afzelius BA: The occurrence and structure of microbodies: a comparative study. J Cell Biol 26:835, 1965
2. Bennett HS: Morphological aspects of extracellular polysaccharides. J Histochem Cytochem 11:14, 1963
3. Biava C: Identification and structural forms of human particle glycogen. Lab Invest 12:1179, 1963
4. Bloom W, Fawcett DW: A Textbook of Histology, 10th ed. Philadelphia, WB Saunders, 1975
5. Burnside MB: Possible roles of microtubules and actin filaments in retinal pigmented epithelium. Exp Eye Res 23:257, 1976
6. Caro LG: Electron microscopic radioautography of thin sections: the Golgi zone as a site of protein concentration in pancreatic acinar cells. J Biophys Biochem Cytol 10:37, 1961
7. Dalton AJ: Golgi apparatus and secretion granules. In Brachet J, Mirsky EA (eds): The Cell: Biochemistry, Physiology, Morphology, vol 2. New York, Academic Press, 1961, pp 603–619
8. deDuve C: Lysosome, a new group of cytoplasmic particles. In Hayashi T (ed): Subcellular Particles. New York, Ronald Press, 1959, pp 128–159
9. DeRobertis, EDP, Saez FA, DeRobertis EMF Jr: Cell Biology, 6th ed. Philadelphia, WB Saunders, 1975
10. Ericsson JLE, Trump BF: Electron microscopic studies of the epithelium of the proximal tubule of the rat kidney. III. Microbodies, multivesicular bodies, and the Golgi apparatus. Lab Invest 15:1610, 1966
11. Ericsson JLE, Trump BF, Weibel J: Electron microscopic studies of the proximal tubule of the rat kidney. II. Cytosegrosomes and cytosomes: their relationship to each other and to the lysosome concept. Lab Invest 14:1341, 1965
12. Gahan PD: Histochemistry of lysosomes. Int Rev Cytol 21:1, 1967
13. Ham AW: Histology, 7th ed. Philadelphia, JB Lippincott, 1974
14. Ishikawa T, Pei YF: Intramitochondrial glycogen particles in rat retinal receptor cells. J Cell Biol 25:402, 1965
15. Luna LG (ed): Manual of Histologic and Special Staining Technics, 3rd ed. New York, McGraw-Hill, 1968
16. Munn EA: The Structure of Mitochondria. New York, Academic Press, 1974, pp 44, 48, 65
17. Palade GE: A small particulate component of the cytoplasm. In Palay SL (ed): Frontiers in Cytology. New Haven, Yale University Press, 1958
18. Palade GE, Siekevitz, P: Pancreatic microsomes: an integrated morphological and biochemical study. J Biophys Biochem Cytol 2:671, 1956
19. Palay SL: The morphology of secretion. In Palay SL (ed): Frontiers in Cytology. New Haven, Yale University Press, 1958
20. Paluello M, Rosati G: The influence of fixation and dehydration on the isolated glycogen. J Microsc 7:275, 1968
21. Parsons DF: Recent advances correlating structure and function in mitochondria. Int Rev Exp Pathol 4:1, 1965
22. Pearse AGE: Histochemistry, Theoretical and Applied, 2nd ed. Boston, Little, Brown, 1960
23. Porter KR, Claude A, Fullam EF: A study of tissue culture cells by electron microscopy: methods and preliminary observations. J Exp Med 81:233, 1945
24. Revel JP: Electron microscopy of glycogen. J Histochem Cytochem 12:104, 1964
25. Rhodin J: Correlation of Ultrastructural Organiza-

tion and Function in Normal and Experimentally Changed Proximal Convoluted Tubule Cells of the Mouse Kidney. Stockholm, Godvil, 1954

26. Robertson JD: Unit membranes: a review with recent new studies of experimental alterations and a new subunit structure in synaptic membranes. In Locke M (ed): Cellular Membranes in Development. New York, Academic Press, 1964, p 1

27. Siekevitz P, Palade GE: A cytochemical study on the pancreas of the guinea pig. V. In vivo incorporation of leucine-1-C^{14} into the chymotrypsinogen of various cell fractions. J Biophys Biochem Cytol 7:619, 1960

28. Singer SJ, Nicholson GL: The fluid mosaic model of the structure of cell membranes. Science 175: 720, 1972

29. Trump BF: An electron microscopic study of the uptake, transport, and storage of colloidal materials by the cells of the vertebrate nephron. J Ultrastruct Res 5:291, 1961

30. Yanoff M, Fine BS: Ocular Pathology: A Text and Atlas. Hagerstown, Maryland, Harper & Row, 1975

chapter 3

CELL INTERRELATIONS

THE INTERCELLULAR SPACE   33
THE DESMOSOME (MACULA ADHERENS)   33
THE TERMINAL BAR (ZONULA ADHERENS AND
          ZONULA OCCLUDENS)   33
THE GAP JUNCTION   34

THE INTERCELLULAR SPACE

In electron micrographs the intercellular space is seen as a rather uniform (~150 A wide) lucent space between the dense plasma membranes of adjacent cells (3) (Fig. 3–1). Except for some modification (*e.g.,* nonpigmented ciliary epithelium) in normal tissues and much more gross exaggerations in pathologic tissues (18, 19), this space is remarkably uniform and probably represents the *in-vivo* situation closely.

THE DESMOSOME

In any plane from apex to base (Fig. 3–2), focal densities (desmosomes) (9, 11–13) may connect adjacent cells, especially in certain epithelia (*e.g.,* epidermis [11], corneal epithelium, neuroepithelial layers). Long appreciated by light microscopists as small attachment foci on the intercellular bridges of the epidermal prickle or squamoid cell layer (as seen with iron hemotoxylin stain), the desmosomes partially occlude the intercellular space with a cement substance and function as strong focal attachments between adjacent cells. The attachments are so strong that the cell generally ruptures long before the desmosome can be made to separate by mechanical means.

On electron microscopic examination, a desmosome in cross section consists of apposing plasma membranes that are rather rigidly held and more widely separated than in a normal intercellular space by the presence of an intercellular cement of moderate electron density (Fig. 3–3). A dense plaque (16, 17) lies along the cytoplasmic surface of the trilaminar cell unit membrane or plasmalemma. Loops of cytoplasmic filaments or **tonofilaments** are attached to the plaques (Fig. 3–4). The coarser appearance of clusters of tonofilaments observed by light microscopists are called **tonofibrils.**

In three dimensions desmosomes appear as small ovoid plaques, and in the terminology of

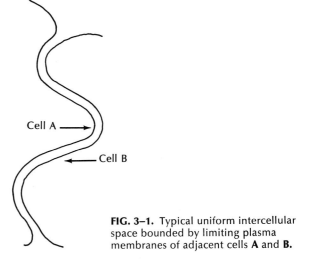

FIG. 3–1. Typical uniform intercellular space bounded by limiting plasma membranes of adjacent cells **A** and **B.**

widest current usage, they are also called **maculae adherentes** (2).

THE TERMINAL BAR

Attachment densities lying in a single plane near the lumen of various epithelia (*e.g.,* intestinal epithelium, retinal pigment epithelium) have long been appreciated by light microscopists, especially in sections stained with iron hematoxylin. The attachment zones form complete encircling girdles around the epithelial cells so that on surface view they often resemble chickenwire and were once called **fenestrated membranes.** The outer limiting membrane of the retina (Fig. 6–39 and 6–40) is a good example of such a "fenestrated membrane." The girdle-like attachments resemble desmosomes in that they attach adjacent cells to each other, but they differ somewhat from desmosomes in their location, which is always apical, and in their electron microscopic structural appearance (Fig. 3–5).

The terminal bar region seen by light microscopy to be characteristic of various epithelia can be shown by electron microscopy to consist of two parts. The basilar portion **(zonula adherens)** closely resembles a desmosome in cross section except for its slightly narrower intercellular space and its encircling arrangement (Fig. 3–6). The apical portion **(zonula occludens)**, not visible by light microscopy, consists of dense adjacent cell membranes so closely apposed that the intercellular space appears more or less obliterated. No adjacent cytoplasmic densities accompany this apical part of the terminal bar.

The term **junctional complex** is often used in a nonspecific way for the apical attachment zones and may include a third part, a typical desmosome or macula adherens, on the basilar side of the bipartite arrangement. Then the complex becomes a tripartite arrangement.

These arrangements may have some variability (compare the fenestrated membrane of the retinal pigment epithelium and the fenestrated or external limiting membrane of the retina; Ch. 6).

THE GAP JUNCTION

On the basis of electron microscopic appearance, a further distinction can be made for the apical part of a terminal bar. If the outer leaflets of adjacent cell *unit membranes* (15) (Fig. 3–7) can be demonstrated to fuse (*i.e.*, to form a pentalaminar configuration), the junction is truly occlusive functionally as well as anatomically.* If, however, the outer leaflets of adjacent cell unit membranes come very close together but do not fuse, the intercellular space is not completely obliterated (*i.e.*, a gap of 20–30 A persists). The term **gap junction** (1, 5, 6), **nexus,** or **macula communicans** is then applied to this seven-layered configuration, and the space that is observed also represents morphologically some functional continuity with the adjacent intercellular space. Gap junctions have been observed between pigment epithelial cells (8), ependymal cells, between astrocytes, and between some electrically coupled neurons (1). Junctions that persist with more than one method of fixation are considered to be more "real" than "tight" junctions seen with only one method of fixation. Some of the spurious tight junctions are considered to be mere apposi-

---

* Tight junctions in vertebrate epithelia appear to be functionally analogous to septate junctions in invertebrate epithelia (10).

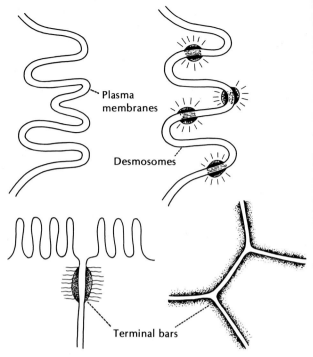

FIG. 3–2. Schematic drawing showing a typical intercellular space, desmosomes distributed along the intercellular space, and, at bottom, an apical terminal bar attachment in cross-section on the left and tangentially on the right.

FIG. 3–3. Schematic drawing of typical desmosome (macula adherens). **I C**, intercellular cement.

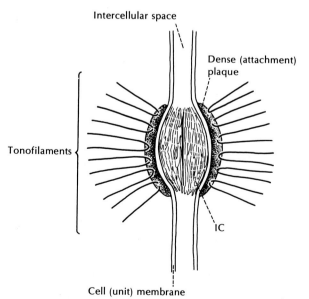

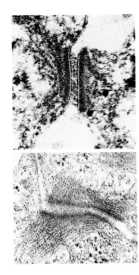

FIG. 3–4. Top. Desmosome from corneal epithelium. Trilaminar plasmalemma, intercellular cement, and dense cytoplasmic plaques can be seen. (× 72,000) Bottom. Desmosome from nonpigmented ciliary epithelium. Tonofilaments are clearly evident. (× 31,000)

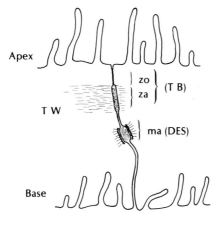

FIG. 3–5. A junctional complex consists of a complete terminal bar (**TB**) composed of zonula occludens (**zo**) and zonula adherens (**za**), together with associated desmosome (**DES**), *i.e.*, macula adherens (**ma**). **TW**, terminal web.

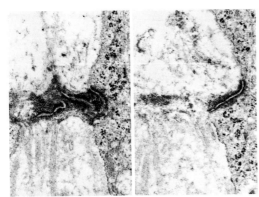

FIG. 3–6. Terminal bar of neural retina (foveal region). Narrow intercellular space and adjacent cytoplasmic densities are seen cut in cross section (**right**) and obliquely (**left**). (× 15,800)

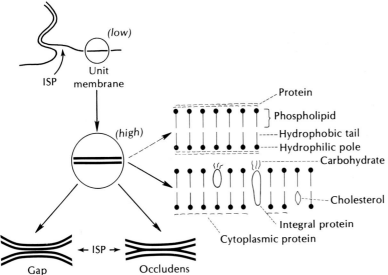

FIG. 3–7. Schematic drawing showing trilaminar appearance of unit membrane at high magnification. An occludens junction is pentalaminar; a gap junction septilaminar. **ISP**, intercellular space. On the right, the classic concept of cell membrane structure (**broken arrow**) has been modified to include structural proteins, carbohydrate, and even cholesterol (**solid arrow**) (see Ch. 2).

tions of adjacent cell membranes and are called **labile appositions** (1).

More recently, using the method of freeze-fracture etching (*e.g.*, Fig. 6–15) it is found that in many zonulae occludentes, the adjacent cell membranes are not uniformly fused but only where matching plasmalemmal ridges meet. The more ridges and the more complex their distribution, the better the seal of the intercellular space.

Gap junctions are widely believed to represent the site of electrotonic coupling (*i.e.*, site of low electrical resistance) between adjacent cells. Occasionally, a desmosome is seen joining two parts of the same cell. Gap junctions may also be observed connecting two parts of the same cell. The term "reflexive" gap junction (7) has been proposed for the latter.

Attachments that resemble short segments of a zonula occludens or a zonula adherens are termed **fascia occludens** or **fascia adherens** respectively.

Short attachments resembling desmosomes (4) but lacking the enlarged intercellular space as well as most of the associated cytoplasmic filaments are called **puncta adherentes** (14). A punctum adherens appears to act much like a desmosome and is the desmosomal equivalent in the central nervous system (see sections on the retina, Ch. 6; optic nerve, Ch. 12).

REFERENCES

1. Brightman MW, Reese TS: Junctions between intimately apposed cell membranes in the vertebrate brain. J Cell Biol 40:648, 1969
2. Farquhar MG, Palade GE: Junctional complexes in various epithelia. J Cell Biol 17:375, 1963
3. Fawcett DW: Structural specializations of the cell surface. In Palay SL (ed): Frontiers in Cytology. New Haven, Yale University Press, 1958
4. Fine BS, Zimmerman LE: Müller's cells and the "middle limiting membrane" of the human retina. Invest Ophthal 1:304, 1962
5. Friend DS, Gilula NB: Variations in tight and gap junctions in mammalian tissues. J Cell Biol 53:758, 1972
6. Goodenough DA, Revel JP: A fine structural analysis of intercellular junctions in the mouse liver. J Cell Biol 45:272, 1970
7. Herr JC: Reflexive gap junctions—gap junctions between processes arising from the same ovarian decidual cell. J Cell Biol 69:495, 1976
8. Hudspeth AJ, Yee AG: The intercellular junctional complexes of retinal pigment epithelia. Invest Ophthalmol 12:354, 1973
9. Kelly DE: Fine structure of desmosomes, hemidesmosomes and an adepidermal globular layer in developing newt epidermis. J Cell Biol 28:51, 1966
10. Lord BAP, Di Bona DR: Role of the septate junction in the regulation of paracellular transepithelial flow. J Cell Biol 71:967, 1976
11. Odland GF: The fine structure of the interrelationship of cells in the human epidermis. J Biophys Biochem Cytol 4:529, 1958
12. Overton J: Desmosome development in normal and reassociating cells in the early chick blastoderm. Dev Biol 4:532, 1962
13. Overton J: Selective formation of desmosomes in chick cell reaggregates. Dev Biol 39:210, 1974
14. Peters A, Palay S, Webster H deF: The Fine Structure of the Nervous System: The Neurons and Supporting Cells. Philadelphia, WB Saunders, 1976
15. Robertson JD: Unit membranes: a review with recent new studies of experimental alterations and a new subunit structure in synaptic membranes. In Locke M (ed): Cellular Membranes in Development. New York, Academic Press, 1964, p 1
16. Skerrow CJ, Maltoltsy AG: Isolation of epidermal desmosomes. J Cell Biol 63:515, 1974
17. Skerrow CJ, Maltoltsy AG: Chemical characterization of isolated epidermal desmosomes. J Cell Biol 63:524, 1974
18. Yanoff M, Fine BS: Ocular pathology: a text and atlas. Hagerstown, Harper & Row, 1975
19. Zimmerman LE, Fine BS: Production of hyaluronic acid by cysts and tumors of the ciliary body. Arch Ophthal (Chicago) 72:365, 1964

chapter 4

EXTRACELLULAR MATERIALS

FIBROUS MATERIALS   39
  COLLAGEN AND RETICULIN
  ELASTIC TISSUE
    MICROFIBRILS AND ELASTIN
MUCINOUS MATERIALS   41
  POLYSACCHARIDES
  GLYCOPROTEINS
CRYSTALLINE MATERIALS: MINERALS   42
BASEMENT MEMBRANES   42
  THIN
  THICK
    HOMOGENEOUS, VACUOLATED
    BANDED: ORDERED, DISORDERED
    FILAMENTOUS/FIBROUS
  MULTILAMINAR

An aggregate of cells together with their extracellular materials constitutes a tissue (Fig. 4–1). The extracellular materials are separable morphologically into at least three groups: fibrous materials (e.g., collagen, elastic tissue), mucinous materials (e.g., mucins, mucopolysaccharides, glycoproteins), and crystalline materials (e.g., calcium, bone). Basement membranes are sometimes considered as a special form of fibrous material (i.e., collagen).

FIBROUS MATERIALS: COLLAGEN AND RETICULIN

The fibrous components of ocular tissues consist of bundles of macromolecules composed of linear arrangements of amino acids. Amino acids, having rather rigid "backbones" to their molecules, produce, in turn, rigid macromolecules that in aggregates form rigid filaments, fibrils, and fibers (Fig. 4–2).

Collagen is the most ubiquitous fibrous component (Greek *kolla*, glue, plus Greek *gennan*, to produce). It is characterized by its morphology, its x-ray diffraction pattern, its amino acid composition (especially its content of hydroxyproline and hydroxylysine), and its structural content of sugar (12).

X-ray diffraction studies show that "native" collagen (i.e., that which is derived from natural sources such as tendons in contradistinction to collagen produced in vitro) produces a repeating pattern of ~640 A. The pattern is almost identical, with a periodicity (**banding**) observed in the fibrils by electron microscopy (Fig. 4–3), a periodicity that has come to be considered characteristic of "mature" collagen. Further subdivision of the periodic bands (intraperiod banding) can also be observed.

Fibrous structures of smaller diameter often are seen in fetal tissues, in cultures of young fibroblasts, and in the vitreous body. Although they all possess a smaller periodicity (~220 A), their amino acid composition is appropriate for collagen. The smaller diameter structures may

be termed filaments of embryonic, fetal, or "young" collagen.

The smallest basic unit of a collagen fibril or filament is the collagen molecule (12). It measures ~15 A in diameter and 2800–3000 A in length in its hydrated state. The molecule is composed of three similar polypeptide chains called alpha (α) chains arranged in the form of a three-stranded or triple helix. Two of the amino acids, hydroxyproline and hydroxylysine, are considered highly characteristic of the collagen molecule, as they are not found elsewhere in significant concentration. The collagen molecule is intimately associated with a small amount of sugar, mainly glucose, from which it cannot be completely separated. The small amount of sugar is considered an integral part of the collagen molecule. Collagen is therefore a glycoprotein. The collagen molecules align themselves to produce increasingly visible filaments and fibrils of varying diameters and lengths. In cross section, collagen fibrils often show zones of axial lucency, as well as cross sections of uniform density. These observations suggest a structure not unlike a stalk of bamboo.

In the production of collagen, three pro-alpha polypeptide chains are synthesized and cross-linked within the cell to form a molecule slightly longer than a collagen molecule. This is called the **procollagen** molecule. The highly soluble procollagen molecule cannot polymerize and is converted into collagen presumably by enzymatic (endopeptidase) activity, which shortens the molecule by ~15% by removing coordination peptides located at the N terminal end of the polypeptide chains. Such conversion from pro-alpha to alpha chains is rapid and probably occurs at or near the site of transport of the molecule across the cell membrane. The newly converted molecule is also called tropocollagen and can polymerize readily. Outside the cell the collagen molecules assemble into filaments, fibrils, and fibers of varying diameters. Very little, if any, procollagen can be found outside the cell (see section on basement membranes).

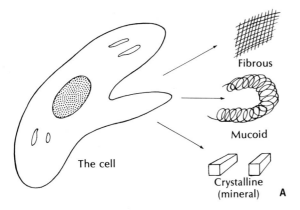

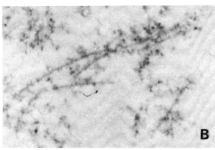

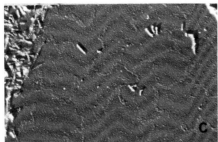

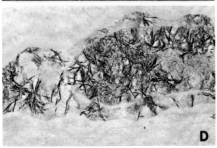

FIG. 4–1. Components of tissue. A. Tissue consists of cells surrounded by extracellular materials. B, C, D. Electron microscopy visualizes fibrous extracellular materials as filaments (**B**) or fibrils (Fig. 4–3); mucinous materials as fluffy aggregates in thin sections (**B**) or as irregular drying patterns in shadow-cast preparations (**C**), and minerals as crystalline structures (**D**). (**B,** × 32,000; **C,** × 16,000; **D,** × 21,000)

The best characterized collagen is that derived from skin, bone, tendon, and cornea (8). It contains three polypeptide chains (α chains) arranged in a triple helix. This collagen (called type I)* has two identical chains α 1 (I) and one similar but not identical chain, α 2. Each collagen has a unique amino acid sequence. The chain composition is therefore $[\alpha\,1\,(I)]_2\,\alpha\,2$. The other known vertebrate collagens consist of three identical chains. Type II* collagen is found in hyaline cartilage, vitreous body, neuroretina, and notochord (*i.e.*, chain composition $[\alpha\,1\,(II)]_3$). Type III* collagen is abundant in fetal tissue and is found in skin, blood vessels, and intestine (*i.e.*, chain composition $[\alpha\,1\,(III)]_3$). Type IV* is located in basement membranes (*i.e.*, chain composition $[\alpha\,1\,(IV)]_3$).

In ocular tissues, the term **fibril** has been reserved for those collagens that are of sufficient diameter to bear the 640-A periodicity (e.g., as in the cornea, uvea, and sclera). The term **filament** is used for the finer structures characteristic of vitreous framework, and the term **fiber** is used for the more grossly visible structures such as the zonule of the lens.

Reticulin is a term for the hypothetic structural component of a *reticulum* (e.g., liver reticulum), a delicate network observed around a variety of cells (11). Currently, a reticulum or its "reticulin" is demonstrated by the deposition of silver salts on the delicate extracellular network. By electron microscopy, the fibrous component of the network is seen to vary from "typical' 640-A period collagen *fibrils* (e.g., iris stroma) to "atypical" 220-A period collagen *filaments* (e.g., vitreous framework). That the densely packed typical collagen fibrils in the corneal stroma, which stain poorly for reticulin, can be made to stain well if foci of the stroma are mechanically disrupted indicates that reticulin is but a mechanically looser arrangement of various collagen fibrils or filaments.

ELASTIC TISSUE: MICROFIBRILS, ELASTIN

Elastic tissue is best observed when it occurs in quantity (*i.e.*, ligamentum nuchae or the internal elastic lamina of larger arteries). It is generally identified in light microscopy by special staining methods (e.g., Verhoeff's or Weigert's stains).

* Based on characteristic amino acid composition of the molecule.

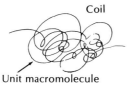

Mucoid molecules

Coil

Unit macromolecule

Fibrous molecules

Bundle

Unit macromolecule

FIG. 4–2. Schematic drawing of unit macromolecules and their aggregate forms.

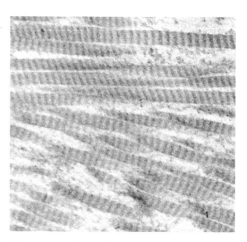

FIG. 4–3. Collagen fibrils as seen by electron microscopy in thin section. Cross-striation or periodicity of ~640 A is characteristic of most collagen fibrils. (× 25,000)

Chemically it differs from collagen by its lower content of hydroxyproline, by the absence of hydroxylysine, by its higher valine content, and by its relative chemical inertness (*i.e.,* resistance to hydrolysis by mild acid or alkali). By electron microscopy (see Fig. 10–34A, 73, 12–22) it is characterized by two components (6, 14), the fibrillar part or *microfibrils* (~110 A diameter), and the homogeneous part, *elastin.* It appears to originate early in life in a manner similar to collagen, as recognizable extracellular filaments or microfibrils lying adjacent to the plasma membranes of the synthesizing cells (*e.g.,* fibroblasts, smooth muscle cells). The homogeneous component, elastin, appears later, within the bundle of microfibrils, producing the composite structure *elastic tissue.* The microfibrils and the elastin differ considerably from each other in their chemical composition. Elastin contains the amino acids desmosine and isodesmosine, which are responsible for crosslinking the polymers to produce a special elastic syncytium. The microfibrils lack these two amino acids and are considered to act as a sort of scaffolding, which serves to shape the homogeneous deposits of elastin into fibrous or sheetlike, fenestrated arrangements (*e.g.,* in ligaments or in elastic arteries).

MUCINOUS MATERIALS: POLYSACCHARIDES AND GLYCOPROTEINS

Considerable confusion exists in the literature concerning the exact meaning of the terms mucins, mucoids, mucinous substances, mucosubstances, mucoproteins, mucopolysaccharides, acid mucopolysaccharides, and glycoproteins. All these substances are amino-sugar-containing compounds. Except for glycogen and the nucleic acids, all carbohydrate polymers of higher animals contain amino sugars. For the sake of simplicity, the following terminology will be used in this discussion:

Polysaccharide. A macromolecule composed of monosaccharide units with or without protein attachments

Homopolysaccharide. A macromolecule composed of many monosaccharide units generally not linked to proteins, *e.g.,* glycogen

Heteropolysaccharide. A macromolecule composed of a mixture of constituent building blocks, *e.g.,* amino sugars and hexuronic acids in acid mucopolysaccharides. The heteropolysaccharides may be weakly linked to proteins.

Glycoprotein (15, 17). A saccharide, usually an oligosaccharide, that is strongly attached to a protein and forms an integral part of the protein molecule. Examples are basement membranes (lens capsule, Descemet's membrane) and collagen (reticulin).

Acid mucopolysaccharides (AMP). Heteropolysaccharides containing amino sugars and hexuronic acids or sulfate esters or both (3, 9, 10, 21).

In their native state AMP are thought to be

associated with proteins by weak ionic linkages or labile covalent bonds. They differ, therefore, from glycoproteins in containing hexuronic acids or sulfate esters or both and in not having oligosaccharide units or firm linkage by covalent bonds to protein. Since AMP are composed of amino sugars and hexuronic acids, they have little intrinsic strength and so lie coiled up within a jacket of water. In tissue, therefore, they form a slippery, loose, watery network between collagen fibrils and filaments, best exemplified in the vitreous body. These networks appear morphologically as indistinct "fluffy" patches on fibrous structures when seen in thin electron microscopic sections (Fig. 4–1B and 4–2). On the surface of shadow-cast, thicker sections, from which only the water and various ions have been removed, they appear as "drying patterns" (Fig. 4-1C).

Another characteristic of AMP is that they contain a large number of negatively charged groups or ions. They are, therefore, polyanionic and have to carry an equivalent number of cations, usually sodium, called **counterions.** Use is made of the polyanionic nature of AMP in a number of histochemical techniques. The colloidal iron method utilizes a trivalent ferric cationic complex that attaches to the anions of AMP and then is made visible by staining with ferrocyanide (the Prussian blue reaction). Alcian blue is a tetravalent cationic complex that attaches to polyanionic substances and directly colors the material blue. Another histochemical technique that utilizes the polyanionic nature of AMP with the additional prerequisite of sulfate esters is the metachromatic staining* achieved with certain cationic dyes (e.g., toluidine blue, methyl violet, crystal violet). Since hyaluronic acid does not contain sulfate esters, it does not exhibit metachromasia.

Acid mucopolysaccharides do not react with the PAS stain (17). For a substance to be PAS-positive, it must have unsubstituted vicinal glycol groups (CHOH-CHOH). The periodic acid oxidizes the groups to dialdehydes (CHO-CHO). The Schiff reagent (leucofuchsin) then reacts with the dialdehydes. The Schiff reagent-dialdehyde complexes range in color from red to magenta and are easily identified in tissue

sections. The homopolysaccharides (e.g., glucose) have abundant vicinal glycol groups along the course of their long-chain monosaccharide units and are, therefore, PAS-positive. Glycoproteins (e.g., lens capsule) also contain many vicinal glycol groups in the large number of unsubstituted sugars located at the ends of their oligosaccharide chains and are also PAS-positive. Glycogen can be differentiated from glycoprotein by applying diastase to the tissue under consideration. The diastase digests out the glycogen so that the PAS method no longer stains glycogen but continues to color glycoprotein. Other groups of compounds that give a PAS-positive reaction include glycolipids (e.g., gangliosides and cerebrosides) and unsaturated lipids and phospholipids (e.g., sphingomyelin and lipofuscins).

The AMP found in the eye are listed in Table 4–1. Hyaluronic acid is the only AMP found in the vitreous body. The AMP associated with rods and cones in bovine eyes contains a mixture of partly sulfated chondroitin and sialoglycan (see Retina, Ch. 6). In human eyes sialic acid may be contributed by the pigment epithelium (5).

CRYSTALLINE MATERIALS: MINERALS

Calcification does not occur in the normal eye (except in aging tissues), but it may occur in pathologic tissues. Figure 4–1D shows hydroxyapatite crystals within a cell. With aging, calcification occurs in Bruch's membrane (Fig. 6–11) as well as in various basement membranes (Fig. 4–10, 10–38B).

BASEMENT MEMBRANES

Associated with, but lying outside, the basal plasma membranes of various epithelia (or endothelia) is the *basement membrane*, a continuous layer of material of moderate electron density. The layer may be so thin (Fig. 4–4) as to be inadequately observable by light microscopy, or so thick (Fig. 4–5, 4–6) that it can be seen with the naked eye. Thin basement membranes,* are separated from the cell plasma

---

* Metachromasia may be defined as the staining of a tissue component so that the absorption spectrum of the resulting tissue dye complex differs sufficiently from that of the original dye, and from its ordinary tissue complexes, to give a marked change in color.

---

* The term **thin basement membrane** is synonymous with the term **basal lamina** (1) used by some anatomists. **Basement membrane** is the preferred term because it is consistent historically with the terms used to describe normal ocular structures, as well as currently for pathologic ocular structures (20).

membrane by a lucent zone (Fig. 6–68, 6–69). When the basement membrane is thick (Fig. 6–65), this zone is absent, suggesting that the lucent zone consists of a watery material, that some juxtacellular material is lost consistently and uniformly during the processing of the tissue, or that this membrane retracts from the cell during processing.

Some thick ocular basement membranes are formed by an interweaving of multiple thin basement membranes, the composite structure being a *multilaminar* basement membrane. The multilaminar basement membranes may themselves be composed of thickened lamellas (*e.g.,* peripheral corneal epithelium or external basement membrane of the ciliary epithelium of the pars plicata) or of thin lamellas (*e.g.,* in-

FIG. 4–4. Typical thin basement membrane (**BM**) normally following contour of cell plasma membrane and separated from it by uniform zone of lucency. In regions of abnormality, thin basement membrane (**BM₁**) may be markedly folded or convoluted. ($\times$ 13,500)

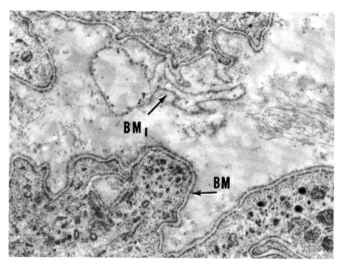

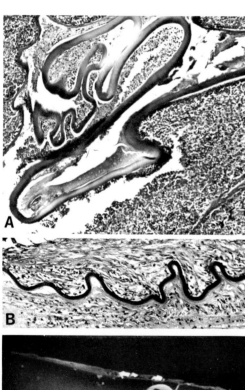

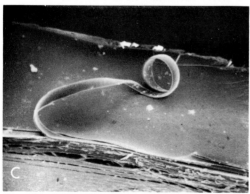

FIG. 4–5. Scanning electron micrograph of broken edge of posterior lens capsule (**arrow**) showing thick, sheetlike basement membrane. ($\times$ 57)

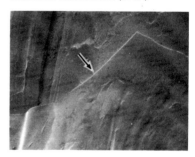

FIG. 4–6. Marked folding of disrupted thick basement membranes. A. Membrane from rabbit lens capsule. (PAS, $\times$ 100) (AFIP Neg. 66-8918) B. Descemet's membrane from rabbit cornea. (PAS, $\times$ 100) (AFIP Neg. 66-8919). C. Scanning electron micrograph of anterior lens capsule. Detached strip of capsule lies coiled on the free surface ($\times$ 30).

Table 4–1. Acid Mucopolysaccharides of the Eye

Acid mucopolysaccharide	Amino sugar	Uronic acid	Sulfate groups	Characteristic			Main location
				Alcian blue after testicular hyaluronidase	Alcian blue after streptococcal hyaluronidase	Metachromasia	
Hyaluronic acid	Glucosamine	Glucuronic acid	0	Negative	Negative	Negative	Vitreous, cornea, sclera
Chondroitin sulfate A	Galactosamine	Glucuronic acid	1	Negative or weakly positive	Positive	Positive	?Cornea, sclera
Chondroitin sulfate B	Galactosamine	Iduronic acid	1	Positive	Positive	Positive	?Cornea, sclera
Chondroitin sulfate C	Galactosamine	Glucuronic acid	1	Negative or weakly positive	Positive	Positive	?Cornea, sclera
Chondroitin	Galactosamine	Glucuronic acid	0	Negative	Negative	?	Cornea
Keratosulfate	Glucosamine	(Galactose)	1	?	?	Positive	Cornea
Heparin	Glucosamine	Glucuronic acid, iduronic acid	2.5	Positive	Positive	Positive	Mast cells
Heparin monosulfuric acid	Glucosamine	Glucuronic acid, iduronic acid	1	Positive	Positive	Positive	Mast cells
Retinal receptor AMP	?	?	?	Positive	Positive	Positive	Space between retinal receptors

ternal basement or limiting membrane of the ciliary epithelium).

The thicker ocular basement membranes have long been appreciated by histologists and known by the synonyms "glass membranes" or "cuticular membranes." Many of their chemical and physical properties can be determined from light and electron microscopic studies of the normal and abnormal basement membranes as well as from direct clinical observation *in vivo* (*e.g.*, their transparency).

Because basement membranes are glycoproteins (2) and have abundant vicinal hydroxyl groups (see glycoproteins), they stain vividly with the PAS method (Fig. 4–6). The membranes are perhaps best appreciated as a two-phase system (16) in which the fibrous component consists of collagen in exceedingly fine filamentous to microfilamentous form (even to the procollagen molecule level) embedded in a matrix of various polysaccharides (up to 10% of their weight).* Some basement membranes (*e.g.*, lens capsule) show a distinct filamentous composition, while others (*e.g.*, kidney glomerulus) are less distinct.

From histopathologic and clinical observations it is clear that the thicker basement membranes are transparent and remain so, are relatively indigestible, possess the elastic properties of retracting and folding when disrupted (Fig. 4–6), and are elaborated by the cells that lie upon them (*i.e.*, epithelium or endothelium). When the known properties of thick basement membranes are extrapolated to the thin basement membranes, the properties of the latter can be better understood—their relative indigestibility, their folding (Fig. 4–4) and elastic-like retraction when broken, and their elaboration by the cells that lie upon them.

The free surfaces of such thick glasslike basement membranes are smooth (see Fig. 8–7, 8–11) and highly reflecting. This accounts for the shining surfaces of such membranes as Descemet's, the lens capsule, or the normal internal limiting membrane of the human retina. As the structural macromolecules slowly alter with age (*e.g.*, increasing polymerization), some of the

---

* Although type IV collagen has been prepared from some basement membranes (7), it has not yet been well characterized. The morphologic differences from filamentous to fibrous composition in normal and pathologic ocular basement membranes indicates that a wide variety of basement membranes can be formed. Variants of type IV collagen may, therefore, also occur.

physical and morphologic properties of these basement membranes presumably are altered. They therefore may become less reflecting, as in the lens capsule or the internal limiting membrane of the retina, or may show foci of rarefaction and densification, as in the internal limiting membrane of the retina or the basement membranes of retinal blood vessels.

CLASSIFICATION:

Thin 300–500 A (30–50 nm) thick, generally separated by a lucent space from the cell basal plasmalemma and appears as a homogeneous to finely filamentous (feltwork-like) material (Fig. 4–7A).

FIG. 4–7. A. Typical thin basement membrane following basal plasmalemmas of cells (basement membrane of nonpigmented ciliary epithelium or internal basement membrane of the ciliary epithelium). (× 14,000) B. Thin basement membrane (**on left**) sectioned tangentially (**on right**) to show its microfilamentous (>50 A diameter) or feltwork-like construction. (Rh fovea, internal limiting membrane, × 28,000)

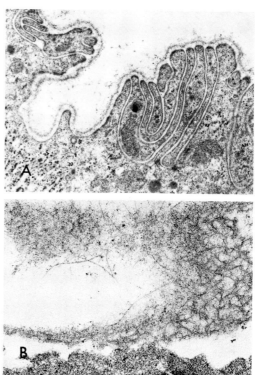

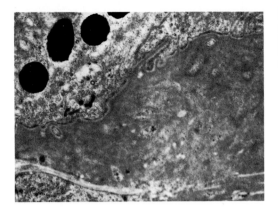

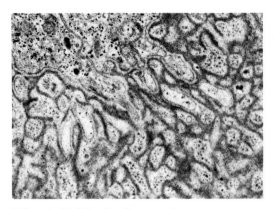

FIG. 4–8. Thick basement membrane applied to basal plasmalemmas of pigment epithelial cells of pars plana ciliaris (external basement membrane of the ciliary epithelium (× 17,600)

Thick > 500 A (50 nm) in thickness, applied directly to the cell basal plasmalemma (Fig. 4–8) and varying in appearance from homogeneous (or vacuolated) to filamentous or banded. The latter have an ordered periodicity of either 500 or 1000 A* (50 or 100 nm) or may appear disordered (without periodicity) (see Figs. 4–12).

Multilaminar Composed of thin basement membranes superimposed in the fashion of a honeycomb (Fig. 4–9). Each lamella may be either thin or thick.

In pathologic tissues (20), the characteristics are grossly exaggerated, modified or altered. The normal or altered structure of the basement membranes undoubtedly mirrors the biochemical activities conducted by the producing cell (*i.e.*, more carbohydrate → more homogeneous basement membrane (19), more collagen → more filamentous-to-fibrous basement membrane [18]).

Embryonically, all basement membranes commence as the thin variety. With growth and

FIG. 4–9. Multilaminar basement membrane applied to basal plasmalemmas of pigmented ciliary epithelium of the pars plicata ciliaris (external basement membrane of the ciliary epithelium)-(TSC, × 22,400)

FIG. 4–10. Base of pigment epithelial cell of the retina. Patches of banded (~1000 A) basement membrane (**b**) produced within basilar infoldings of the cell are undergoing calcification (**arrows**); **bm,** normal thin basement membrane of cell. (× 17,000)

* The basement membrane with 1000-A periodicity should not be confused with the 2000-A to 3000-A periodic collagen fibril, which can be produced *in vitro* by reconstitution of separated collagen molecules. Measurements of periodicity similar to those *in vitro* or reconstituted collagen fibrils have not yet been observed in normal ocular tissues. *In-vitro* collagen fibrils are formed by dissolution of normal or "native" collagen into basic collagen molecules (dimension ~15 by 2800–3000 A). Their subsequent reconstitution *in vitro,* achieved by manipulating their milieu, produces a true native type of periodic collagen *fiber* (*i.e.*, with 640-A axial periodicity), a non-native fibrous long-spacing *fiber* (*i.e.*, with ~2800-A axial periodicity), or non-native *segments*, called segment long-spacing (*i.e.*, ~2800 A in *length*) structures.

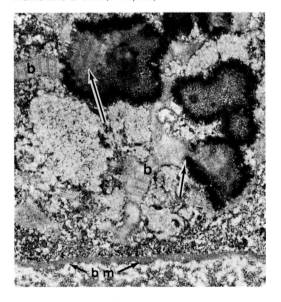

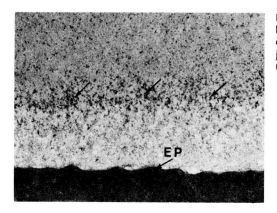

FIG. 4–11. Siderosis lentis. Iron particles have penetrated through anterior lens capsule, forming a distinct band (**arrows**) just anterior to lens epithelium (**EP**). (× 25,500)

aging, the thicker and more complex varieties are produced in a controlled manner. Deposition of pathologic materials, e.g., calcium (see Fig. 4–10, 6–11, 10–38B), fibrin, or amyloid, or the addition of metallic substances not normally present, e.g., silver, copper, or iron (Fig. 4–11), produces more complex basement membranes (20).

Although it is not our intent to discuss pathologic tissues here, it is difficult to completely avoid them because "the pathologic is often an aberration of the normal," a phrase most aptly applied to any discussion of basement membranes. The "physiologic" changes of aging provide the most suitable bridge to examine, lying between the "normal" (*i.e.*, young adult) the aged adult, and the abnormal.

In the aging eye a variety of basement membranes are produced (Fig. 4–12); structures that are not common or are even absent in the young adult become more noticeable with age, e.g., banded, filamentous/fibrous, filamentous-banded (Fig. 4–12A) or vacuolated basement membranes (Fig. 4–12D); and even more prominent in conditions considered pathologic (*e.g.*, cornea guttata or Fuchs' combined dystrophy of the cornea [Fig. 4–12F]). On the other hand, abnormal cells produce such a variety and quantity of basement membranes (4, 13, 18–20) (Fig. 4–12E) that the gross exaggerations so produced provide us with additional insight into the mechanisms of basement membrane (or even collagen) formations by the normal cell.

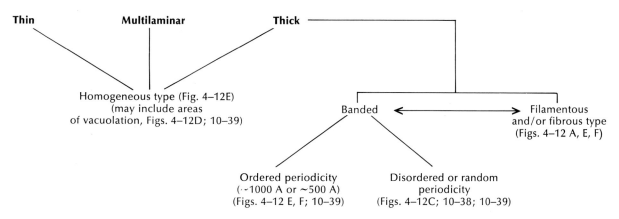

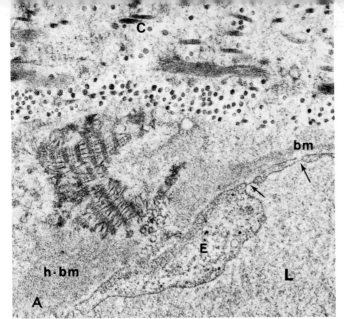

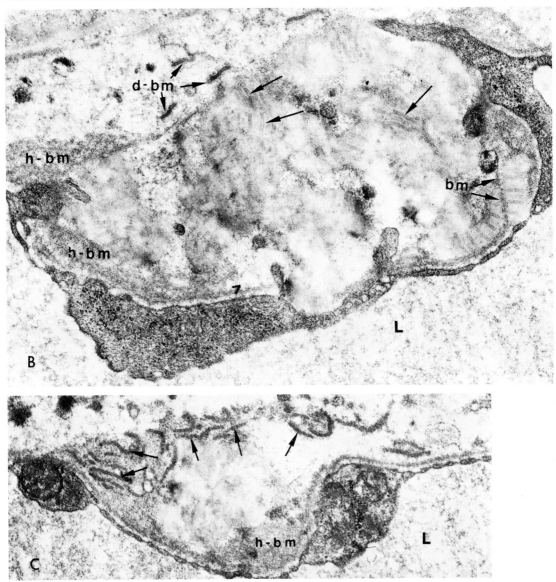

FIG. 4–12. A. Choriocapillaris, region of fovea. Note fenestrae (**arrows**) in endothelial (**E**) cell. Thin basement membrane (**bm**) at right is altered into a patch of homogeneous basement membrane (**h-bm**) at left. A patch of filamentous banded (~1000 A) basement membrane has formed within the patch of homogeneous basement membrane. **C,** collagen fibrils within Bruch's membrane; **L,** lumen of choriocapillaris. (TSC, × 29,000) B. Choriocapillaris, fovea, 18-year-old subject. Endothelium has produced an excess ("druse") of basement membrane in a variety of forms. Note attenuation of thin basement membrane (**bm**) into a mass of banded (~1000 A) basement membrane. Patches of similar banded basement membrane are present within ▶

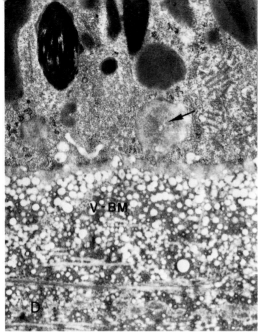

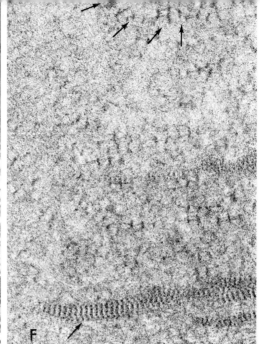

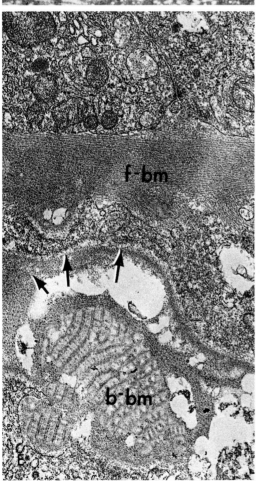

the nodule. Note "double-walled"
structure characteristic of banded
basement membrane (**arrows**). Similar
double-walled structures lie freely near
by (disordered, banded basement
membrane, **d-bm**). Patches of
homogeneous basement membrane
(**h-bm**) are in continuity with the thin
basement membrane. **L,** lumen of
choriocapillaris. ($\times$ 31,000) C.
Choriocapillaris, fovea, 18-year-old
subect. Nodules of homogeneous
basement membrane (**h-bm**) formed by
endothelial cell. Disordered banded
basement membrane (**arrows**) is present
within one of the homogeneous masses.
L, lumen of choriocapillaris. ($\times$ 31,000)
D. Vacuolated basement membrane
(**v-bm**) produced by pigment epithelium
in foveal region of 76-year-old subject.
Basement membrane lining basal
plasmalemma is homogeneous, as is a
similar nodule formed within an
infolding of the plasmalemma (**arrow**).
(See Drusen Ch. 10). ($\times$ 18,000)
E. Basement membranes secreted by
irritated pigment epithelial cells. Note
transition of normal thin basement
membranes into wider area of
homogeneous basement membrane
(**arrows**). Upper region of basement
membrane is clearly filamentous (**f-bm**),
while lowermost region is composed of
ordered banded basement membrane
(**b-bm**) ($\sim$1000 A). ($\times$ 20,000) (From
Yanoff M, Fine BS: Ocular Pathology.
Hagerstown, MD, Harper & Row, 1975)
F. Basement membranes (cornea guttata)
secreted by abnormal corneal
endothelial cells. Ordered banded
($\sim$1000 A) basement membrane is
present (**arrows**) as well as $\sim$500 A
banded basement membrane (**single
arrow**). ($\times$ 28,000)

REFERENCES

1. Bloom W, Fawcett DW: A Textbook of Histology, 10th ed. Philadelphia, WB Saunders, 1975
2. Dische Z: The glycans of the mammalian lens capsule—a model of basement membranes. In Siperstein M (ed): Small Blood Vessel Involvement in Diabetes Mellitus. Washington DC, American Institute of Biological Science, 1964
3. Dorfman A: Polysaccharides of connective tissue. J Histochem Cytochem 11:2, 1963
4. Fine BS, Yanoff M, Pitts RE, Slaughter FD: Meesmann's epithelial dystrophy of the cornea: report of two families with discussion of the pathogenesis of the characteristic lesion. Am J Ophthalmol 83: 633, 1977
5. Font RL, Zimmerman LE, Fine BS: Adenoma of the pigment epithelium: histochemical and electron microscopic observations. Am J Ophthalmol 73:544, 1972
6. Greenlee TK, Jr, Ross R, Hartman JL: The fine structure of elastic fibers. J Cell Biol 30:59, 1966
7. Kefalides NA: Structure and biosynthesis of basement membranes. Int Rev Connect Tissue Res 6:63, 1973
8. Martin GR, Byers PH, Piez KA: Procollagen. In Meister A (ed): Advances in Enzymology, vol 42. New York, John Wiley & Sons, 1975, p 167
9. Meyer K: Chemistry and biology of mucopolysaccharides and glycoproteins. Cold Spring Harbor Symp Quant Biol 6:91, 1938
10. Meyer K, Davidson E, Linker A, Hoffman P: The acid mucopolysaccharides of connective tissue. Biochem Biophys Acta 21:506, 1956
11. Puchtler H: On the original definition of the term "reticulin." J Histochem Cytochem 12:552, 1964
12. Ramachandran GN, Reddi AH (eds): Biochemistry of Collagen. New York, Plenum Press, 1976
13. Rodrigues MM, Fine BS, Laibson PR, Zimmerman LE: Disorders of the corneal epithelium—a clinicopathologic study of dot, geographic and fingerprint patterns. Arch Ophthalmol 92:475, 1974
14. Ross R, Bornstein P: The elastic fiber. I. The separation and partial characterization of its macromolecular components. J Cell Biol 40:366, 1969
15. Sharon N: Glycoproteins. Sci Am 230:78, 1974
16. Slayter G: Two-phase materials. Sci Am 206:124, 1962
17. Spiro RG: Glycoproteins: their biochemistry, biology, and role in human disease. New Engl J Med 281: 1043, 1969
18. Waring GO, Font RL, Rodrigues MM, Mulberger RD: Alterations of Descemet's membrane in interstitial keratitis. Am J Ophthalmol 81:733, 1976
19. Weiter J, Fine BS: A histologic study of regional choroidal dystrophy. Am J Ophthalmol 83:741, 1977
20. Yanoff M, Fine BS: Ocular Pathology: A Text and Atlas, Hagerstown, Harper & Row, 1975, p 638
21. Zugibe FT: Mucopolysaccharides of the arterial wall. J Histochem Cytochem 11:35, 1963

chapter 5

ARRANGEMENT OF TISSUES AND CELLS

EPITHELIA, ENDOTHELIA, AND MESOTHELIA   53

EFFECT OF CELL GROWTH AND
      DIFFERENTIATION ON CONFIGURATION
      OF CELL MEMBRANE   54

CONNECTIVE TISSUE   55

MUSCLE   55

NERVE TISSUE   55

CONVENTIONS USED IN DESCRIBING THE
      EYE   55

  THE THREE-COAT (TRILAMINAR)
      ARRANGEMENT   55

  DIRECTIONS   56

  ORIENTATION   56

  THE THREE-TISSUE ARRANGEMENT   57

EPITHELIA, ENDOTHELIA, AND MESOTHELIA

When epithelium or endothelium lines a lumen or a free surface, each cell has a free end and an attached end (Fig. 5–1). The free end of the cell is called the *apex,* and the attached end the *base.* In highly oriented or *polarized* cells there are *apical* plasma membranes, *basilar* plasma membranes, and *lateral* plasma membranes or plasmalemmas.

Lying outside the basilar plasmalemmas of epithelia or endothelia is a continuous thick or thin layer of homogeneous-appearing extracellular material, the basement membrane (see Ch. 4). On the other side of the basement membrane is the *connective tissue,* usually collagenous fibrils, which also may be *thick* or *thin, i.e.,* fibrils or filaments. Other interfibrillar materials may be present. As in retinal blood vessels, the connective tissues occasionally may be replaced by another basement membrane and its associated cell.

Ocular epithelia are derived from surface *ectoderm* or *neuroectoderm.* The epithelia may undergo the usual modifications of epithelia elsewhere and may produce apical villi and cilia, glands that secrete mucinous materials, as well as melanin granules. The cells may vary in shape from the flattened *squamous* cell of the corneal epithelial surface through the *cuboidal* cells of the lens epithelium or retinal pigment epithelium to the *columnar* cells of the nonpigmented epithelial layer of the posterior pars plana.

The cells that form the innermost lining of the blood vessels and lymphatics are called **endothelial** cells. They are derived from mesoderm.

The cells that line body cavities other than those of the vascular-lymphatic system (*i.e.,* pleural, pericardial, peritoneal, and anteriormost boundary of the aqueous compartment) are called **mesothelial cells.**

According to one authority (3), the term epithelium is used in the context of its *appearance* and *function.* The term endothelium and mesothelium refer to their mesodermal origin.

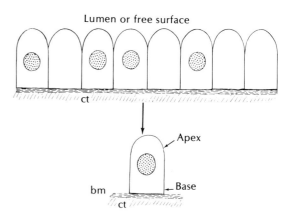

Lumen or free surface

Apex

Base

FIG. 5–1. Schematic drawing of highly oriented or polarized epithelia or endothelia lining a lumen or a free surface, showing basic relation of a cell to its basement membrane (**bm**) and adjacent connective tissue (**ct**).

Morphologically, endothelial cells are but a modification of epithelial cells. The cell body is the site of the nucleus and therefore protrudes with the apical cytoplasm into the lumen. To form an endothelial tube, the lateral cytoplasm near the base of the cell is drawn out into large sheets, which adhere to neighboring cells by an attachment girdle (terminal bars) common to various epithelia (see Fig. 6–77). A basement membrane outside this elongated basilar plasma membrane completely envelops the endothelial tube.

The term **mesothelium** refers to cells having the ability to act like connective tissue cells in various pathologic conditions. Mesothelia closely resemble epithelia, are generally cuboidal and one-cell-layer thick, interdigitate laterally with neighboring cells, and may have an apical junctional complex and a moderate to very thick basement membrane (e.g., corneal "endothelium" with its Descemet's membrane) (see Ch. 4).

Embryologically the mesodermal portion of the primitive trilaminar structure gives rise to the musculoskeletal system and supporting connective tissues. The mesodermal tissues, therefore, are derived from the developing somites and other paraxial mesoderm. Recently it has been pointed out (4) that the primitive mesoderm becomes organized into various epithelial units, best represented by the somites which have lumens and basement membranes. The primitive mesoderm is called "primary mesenchyme," using the term **mesenchyme** as a general one to refer to embryonic and mesodermal connective tissues from all sources, including those from the neural crest. The luminal somites break up generally to form nonepithelial mesenchyme, called the **secondary mesenchyme.**

In the human, the head region does not form somites, and the primitive mesoderm appears as loosely arranged cells or sheets without lumens. The mesenchyme of the head and neck region is provided in large part by the neural crest so that the connective tissues of the head and neck are mostly mesectoderm (5, 6) (or ectomesenchyme). Mesodermal mesenchyme, however, still supplies the extraocular muscles and the orbital vascular components. Thus, the intraocular supporting structures, such as uveal cells, intraocular vascular pericytes, ciliary smooth muscle, keratocytes and corneal endothelial cells are now believed to be derived from neural crest mesenchyme.

The formation of tumors within the eye, wherein there is confusion by light microscopy between schwannomas and leiomyomas highlights these new embryologic concepts (5, 6, 9). Electron microscopic examination may be helpful and even necessary in establishing a firm diagnosis in such instances. The finding of striated muscle cells within a tumor of apparently neuroepithelial origin would not be as startling with this concept in mind.

EFFECT OF CELL GROWTH AND DIFFERENTIATION ON CONFIGURATION OF CELL MEMBRANE

With growth, a cell increases in volume and its ratio of volume to surface area changes (Fig. 5–2). However, since the surface area of the cell plasma membrane limits the relations (1), the cell has only a few alternatives: 1) it may cease to grow larger; 2) it may divide into two daughter cells; 3) it may increase its surface area by developing surface infolding and/or *villi*; 4) it may increase its surface area by simple elongation into a "straplike" flattened cell; 5) it may combine the last two alternatives so that the inner half of the cell consists of a stout elongated portion with many small delicate side projections and the outer half consists of large delicate cytoplasmic leaflets with much surface area. This last response is best exemplified by the Müller (glial) cell of the retina (see Ch. 6). Examples of other responses to cell growth are epithelial cells that show marked infoldings of their surfaces, lens and corneal stroma cells that undergo remarkable flattening and elongation into straplike formations, vascular endothelia that flatten into wide sheets, and neurons that produce enormous elongated cell extensions.

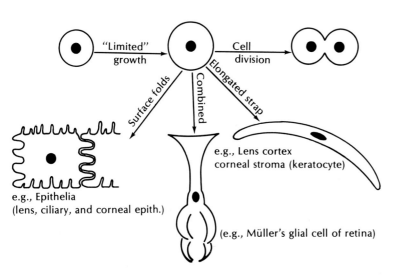

FIG. 5–2. Schematic drawing illustrating effect of cell growth on configuration of plasma membrane.

"Limited" growth

Cell division

Surface folds

Combined

Elongated strap

e.g., Lens cortex
corneal stroma (keratocyte)

e.g., Epithelia
(lens, ciliary, and corneal epith.)

(e.g., Müller's glial cell of retina)

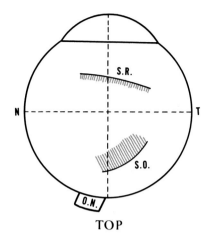

TOP

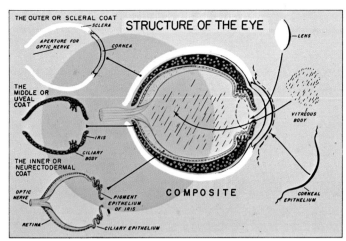

FIG. 5–3. Three-coat (trilaminar) arrangement of eye.

FRONT

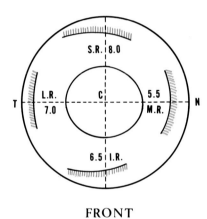

BACK

FIG. 5–6. Landmarks of front, back, and top of enucleated right eye. Tendons are shown in *green*, muscles in *brown*, nerves in *yellow*, arteries in *red*, veins in *blue*. **M.R., I.R., L.R., S.R.,** medial, inferior, lateral, and superior rectus muscles, respectively; **I.O.,** inferior oblique muscle; **S.O.,** superior oblique muscle; **V,** various vortex veins; **O.N.,** optic nerve; **L.P.C.A.,** long posterior ciliary artery; **L.C.N.,** long ciliary nerves. (Modified from Salzmann M: The Anatomy and Histology of the Human Eyeball in the Normal State: Its Development and Senescence. Chicago, University of Chicago Press, 1912)

CONNECTIVE TISSUE

A connective tissue consists of cells embedded in a matrix of extracellular materials. (The extracellular substances are described in Ch. 4.) Connective tissues vary in density from the extreme delicacy of the vitreous body to the marked density of cornea and sclera.

The most common cell type in connective tissue is the fibroblast, which, as the name implies, produces much of the fibrous as well as mucinous extracellular materials. In ocular tissues some of these cells have been given special names (*e.g.*, the *keratocyte* of the cornea). **Histiocytes,** which also may be present, have large, ovoid nuclei and are not readily identified until they have engulfed some foreign material. Then they are known as **macrophages** (as distinguished from the **microphages** of the bloodstream, more commonly known as **polymorphonuclear leukocytes**). The composition of the material engulfed (*e.g.*, blood-filled macrophages, melanin-filled macrophages, lysed lens-material–filled macrophages) determines the cytologic appearance of macrophages.

Mast cells are large cells that may be found in various connective tissues. In the eye they have been well demonstrated in the loose vascular connective tissue at the limbus and in the uveal tract. Their cytoplasm is almost filled with large *metachromatic* and PAS-positive granules containing *heparin* (see Fig. 9–45).

Among other cells that may be found in the connective tissue or may invade from the bloodstream are the plasma cells, which may be identified by their enormous amount of granular endoplasmic reticulum; the red blood cells themselves; the polymorphonuclear leukocytes, with cytoplasmic granules that differ in appearance from all the others; the eosinophils with their characteristic crystal-containing granules; the basophils; the monocytes; the lymphocytes; and the platelets.

MUSCLE

For discussion of the structure of striated muscles (of which the extraocular muscles are a good example), the reader is referred to Chapter 13, Orbit, as well as to standard texts on histology (2, 3). Smooth muscles (ciliary muscles, dilator and sphincter muscles of the iris) are discussed with the ciliary muscle of the ciliary body region (Ch. 10).

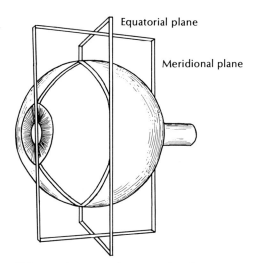

FIG. 5–4. Diagram of equatorial and meridional planes of the eye. (Scheie HG, Albert DM: Adler's Textbook of Ophthalmology. Philadelphia, WB Saunders, 1969)

NERVE TISSUE

The structure of typical and atypical neurons is described in Chapter 6. Current concepts of the morphology of the glia are discussed in Chapters 6 and 12.

CONVENTIONS USED IN DESCRIBING THE EYE

THE THREE-COAT (TRILAMINAR) ARRANGEMENT

Classically, the globe is described as three-layered (Col. Fig. 5–3). The outer, tough, collagenous, protective, or "skeletal" coat is opaque sclera, except anteriorly, where it becomes the transparent cornea. The innermost coat, the neuroectodermal layer, is a double layer of cells derived from an outpouching of the lateral wall of the primitive forebrain. It consists of the sensory neural retina with its pigment epithelium posteriorly and anterior extensions to form the double-layered epithelium of the ciliary body and iris. The primitive neural epithelium is sometimes called the medullary epithelium. Between the outer and inner layers of the eye lies the vascular and heavily pigmented uveal tract, which is subdivided topographically into three parts: the iris stroma anteriorly, the choroid posteriorly, and the ciliary body in between.

DIRECTIONS

The two principal planes in the eye are the equatorial and the meridional (Fig. 5–4). The **equatorial plane** lies midway between the anterior and posterior poles and is perpendicular to the meridional plane. Planes parallel to the equatorial plane (*i.e.,* anterior or posterior to it) are called transverse, coronal, frontal, or radial planes. The **meridional plane** passes through the anterior and posterior poles of the eye. Meridional planes may be horizontal, vertical, or oblique. Planes parallel to the meridional plane but *not* passing through the anterior and posterior poles are called **sagittal planes.**

ORIENTATION

The anatomic (ophthalmologic) orientation of the eye for descriptive purposes is such that the cornea is up and the optic nerve down (Fig. 5–5). The directional terms *anterior* and *posterior* are derived from this orientation. The terms *internal* and *external* (or lateral) are applied to directions proceeding *toward* and *away from* the geometric center of the globe.

The posterior view of the globe is the most useful in determining whether an enucleated eye (globe) is right or left (back view, Col. Fig. 5–6). The optic nerve and the adjacent fleshy attachment for the inferior oblique muscle are two of the most important landmarks in this view.

The optic nerve exits from the posterior aspect of the globe through a 3-mm diameter scleral canal 3 mm nasal to and 1 mm superior to the posterior pole. It can be readily observed lying within its meningeal sheaths. The temporal side of the eye from optic nerve to limbus features a longer arc than does the nasal side. The horizontal meridian is easily identified by two prominent blue lines radiating anteriorly in opposite directions from points near the optic nerve. The lines are the pathways of the long posterior temporal and long posterior nasal ciliary arteries and the accompanying long ciliary nerves. Once this horizontal meridian is identified, the superior, inferior, temporal, and nasal quadrants of the posterior pole of the eye can be easily determined from the insertions of the oblique muscles. The inferior oblique is the only one of the six extraocular muscles that inserts into the globe via a muscular (or at the most a very short tendinous) attachment. The attachment is easily identified temporal to the

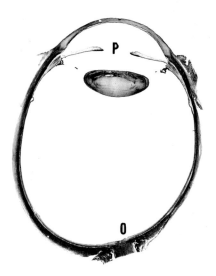

FIG. 5–5. Horizontal meridional section of an eye oriented in ophthalmic manner, with cornea *up* and optic nerve *down.* Note that section passes through both pupil (**P**) and optic nerve head (**O**). Such a section is sometimes called a **PO** section. (H & E stain, × 3) (AFIP Neg. 70-7292)

optic nerve and is inserted almost precisely along the horizontal meridian. Because the fibers of the inferior oblique muscle course downward, the inferior part of the globe can be identified. The fovea lies within the eye anterior to the nasal portion of the muscular insertion. Thus, by examining the posterior aspect of the globe, aligning the silhouettes of the two ciliary vessels into the horizontal meridian, and finding the muscular insertion of the inferior oblique, a right or left globe can be readily identified. The identification may be confirmed by seeking the tendinous insertion of the superior oblique muscle, which attaches to the sclera in the upper temporal quadrant (Fig. 5–6, top view).

Frequently, the vortex veins, usually four in number, are prominent. The position of these veins may vary considerably. In general, two lie above the optic nerve and two below. Each pair straddles the vertical meridian with the upper approximately 7 or 8 mm behind the equator and the lower ∼2 mm closer to it. Although the remnant insertions of the four rectus muscles are in a regular but varying relation to the limbus, they generally are not as useful as other landmarks for identifying a right or left eye. The short curved lines that mark the attachments of the rectus muscles do, however, spiral round the cornea in such a way that the medial rectus lies closest to the corneal margin (limbus) and the superior rectus lies the farthest away (Fig. 5–6, front view). A line connecting the insertions of the four rectus muscles forms the **spiral of Tillaux.** Many short posterior ciliary arteries and short ciliary nerves enter the sclera in a cluster around the optic nerve, but they are difficult to identify without the aid of a dissecting microscope. Because the cornea is oval, with the horizontal meridian larger than the vertical one, the horizontal meridian of the eye sometimes can be identified from the anterior view of the globe.

THE THREE-TISSUE ARRANGEMENT

The parts of the globe may also be described in terms of their predominant tissue component: those composed almost entirely of cells (e.g., lens, retina, and its pigment epithelium, and anterior extensions of ciliary and iris epithelium); those composed almost entirely of extracellular materials (e.g., corneosclera, vitreous body); and those composed of an even mixture of cells and extracellular materials (e.g., uveal tract). This classification is particularly appropriate to descriptions of ocular tissue studied by electron microscopy, and it is the one used in the succeeding chapters of this book.

REFERENCES

1. Asimov I: The Well Springs of Life. New York, New American Library, 1960
2. Bloom W, Fawcett DW: A Textbook of Histology, 10th ed. Philadelphia, WB Saunders, 1975
3. Ham AW: Histology, 7th ed. Philadelphia, JB Lippincott, 1974
4. Hay ED: Organization and fine structure of epithelium and mesenchyme in the developing chick embryo. In Fleischmajer R, Billingham R (eds): Epithelial-Mesenchymal Interactions. Baltimore, Williams & Wilkins, 1968, pp 31–55
5. Jakobiec FA, Font R, Tso MOM, Zimmerman LE: Mesectodermal leiomyoma of the ciliary body: a tumor of presumed neural crest origin. Cancer 39: 2102, 1977
6. Jakobiec FA, Tannenbaum M: Embryologic perspectives on the fine structure of orbital tumors. In Duane TD (ed): Clinical Ophthalmology, Vol 2. Hagerstown, Harper & Row, 1976, pp 1–15
7. Salzmann M: The Anatomy and Histology of the Human Eyeball in the Normal State: Its Development and Senescence. Brown EVL (trans). Chicago, University of Chicago Press, 1912
8. Scheie HG, Albert DM: Adler's Textbook of Ophthalmology. Philadelphia, WB Saunders, 1969
9. Yanoff M, Fine BS: Ocular Pathology: A Text and Atlas. Hagerstown, Harper & Row, 1975

chapter 6

THE RETINA

EMBRYOLOGY   61

THE PIGMENT EPITHELIUM   61

THE NEURAL (SENSORY) RETINA   70

  THE NEURONAL SYSTEM   71

    RODS AND CONES

    EXTERNAL LIMITING MEMBRANE

    OUTER NUCLEAR LAYER

    OUTER PLEXIFORM LAYER AND HENLE'S FIBERS

    INNER NUCLEAR LAYER

      BIPOLAR

      ACCESSORY NEURONS

    INNER PLEXIFORM LAYER

    GANGLION CELL LAYER

    NERVE FIBER LAYER

    INTERNAL LIMITING MEMBRANE

  THE GLIAL SYSTEM   99

    THE MÜLLER CELL

    ACCESSORY GLIA

  THE VASCULAR SYSTEM   103

  TOPOGRAPHIC VARIATIONS   111

    AREA CENTRALIS

    FOVEA (CENTRALIS)

    FOVEOLA

  MACULA (LUTEA)

  THE SUBRETINAL SPACE

    ORA SERRATA AND ANTERIOR SUBRETINAL

      CUL-DE-SAC

    POSTERIOR SUBRETINAL CUL-DE-SAC

In terms of the three-tissue classification described in Chapter 5, the retina is a tissue composed chiefly of cells.

EMBRYOLOGY

The *neuroectodermal cells* lining the floor of the primitive forebrain proliferate outward as a blind diverticulum (Fig. 6–1) (55). The proliferation continues until the diverticulum lies beneath the laterally extended *ectoderm* (the *surface* ectoderm), where it balloons out to form a large single-layered vesicle, the (primary) **optic vesicle,** connected to the forebrain vesicle by the *optic stalk*. Invagination of the vesicle produces a two-layered structure, the **optic cup** (or secondary optic vesicle), which almost obliterates the lumen of the optic vesicle. The cells contained in these two primitive neuroectodermal layers therefore come to lie in apposition, apex-to-apex (Fig. 6–2). The outer layer remains upright and develops heavy pigmentation. It continues into maturity as a single layer of epithelium and becomes the definitive pigment epithelium of the retina and ciliary body and the anterior pigment epithelial layer of the iris. Posteriorly, the cells of most of the inverted *inner* neuroectodermal layer multiply repeatedly to produce the final mature, many-layered neural (or sensory) retina (Fig. 6–3, 6–4). Anteriorly, beyond the *ora serrata*, the inner neuroectodermal layer continues as a single layer of epithelium, the nonpigmented epithelium of the ciliary body and the posterior layer of iris pigment epithelium (see Ch. 10).

THE PIGMENT EPITHELIUM

Like all epithelial and endothelial cells, the pigment epithelial cells have apexes and bases (Fig. 6–5). Lying apposed to the basal plasma membranes of these cells is a thin basement membrane (Fig. 6–6).

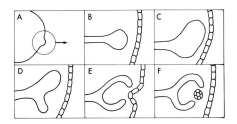

FIG. 6–1. Embryonic development of retina. Evagination of primitive forebrain (**A**) extends outward to lie beneath surface ectoderm (**B**) as a vesicle (**C**) which subsequently invaginates (**D**) to form optic cup (**E**). Lens vesicle forms from surface ectoderm (**E, F**).

The thin basement membrane as observed by electron microscopy is interpreted most usefully as the equivalent of the cuticular portion ("lamina vitrea") of Bruch's membrane (68, 79), as seen either grossly or by light microscopy. Bruch originally described a continuous shiny cuticular surface which could be best observed grossly by careful removal of the pigment epithelial cell layer (Fig. 6–7, 6–8). With subsequent examination by light microscopic techniques, the full thickness of tissue lying between pigment epithelium and the plane of the choriocapillaris appeared homogeneous and assumed the designation of "the membrane of Bruch," which was then synonymous with lamina vitrea. This zone was later subdivided into two parts: an inner cuticular portion and a more fibrillary outer portion. The latter portion stained prominently with orcein or Weigert's elastic tissue stain, hence the name lamina elastica. On electron microscopic examination, this bipartite region may be subdivided into numerous parts, depending upon the age and location of the tissue examined. A layer of true elastic tissue is present in the midzone of the collagenous layer (Fig. 6–9). Posteriorly the *elastic lamina* is thin and interrupted. Anteriorly it becomes very prominent as the elastic lamina of the ciliary body (see Ch. 10).

The structures between the fenestrated *choriocapillaris* and the pigment epithelium in young tissue (96) form a trilaminar arrangement, consisting of two basement membranes, one belonging to the

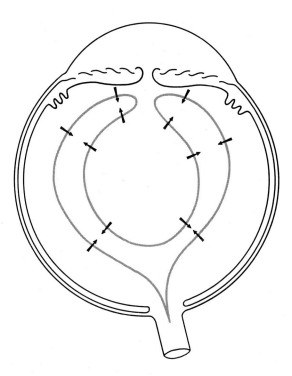

FIG. 6–2. Development of retina. Embryonic invagination to produce optic cup results in two epithelial layers applied to one another with cells arranged apex-to-apex (**arrows**).

FIG. 6–3. Development of retina. With maturation, specialization takes place in various regions of the two-layered neuroepithelium. **Dotted lines** indicate those parts that develop pigmentation or neuroepithelial muscles of iris (dilator and sphincter). **Gray regions** represent persisting nonpigmented cell layers.

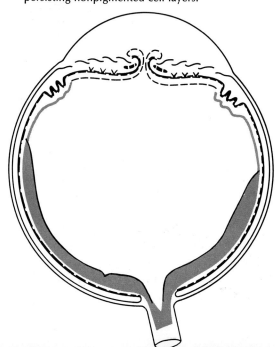

FIG. 6–4. Development of retina. With inversion, neural retina develops basement membrane (**bm**) and associated connective tissue (**ct**) on its anterior surface. Apposing apical regions develop terminal bar attachment girdles (**2, 3**). Further modifications occur. One basement membrane (**1**) becomes thick (internal limiting membrane), while the other basement membrane (of pigment epithelium) remains thin (**4**). Connective tissue associated with internal limiting membrane is composed of thin collagenous filaments (vitreous), while that associated with the basement membrane of pigment epithelium is composed of thick collagenous fibrils (lamina elastica). (Modified from Fine BS: Arch Ophthalmol 66:847, 1961)

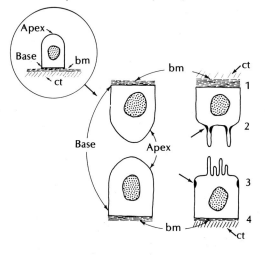

FIG. 6–5. Schematic drawing of pigment epithelial cells, their attachments, associated basement membrane, and connective tissues. Terms commonly used in light microscopy are shown at left and the equivalent cytologic terms at right in the figure.

Proc., apical cell processes
fm, fenestrated membrane
vm, Verhoeff's membrane
Cut. Bruch's, cuticular portion of Bruch's membrane

tb, terminal bar
zo, zonula occludens
za, zonula adherens
bm, basement membrane
ct, connective tissue

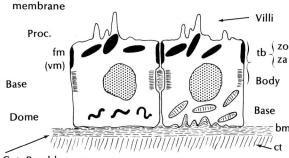

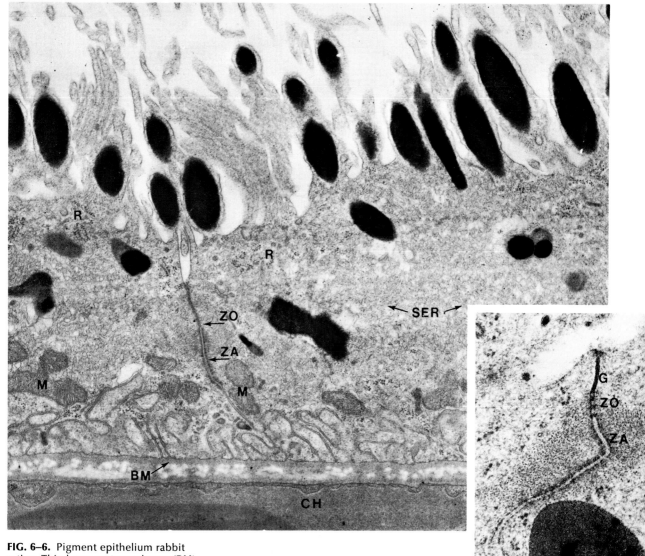

FIG. 6–6. Pigment epithelium rabbit retina. Thin basement membrane (**BM**) is present along base of cell. Most melanin granules are localized to apical cytoplasm and apical villi. Present between adjacent cells is terminal bar attachment girdle consisting of both a zonula occludens (**ZO**) and a zonula adherens (**ZA**) portion. Mitochondria (**M**) are present in basilar cytoplasm. A few clusters of free and attached ribosomes (**R**) are present in apical cytoplasm. Entire cell is permeated by agranular endoplasmic reticulum (**SER**). **CH,** choriocapillaris. (× 22,500) (Modified from Fine BS: In McPherson A (ed): New and Controversial Aspects of Retinal Detachment. New York, Hoeber, 1968) **Inset.** Terminal bar of rhesus monkey pigment epithelium to show regions of gap junction (**G**), zonula occludens (**ZO**), and zonula adherens (**ZA**) (× 45,000)

FIG. 6–7. Scanning electron micrograph of free surface of pigment epithelial basement membrane (**BM**) in parafoveal area. **Arrows,** terminal bar (fenestrated) membrane of pigment epithelium. (× 1500)

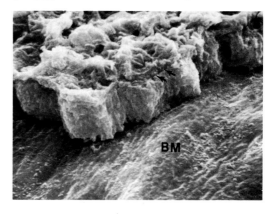

pigment epithelium and the other to the endothelium of the choriocapillaris, separated by a zone of connective tissue. Between adjacent segments of choriocapillaris, however, the basement membrane of the endothelium no longer participates in this trilaminar arrangement, and it becomes bilaminar. The connective tissue portion is exaggerated into "pillars" between the segments of the choriocapillaris by the addition of large quantities of disordered banded basement membrane (Fig. 6–10). The pillars are continuous with the connective tissue of the choroid.

With aging the connective tissue (lamina elastica) portion of Bruch's membrane may take on a basophilia (with hematoxylin and eosin) due to a form of calcification (Fig. 6–11) that is common to the posterior pole. Hypersecretion of various forms of basement membranes either focally, or more rarely, uniformly by the pigment epithelium or the endothelium of the choriocapillaris may occur.

The presence of cells or blood vessels ("subretinal" neovascularization) within the collagenous layer of Bruch's membrane is considered to be abnormal.

From the historic, experimental, and practical points of view, it appears most useful to retain the concept of defining this region, i.e., Bruch's membrane, as two *continuous* layers, the lamina vitrea (basement membrane of the retinal pigment epithelium) and the lamina elastica (the connective tissue layer which contains a variable amount of elastic tissue).

As in other epithelia, the basal plasma membranes often are irregularly infolded (Fig. 6–12). The apexes of the pigment epithelial cells are modified into villi, which generally envelop the impinging tips of the photoreceptor outer segments. Whether these villi are stout or delicate depends upon the location of the cells within the eye and the type of photoreceptor to which they are related (see Rods and Cones; Fovea, later in this chapter). Actin filaments are present within the apical villi and extend into the adjacent apical cytoplasm (10).

The limiting plasma membranes of the villi are separated from those of the adjacent photoreceptor outer segments by a typical intercellular space (30, 34). No specialized attachments are present between the retinal pigment epithelium and the photoreceptors. Near their apexes, the adjacent pigment epithelial cells are attached to one another by terminal bars (Fig. 6–6, 6–13) (1, 2, 14, 30). The terminal bars possess both zonula occludens and zonula adherens portions.

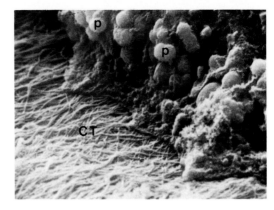

FIG. 6–8. Scanning electron micrograph of torn pigment epithelial cell layer to show the connective tissue (**CT**) underlying the thin basement membrane and a few of the exposed melanin (pigment, **P**) granules. (× 6000)

FIG. 6–9. Region of Bruch's membrane in nasal equator, in 18-year-old subject. The interrupted layer of elastic tissue (**EL**) within the collagenous layer is prominent. (× 18,000)

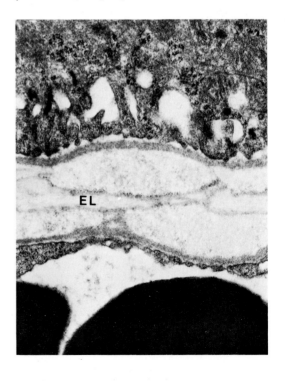

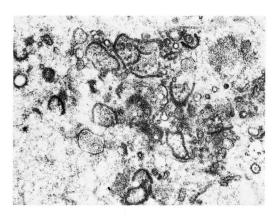

FIG. 6–10. Fovea. Masses of disordered banded basement membrane are added to Bruch's membrane by either the pigment epithelium or the choriocapillaris. (See Choroid) (× 16,800)

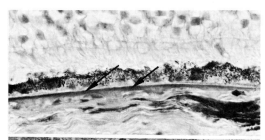

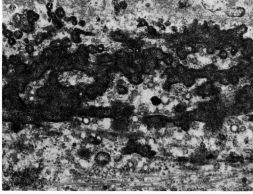

FIG. 6–11. Calcified regions of Bruch's membrane show cylindrical forms (× 49,000). In light micrograph (**at top**), they are basophilic (**arrows**) (H & E stain, × 395). (AFIP Neg. 64-5771)

FIG. 6–12. Markedly infolded basal plasma membrane (**PL**) of pigment epithelium cell. A basement membrane (**BM**) and adjacent connective tissue (**CT**) are present. **M,** mitochondria; **SER,** smooth endoplasmic reticulum. (× 27,000) (Fine BS: In McPherson A (ed): New and Controversial Aspects of Retinal Detachment. New York, Hoeber, 1968)

Using the combined techniques of TEM and freeze-fracture EM, a further subdivision of the terminal bar of the pigment epithelium can be made (42) into an apical gap junction (or macula communicans), intermediate zonula occludens, and a basilar zonula adherens (Figs. 6–14, 6–15B). The apical gap junction functions as the site of electrical coupling of adjacent cells. The zonula occludens is in effect a grouping of maculae occludentes arranged in a girdle (zonule) around the adjoining cells. *Functionally,* the point of obstruction of intercellular passage from the choriocapillaris lies at the apical side of the zonula adherens (Fig. 6–15A), *i.e.,* at the zonula occludens.

The zonula occludens functions as the site of the blood-retinal barrier for passage of extracellular materials between pigment epithelial cells. The pigment epithelial cell itself acts as another blood-retinal barrier. A third blood-retinal barrier is present in the walls of the retinal vessels. It is of interest that the tight junction or zonula occludens of vertebrate epithelia may be functionally analogous to the septate junctions in invertebrate epithelia.

The cytoplasm of the pigment epithelial cell may be subdivided into three zones or layers (35). *All three* are permeated by the interconnecting membranous system of tubules, cisterns, and channels known as the agranular (smooth-surfaced) endoplasmic reticulum. The outer one-third of the cell contains the mitochondria and the prominent infoldings of the

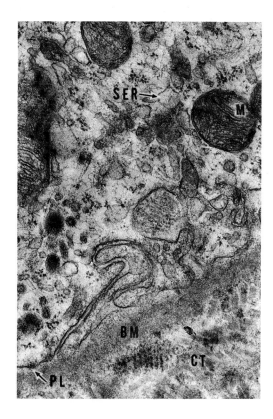

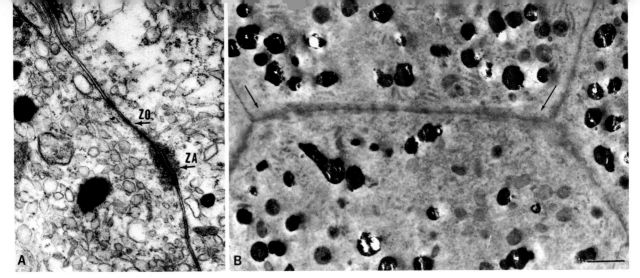

FIG. 6–13. Pigment epithelium. A. Terminal bar attachment girdle in human pigment epithelium. **ZA,** zonula adherens; **ZO,** zonula occludens. (× 27,000) B. Transverse section through retinal pigment epithelium at level of zonula adherens which has been cut along its length (**arrows**), illustrating its circumferential arrangement. (× 12,300) (Fine BS: Arch Ophthalmol 66:847, 1961)

FIG. 6–14. Apical gap junction, zonula occludens (**arrows**) and zonula adherens in retinal pigment epithelium. A. Human. (× 32,000) B. Rhesus monkey. (× 30,000)

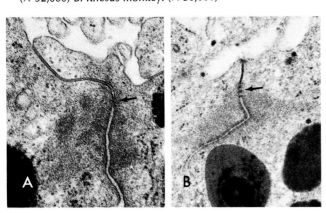

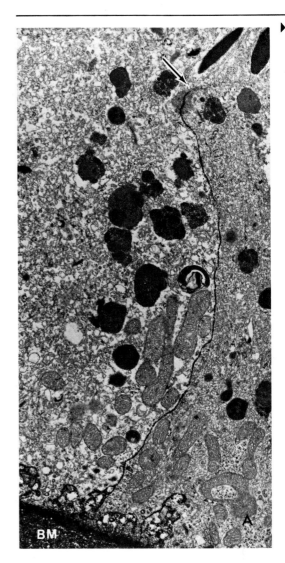

Fig. 6–15 (cont.)

FIG. 6–15. A. Functional obstruction of intercellular passage from choriocapillaris. Obstruction of passage of horseradish peroxidase occurs at apical end of zonula adherens, *i.e.*, at zonula occludens (**arrow**). Note horseradish peroxidase throughout Bruch's membrane (**BM**) and within extracellular spaces of basilar infoldings of pigment epithelial cells. (× 12,000) (courtesy Dr. M.O.M. Tso) B. Junctional complexes between pigment epithelial cells of frog retina. Cell apex is to left and base to right. 1) Frog pigment epithelium as seen by TEM thin section, showing three parts of junctional complex, a gap junction (**GJ**), a zonula occludens (**ZO**), and a zonula adherens (**ZA**) with associated filaments (**F**). **SER,** smooth endoplasmic reticulum; **MB,** myeloid body (× 66,000) 2) Comparable freeze fracture preparation. Gap junction shows cluster of particles on protoplasmic face (**GJ•A**) and arrays of pits on extracellular face (**GJ•B**). Zonula occludens (**ZO**) forms anastomosing grooves on exposed extracellular face. Region of zonula adherens (**ZA**) is indicated by region from which smooth endoplasmic reticulum (**SER**) is displaced. (× 30,000) (Hudspeth AJ, Yee AG: Invest Ophthalmol 12:354, 1973)

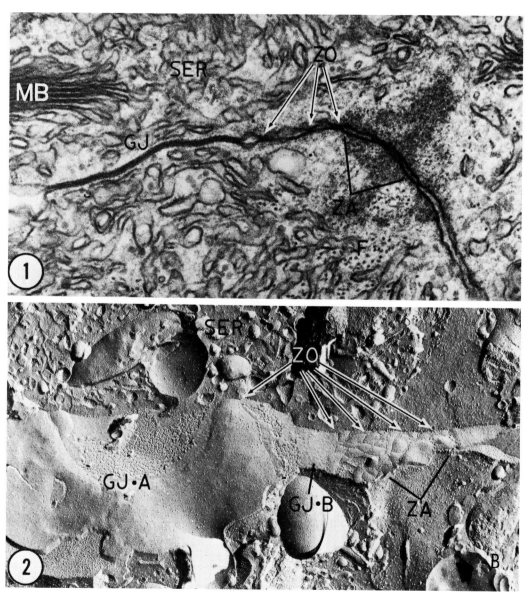

basal plasma membrane. The inner one-third contains most of the melanin (pigment) granules and projects from the apical surface as many villous processes. This zone also contains a few ribonucleoprotein (RNP) particles (ribosomes) lying freely in small clusters ("rosettes") or attached to short segments of granular (rough-surfaced) endoplasmic reticulum. The intermediate zone is relatively free of cell organelles except for the all-pervading agranular reticulum and the nucleus. When granules of lipofuscin are present, they occupy most of this intermediate zone. Glycogen particles are absent.

The pigment (melanin) granules are spherical or ovoid. The spherical granules are present in the apical cell cytoplasm, while the ovoid granules generally are present within the apical villi. The approximately equal ratio of spherical to ovoid granules is in sharp contrast to the predominance of the spherical form in the pigment epithelia of the ciliary body and iris.*

The differences in size and shape of the melanin granules throughout the ocular layers can be readily appreciated by oil-immersion light microscopy (Fig. 2–14). The uveal melanin granules are much smaller, mainly ovoid in form, and therefore easily differentiated. Knowledge of such variation is sometimes useful to the pathologist who wishes to identify the source of the granules in an altered tissue or in a pathologic accumulation.

The spherical and ovoid melanin granules are uniformly dense except for a number of small

* From an examination of human embryonic material (9, 64), development of the large melanin granule of the neuroepithelium can be characterized by the following morphologic classification (modified from others [38, 63, 82]) into the **premelanosome,** which can be observed only by electron microscopy, and the several stages of melanosome (defined here as a developing granule with *any* content of melanin), most of which can be observed but not classified by light microscopy (Fig. 6–19).

Premelanosome. Generally a membrane-enclosed group of highly oriented, weakly electron-dense filaments.

Melanosome. *Early immature (filaments).* Appearance of densification among filaments, varying from a few random spots of densification to complete densification of entire filament. *Late immature (rodlets).* Increase in densification by thickening of filaments into rodlets. *Mature.* Compaction of rodlets into an almost homogeneously dense granule.

These stages are only morphologic guideposts since many variations are seen and many so-called mature granules show regions of incomplete rodlet fusion and small peripheral foci of lucency when examined in very thin sections.

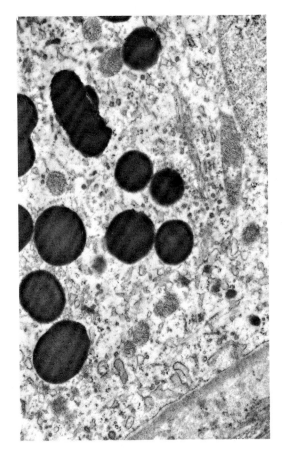

FIG. 6–16. Lipofuscin granules within body of pigment epithelial cell. They are often prominent in region of fovea or in older tissue. (× 21,000)

denser particles or "holes" in their periphery. Many bodies of less dense material are often present adjacent to the melanin granules. These latter bodies represent lipofuscin (Fig. 6–16) or residual bodies. A number of smaller dense melanin granules are frequently found to be embedded in lipofuscin granules (Fig. 6–17A). The latter composite or *compound* granules are commonly observed in the apical and midcytoplasm of older pigmented epithelial cells, and together with lipofuscin granules and residual bodies are prominent in the macular region.

Clinically, in fluorescein angiography (7), the region of the macula (fovea) transmits less of the choroidal fluorescence than other areas. The anatomic basis for this observation appears to lie for the most part with the extent to which each cell is filled from apex to base with opaque granules. Lipofuscin is a yellow-orange colored material, which is as

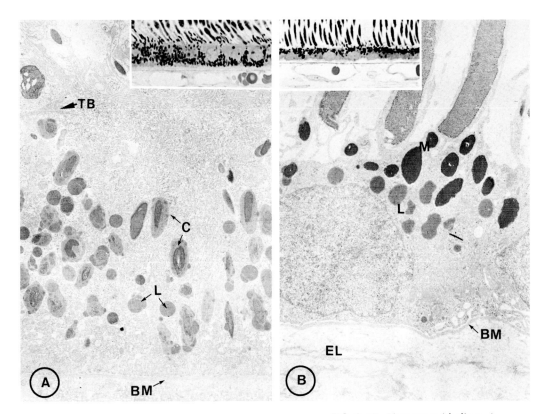

FIG. 6–17. Pigment epithelium. A. Sample of foveomacular pigment epithelium from region similar to inset. Body and base of cell are occupied by lipofuscin (**L**) and compound (**C**) (*i.e.,* melanin embedded in lipofuscin) granules. **BM,** basement membrane of pigment epithelium; **TB,** terminal bar (zonula adherens portion). (× 7400) Inset. Region of foveomacular pigment epithelium. (Epon PD, × 400, AFIP Neg. 71-4896) B. Inset. Pigment epithelium, peripheral retina. (Epon PD, × 400, AFIP Neg. 76-5491) Peripheral pigment epithelial cells contain fewer granules located mostly within apical cytoplasm. Ratio of lipofuscin granules (**L**) to melanin granules (**M**) in the plane of section is also lower here than in the foveomacular region. **BM,** basement membrane of pigment epithelium; **EL,** elastica of Bruch's membrane. (× 7400)

opaque to excited fluorescein, as is melanin. At the posterior pole, the pigment epithelial cells are narrower and taller than peripherally (Fig. 6–17) and are filled from apex to base with a mixture of these pigmented granules. More peripherally the cells contain two or three layers of granules, at most, localized mainly to the apical cytoplasm (Fig. 6–17B). Additional factors that play a role in reducing fluorescence in this area are the yellow pigment contained within the external plexiform (Henle) layer of the macula lutea within the neurosensory retina and, most centrally, the capillary-free zone of the retina (see macula lutea).

Lipofuscin may be identified clinically (ophthalmoscopically) as lighter colored regions of the pigment epithelium that become as opaque as the adjacent melanin when examined by fluorescein angiography (41). It also may accumulate as an orange-colored material overlying some nevi or malignant melanomas of the choroid (39).

Increase in the number of lipofuscin, compound granules, residual bodies, or other unclassified granules can occur readily in the region of the macula not only from aging alone but also from mild, acute or chronic insult (e.g., exposure to various forms of irradiation, diseases of the choroid [109], etc.)

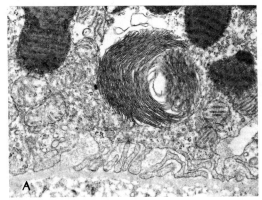
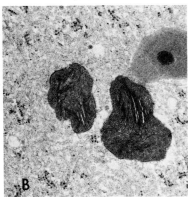

FIG. 6–18. Pigment epithelium. A. Lamellar structure present within basal cytoplasm of pigment epithelial cell. (× 16,000) B. Lamellar structure undergoing later stage of degradation deep in pigment epithelial cell to ultimately produce a residual body. (× 16,800)

Other intracytoplasmic structures that may be present include discrete dense bodies and lamellated bodies (Fig. 6–18). The latter are believed to represent engulfed photoreceptor outer segment material, *phagosomes,* which, on further digestion, produce residual bodies (93, 111–113). *Myeloid bodies* (72, 106), as observed in amphibian retinal pigment epithelium, are lacking in the human. Microperoxisomes, present in human retinal pigment epithelium (77), are tiny bodies (~0.15–0.3 μ diameter), possibly related to lipid turnover, transport, or storage. The Golgi complex of the pigment epithelium is generally not prominent, although on occasion it may be observed dilated with a lucent material (Fig. 6–20), suggesting that this cell may also contribute at least in small measure to the *interreceptor mucoid.* (37).

The pigment epithelial cells vary from the narrow, tall, highly uniform structures in the region of the fovea (Fig. 6–17, A, 6–21) to the wide, low, very irregular structures toward the ora serrata (Figs. 6–17B, 6–22). The latter cells may be less densely pigmented and may be multinucleated.

The pigment epithelial layer regains some of its cuboidal stature at the ora serrata, where it continues as the pigmented ciliary epithelium and finally as the anterior layer of iris epithelium (Ch. 10).

THE NEURAL (SENSORY) RETINA

The neural retina (pars optica retinae) is the innermost layer of the neuroectodermal coat. In the living eye it is a thin, delicate, transparent sheet of tissue containing the special sensory cells (photoreceptors) that convert photic stimuli into nerve impulses and subsequent visual sensations.

The neural retina is ~0.4 mm thick at the margin of the optic nerve, tapering to ~0.15 mm on the nasal side in the region of the ora serrata. Temporarily the retina remains ~0.4 mm thick to the periphery of the fovea where it rapidly thins to ~0.2 mm for a width of ~0.3 mm along the foveal floor (foveola).

Traditionally, the neural retina is subdivided into nine "layers." These are indicated in Figure 6–23. The pigment epithelium is, therefore, the tenth layer.

The neural retina may also be conveniently and usefully classified into three systems: the neuronal, the glial, and the vascular. The neuronal and glial are derived from the primitive neuroectoderm, whereas the vascular is derived from later invasion by mesoderm in the region of the *optic papilla.* The optic papilla generally undergoes atrophy or flattening to become the **nerve head** or **optic disc** (Ch. 12).

The neuronal and glial systems traverse the entire thickness of the neural retina (Fig. 6–24). The three primary connected nerve cells—the neuropithelial photoreceptor, the bipolar cell, and the ganglion cell—form the basic arrangement of the neuronal system. The best known and largest of the cells in the glial system is the Müller cell.

The basic pattern of the neural retina there-

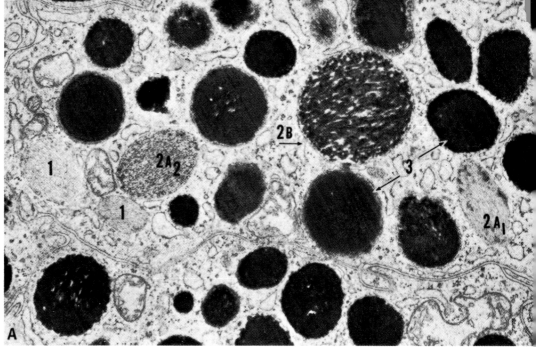

A

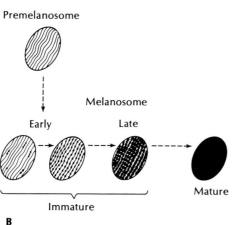

Premelanosome

Melanosome

Early   Late

Immature   Mature

B

FIG. 6–19. Development of melanin granules in human pigment epithelium. A. Melanin granules develop prenatally from premelanosome (1) through immature stages of melanosome 2A$_1$, beginning of early stage; 2A$_2$, later stage; 2B, rodlet stage to mature melanosome (3). Iris pigment epithelium, 16 weeks. (× 8000) B. Schematic drawing showing sequence of melanin granule development. (Mund ML, Rodrigues MM, Fine BS: Am J Ophthalmol 73:168, 1972)

FIG. 6–20. Example of Golgi complex, some of which is dilated with flocculent material (arrows). Golgi complex is not prominent in pigment epithelium (× 16,000)

fore can be most simply understood by superimposing these systems. For completeness, this schema also includes the smaller glia present in the inner layers (fibrous and protoplasmic astrocytes, microglia, and "oligodendrocytes"), the horizontally interconnecting neurons in the bipolar cell layer, the *amacrine* cells on the inner side, and the *horizontal* cells on the outer (Fig. 6–25).

THE NEURONAL SYSTEM

Rods and Cones

The photoreceptor cells are highly specialized neuroepithelial cells analogous to other sensory receptor cells and their special endings

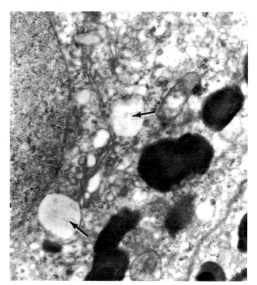

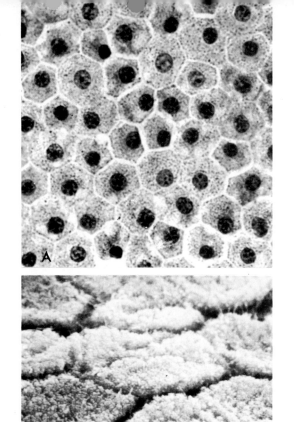

(e.g., Pacini's corpuscles for pressure, Krause's end bulbs for cold, or Meissner's corpuscles for light touch). They, like the remainder of the neural retina, are inverted (Fig. 6–26). The photoreceptor cell outer and inner segments make up the layer of rods and cones. The cell bodies or *perikarya* are located just internal to the plane of terminal bar attachments, known in light microscopy as the external limiting membrane (Fig. 6–23). The apical extensions, *inner*

FIG. 6–21 A. Flat preparation of pigment epithelium in region of Fovea. (H&E stain, ×700) (AFIP Neg. 70-730. Courtesy of Dr. M. O. M. Tso) B. SEM of pigment epithelium, posterior pole of newborn. Myriad apical villi produce the carpet-like appearance. Cell separations are partially artifactitious. (× 3500)

FIG. 6–22 ⟶

FIG. 6–23. Typical section of retina showing its layered arrangement. **ILM,** internal limiting membrane; **NFL,** nerve fiber layer; **GC,** ganglion cell layer; **IPL,** inner plexiform layer; **INL,** inner nuclear layer; **OPL,** outer plexiform layer (**P,** plexiform; **H,** Henle fibers); **MLM,** middle limiting membrane; **ONL,** outer nuclear layer; **XLM,** external limiting membrane; **RC,** layer of rods and cones (**IS,** inner segments; **OS,** outer segments.) Area centralis (Macula) (H&E stain, × 390.) (Modified from Fine BS, Zimmerman LE: Invest Ophthalmol 2:446, 1963)

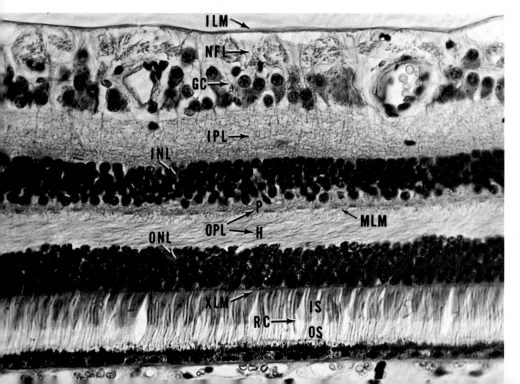

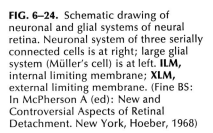

FIG. 6–24. Schematic drawing of neuronal and glial systems of neural retina. Neuronal system of three serially connected cells is at right; large glial system (Müller's cell) is at left. **ILM,** internal limiting membrane; **XLM,** external limiting membrane. (Fine BS: In McPherson A (ed): New and Controversial Aspects of Retinal Detachment. New York, Hoeber, 1968)

FIG. 6–22. Flat preparation of pigment epithelium near region of ora serrata. (H&E stain, × 210) (AFIP Neg. 70-731. Courtesy of Dr. M. O. M. Tso)

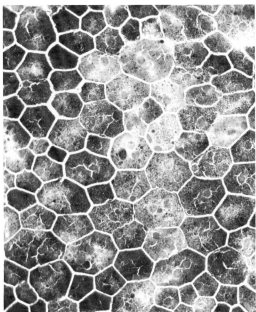

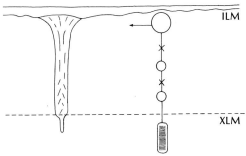

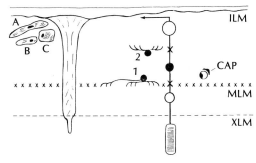

FIG. 6–25. More complete scheme of retinal structure. Included are middle limiting membrane (**MLM**), vascular system represented by its outermost capillary bed (**CAP**), horizontal cells of bipolar layer (**1**), amacrine cells of bipolar layer (**2**), and small glia of inner retinal layers. **A,** fibrous astrocytes; **B,** protoplasmic astrocytes; **C** oligodendrocytes (?).

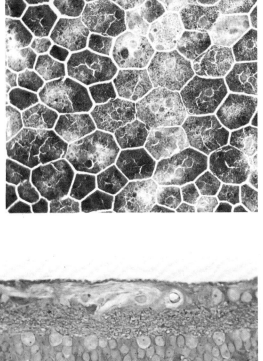

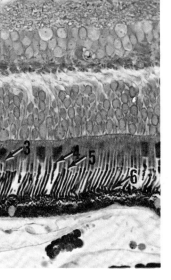

FIG. 6–26. Light micrograph of Epon section of retina. Figures indicate approximate regions illustrated in subsequent micrographs: **1,** Figure 6–27; **2,** Figure 6–28; **3,** Figure 6–29; **4,** Figure 6–31; **5,** Figure 6–33; **6,** Figure 6–37. (PD, × 305) (AFIP Neg. 64-6650. Modified from Fine BS: In McPherson A (ed): New and Controversial Aspects of Retinal Detachment. New York, Hoeber, 1968)

segments, are located just external to this plane. The rod inner segments are cylindrical; those of the cones contain glycogen (Fig. 6–27, 6–34) and are larger and conical, mainly as a result of the great number of mitochondria aggregated at their outer ends.* The inner segments of the photoreceptors contain the prominent Golgi complex (Fig. 6–27, 6–28), whose vesicles usually are filled with a lucent material. The material closely resembles that of the large extracellular space (Fig. 6–29) that extends from the external limiting membrane to the apical surface of the pigment epithelium between the photoreceptor cells. The lucent material has been identified histochemically (37, 117) as containing one or more acid mucopolysaccharides (Col. Fig. 6–30, Fig. 6–31, 6–32).

Berman (8) has chemically separated bovine interreceptor mucoid and has characterized the polysaccharides present as two-thirds "half-sulfated" chondroitin sulfate (which is hyaluronidase-sensitive) and one-third a nonsulfated heteropolysaccharide called sialoglycan (which is hyaluronidase-resistant, but sialidase-sensitive).

Agranular endoplasmic reticulum, free clusters of ribosomes, and lipoidal bodies (see Figs. 6–40, 6–97 B) are also present within the photoreceptor inner segments. Myofilaments are not in evidence, so apparently the segment lacks the myoid portion, unlike the case in certain amphibia.

Projecting from the apex of the inner segment is a highly modified cilium (Fig. 6–31). It lacks central (axial) filaments or microtubules of the more usual 9+2 arrangement of cilia observed elsewhere (e.g., ependyma or respiratory epithelium). The cilium here consists of a 9+0 arrangement: nine microtubules (doublets)† forming a ring, but lacking the two "usual" centrally located microtubules (Fig. 6–33) (97).

The plasma membrane of the cell extends from the apex of the inner segment to form a cup or calyx (Fig. 6–35). The shaft of the cilium covered with plasmalemma projects from the

* Glycogen has been demonstrated actually to lie within the intracristal spaces of mitochondria in rat retinal receptor cells (43). This differs from some misinterpretations that may be made in human material (see legend to Fig. 6–34A).

† In cross section the basal body of the cilium has been described as containing 9 microtubular triplets, the connecting cilium or shaft as containing 9 microtubular doublets; within the outer segment the cilium becomes 9 microtubular singlets (15).

floor of the calyx. Beyond the shaft of the cilium the cell plasmalemma is ballooned outward into a cylindrical or slightly conical sac, the outer segment. In the rod cell, the sac is filled with a stack of superimposed flattened "hollow" discs or double lamellas (membranes) (12, 13, 20, 22, 25, 29, 56, 61, 85, 87, 88, 104, 105, 107). The lamellas (Fig. 6–32, 6–33) are easily separated from one another and are free of attachment to the surface plasma membrane. Each double-membraned disc is also free from attachment to an adjacent disc. The discs possess several clefts at their periphery, where the membranes of the discs occasionally can be observed in continuity with tubules, possibly a vestige of their once completely tubular nature, or an indication of slight tubulovesicular breakdown.* The clefts lie in register forming longi-

* The continuity of lamellas with the surface plasma membrane in the cone (17, 35) implies derivation from this surface membrane. That the rod discs (lamellas or sacs) are similarly derived from the surface plasma membrane has been inferred from developmental studies (22, 66). The PAS-positivity of both rod and cone outer segments (Fig. 6–30) is due to their high content of lipoprotein membranes, as they contain no glycogen (Fig. 6–34A).
The discs or lamellas can easily break down into tubules, an alteration that can be observed as a fixation artifact or as early or chronic pathologic change (100). Proper interpretation then depends on other and/or additional criteria. Bends, loops, bulges, and hooklike formations of the entire photoreceptor outer segments also often occur as artifacts.

FIG. 6–27. Retina. A. Large cone (C) inner segment and adjacent rod (R) inner segment containing their respective Golgi complexes (G). External limiting membrane consists of sectioned terminal bar (i.e., zonulae adherentes) attachment girdles (TB) which unite adjacent photoreceptor and Müller cells (MC). (× 19,000) Inset 1. Random distribution of glycogen between mitochondria in parafoveolar cone inner segment. (TSC-treated) (× 16,000) Inset 2. Müller cell villi (V) project beyond external limiting membrane (TB) for a short distance (× 28,700) (Modified from Fine BS, Zimmerman LE: Invest Ophthalmol 2:446, 1963) B. Scanning electron micrograph of cone isthmus connecting inner segment (above) with outer segment (below). The isthmus contains the connecting cilium. (× 12,500) C. Short tapered calyceal processes (apical villi) surround base of cone isthmus as it leaves cone inner segment (apical cytoplasm). (SEM, × 25,000)

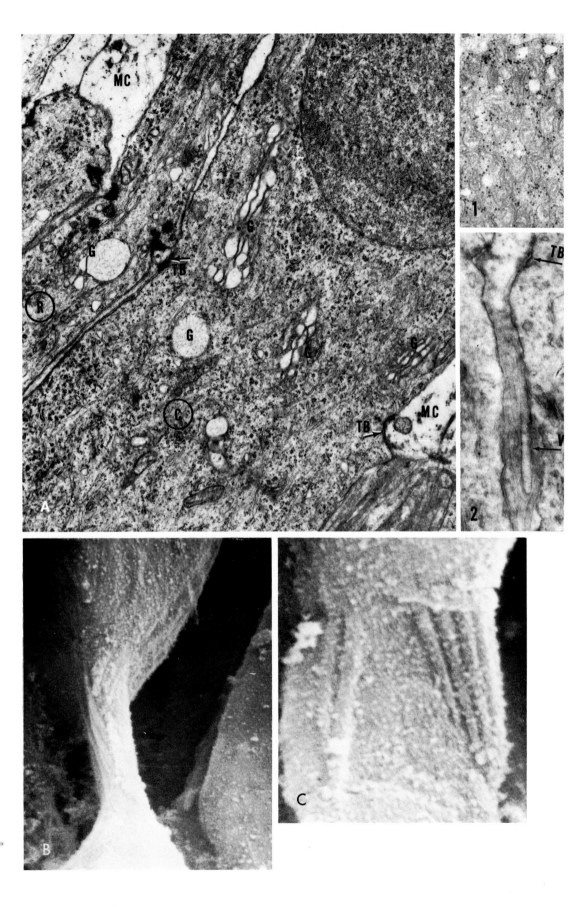

tudinal furrows along the surface of the rod cell outer segments (Fig. 6–33, 6–35).

Differing in many respects from the rod cell outer segment is the cone cell outer segment (Fig. 6–36) (18, 24). Although apparently similar to rod cell lamellas, cone cell lamellas are less easily separated (*i.e.,* the double membranes of each ''disc'' are tightly bound to each other), they possess no peripheral clefts containing groupings of tubules and are in continuity with the surface plasma membrane at least over short segments of their circumference (inset, Fig. 6–31). Their connecting cilia, however, have the 9+0 microtubule arrangement of the rods, pass similarly through a narrow constriction (the isthmus) between inner and outer segments, and possess a basal body and at least two striated rootlets like other cilia. A free centriole generally is observed in the cytoplasm near the basal body.

The rounded, completely enclosed tip of the rod outer segment impinges on the apex of the pigment epithelial cell, which surrounds it with numerous delicate villi as previously mentioned (Fig. 6–37). The attachment between pigment epithelium and rod outer segments appears to be no stronger than that of a usual intercellular space.

The relation of the **extrafoveolar cone** to the pigment epithelium generally differs from that of the rod in that the tapered outer end of the cone falls short of the usual plane of the pigment cell apexes. Long, heavy pigment epithelial villi extend inward to envelop the cone outer segment (95) (Fig. 6–38). The cones are greatly modified in the foveola (see later in this chapter), and toward the ora serrata they are shorter and plumper than elsewhere, have poorly developed outer segments, and increase in number relative to rod outer segments.*

* The presence of considerable inward extension of large numbers of villi from the associated pigment epithelial cell resembles, in some respects, the arrangements present in lower animal forms, such as the amphibian (*i.e.,* frog), in which the interreceptor spaces almost are occupied completely by processes of the pigment epithelial cells. Such observations might be considered to add weight to the contention that the cones (especially extrafoveolar) indeed may represent the more primitive of the two varieties of photoreceptor (101).

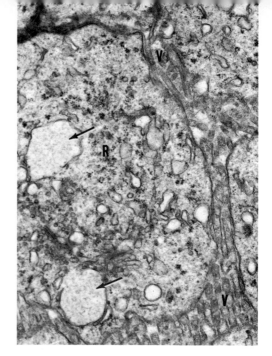

FIG. 6–28. Oblique section of photoreceptor inner segments near external limiting membrane. Dilated Golgi cisternas (**arrows**) are present within segment, as are aggregates of agranular reticulum and clusters of ribosomes (**R**). Villi (**V**) of Müller cells are numerous between inner segments near membrane. (× 18,700)

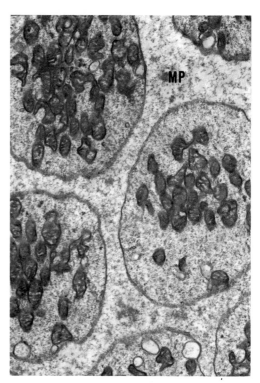

FIG. 6–29. Cross-section of inner segments more distal to Figure 6–28. Note interreceptor mucoid (**MP**), lack of Müller cell villi, and larger aggregates of mitochondria within cell. (× 14,000)

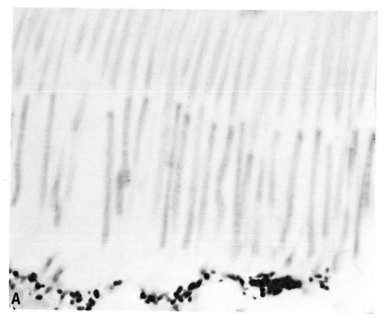

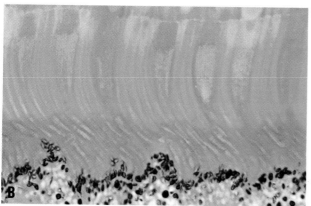

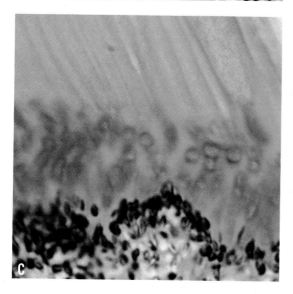

FIG. 6–30. Composition of layer of rods and cones. A. Photoreceptor outer segments are PAS-positive. (PAS-hematoxylin, × 1500) B and C. Spaces between photoreceptor outer segments are positive for acid mucopolysaccharides. Cross-sections of PAS-positive outer segments (in **C**) show size of mucoid-filled extracellular spaces. Note diffuse PAS positivity of cone inner segments, due in part to distribution of glycogen (see Fig. 6–27A, inset 1, and Fig. 6–34). (**B,** PAS, AMP, × 1080; **C,** PAS, AMP, × 2160) (Modified from Fine BS, Zimmerman LE: Invest Ophthalmol 2:446, 1963)

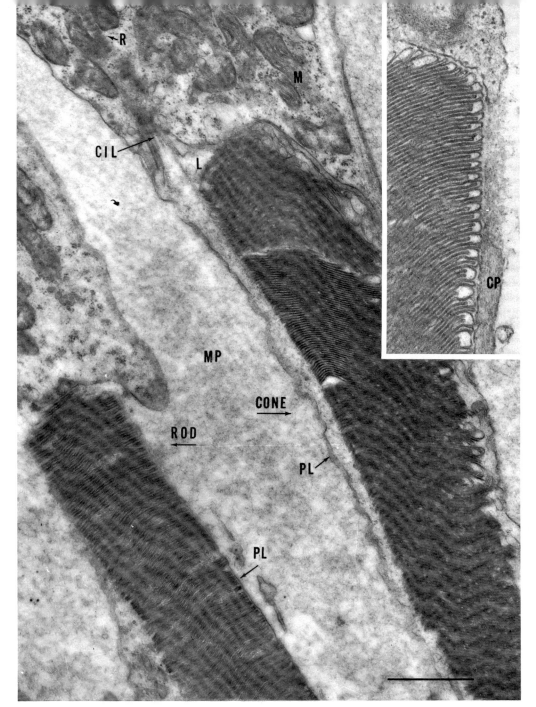

FIG. 6–31. Rod and cone outer segments. Connecting cilium (**CIL**) of cone is shown here. Intercellular mucopolysaccharides (**MP**) are present. Double lamellas of tapering cone outer segment are strongly attached to each other and are connected to others in different plane (see **inset**), as well as to surface plasma membrane. **CP,** calyceal process; **L,** loops of cone outer segment lamellas; **PL,** plasma membrane; **R,** ciliary rootlets. (Main figure, human nasal fovea, × 23,800; inset, monkey cone, fovea, glutaraldehyde fixation, × 40,000) (Modified from Fine BS, Zimmerman LE: Invest Ophthalmol 2:446, 1963)

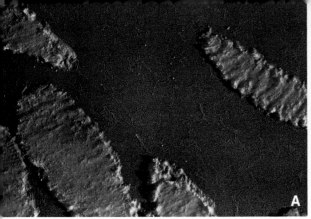

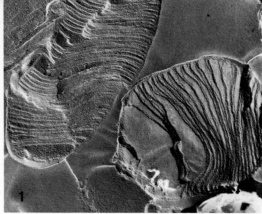

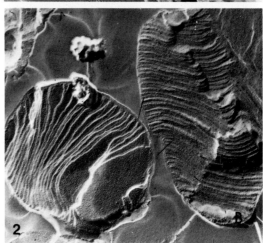

FIG. 6–34. Photoreceptor in fovea. A. Junction of inner segment (**IS**) and outer segment (**OS**). Specimen was initially fixed in glutaraldehyde, accounting for often ''coagulated'' appearance (**free arrows**) of interreceptor mucoid. Section was treated with TSC *only*. Dark (glycogen) particles are widely distributed within inner segment between the mitochondria. Note apparent inclusion of glycogen particles within mitochondrion at **M**. (**Arrow M**₁ indicates a neighboring C-shaped mitochondrion partially enclosing cluster of similar particles. Longitudinal sectioning of latter mitochondrion would give appearance of intramitochondrial glycogen as shown at **M**. (× 15,000) B. Inner segments of cone (**C**) and rod (**R**) cells near the terminal bars (**TB**) of external limiting membrane. The cone inner segment contains TSC-positive particles (glycogen), while those of the rods do not. **N**, nucleus of cell; **MC**, lucent cytoplasm of Müller cell. (Glutaraldehyde-Dalton TSC only, × 15,000.) ▼

FIG. 6–32. Photoreceptor outer ▲ segments. A. Shadow-cast preparation. Interreceptor mucoid is seen as drying patterns between receptor segments. (U-shad, × 12,000) B. Rat photoreceptor outer segments opened by freeze-fracture-etching. Membranes of lamellas have been cleaved (**1** and **2** are mirror images of this cleavage). (× 25,000) (Courtesy of Dr. Russell Steere.)

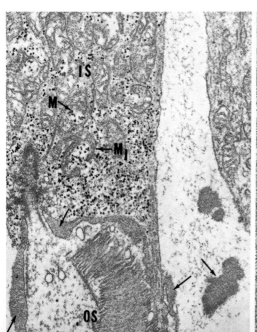

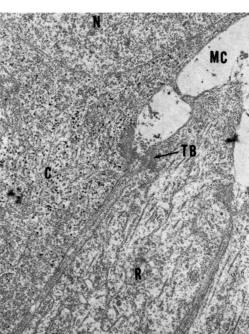

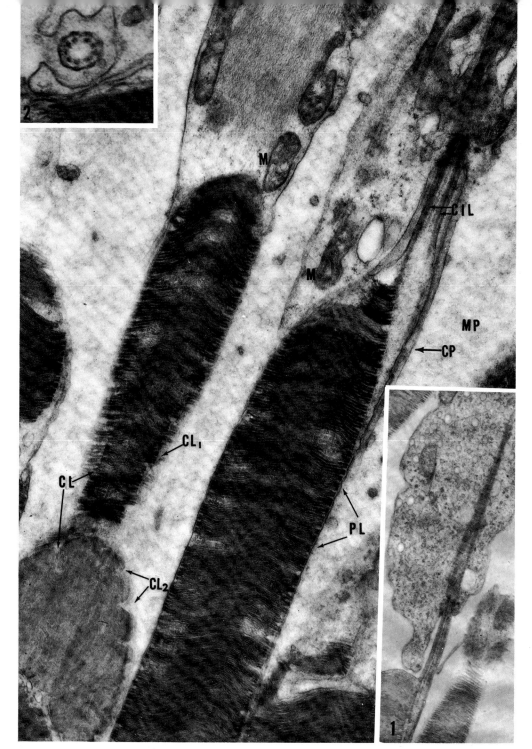

FIG. 6–33. Rod outer segments. Double membranes of discs are loosely attached to each other. Discs are free from one another and from surface plasma membranes, and possess clefts (**CL₂**), which lie in register, forming longitudinal furrows (**CL, CL₁**). A rod-connecting cilium (**CIL**) is present, issuing from calyx of inner segment. A calyceal process (**CP**) extends from inner segment along one side of outer segment. **M,** mitochondria; **MP,** intercellular mucopolysaccharides; **PL,** plasma membrane. (Human nasal fovea, × 25,300) (Fine BS: In McPherson A (ed): New and Controversial Aspects of Retinal Detachment. New York, Hoeber, 1968) Inset 1, from rabbit retina, shows more clearly cross-striations of ciliary rootlets. (× 10,800) Inset 2 shows a cilium cross-sectioned through its shaft. Ciliary filaments are of the 9+0 arrangement. (× 32,000)

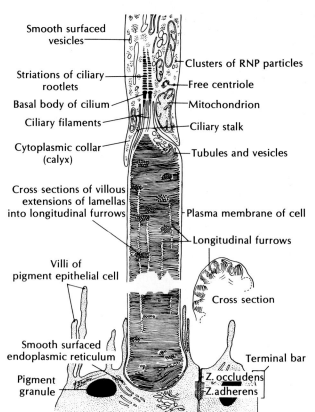

Smooth surfaced vesicles

Clusters of RNP particles

Striations of ciliary rootlets

Free centriole

Basal body of cilium

Mitochondrion

Ciliary filaments

Ciliary stalk

Cytoplasmic collar (calyx)

Tubules and vesicles

Cross sections of villous extensions of lamellas into longitudinal furrows

Plasma membrane of cell

Longitudinal furrows

Villi of pigment epithelial cell

Cross section

Smooth surfaced endoplasmic reticulum

Terminal bar

Pigment granule

Z. occludens
Z. adherens

FIG. 6–35. Schematic drawing of rod outer segment and its relation to pigment epithelial cell and its villi. (Fine BS: In McPherson A (ed): New and Controversial Aspects of Retinal Detachment. New York, Hoeber, 1968)

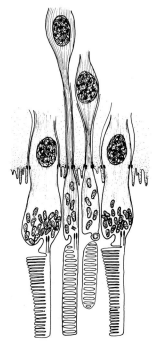

FIG. 6–36. Schematic drawing showing that alignment of rods and cones beyond external limiting membrane is maintained by intervening projections of the Müller cells. Difference in rod and cone cell diameters as well as arrangement of their lamellated outer segments are also illustrated. (Ts'o MOM *et al.*: Am J Ophthalmol 69:350, 1970)

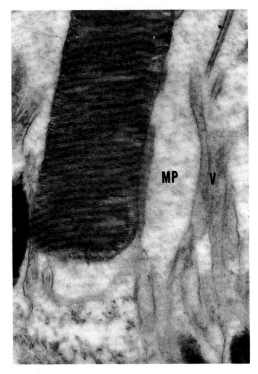

MP V

FIG. 6–37. Rod cell impinging on pigment cell and enveloped by apical villi (**V**) of latter cell. **MP,** interreceptor mucoid. (× 20,000)

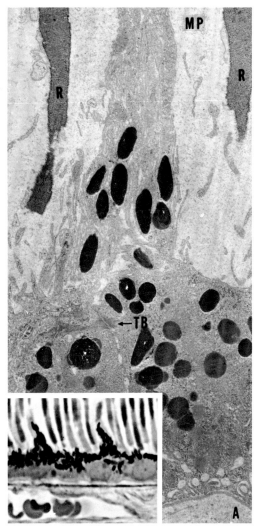

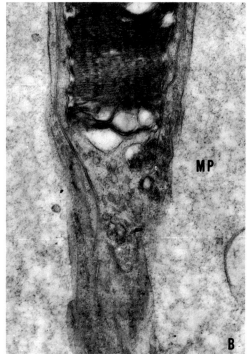

FIG. 6–38. A. Extrafoveolar cone outer segment falls short of the usual plane of pigment epithelium, which sends a mass of pigment bearing villi inward (**inset**) to envelop the outer segment end. **MP,** interreceptor mucoid; **R,** rod outer segments; **TB,** terminal bars. (× 8000; inset, PD, × 820, AFIP Neg. 71-5949) B. Outer end of cone enveloped by pigment epithelial villi some distance inward from the pigmented epithelial cell layer; **MP,** interreceptor mucoid. (× 20,700)

The large extracellular space between photoreceptor outer segments represents the remains of the lumen of the embryonic optic vesicle. The space is filled with a mixture of acid mucopolysaccharides (Fig. 6–30 through 6–32), some of which is sensitive to hyaluronidase.

Separation of the neural retina from its pigment epithelium in the postnatal eye creates, in effect, a gross reappearance of the lumen of the optic vesicle. This is clinically termed a retinal "detachment."

External Limiting Membrane

The external limiting membrane (XLM); (X in Fig. 6–39) is not a true membrane, but rather attachment sites of the adjacent photoreceptor and Müller cells. These attachments are terminal bars (Fig. 6–40) that lack the zonula occludens portion. Thus the intercellular spaces probably are partially limited functionally but are not absent or totally obstructed.

That small molecules can pass easily through the intercellular spaces of the external limiting membrane has been demonstrated recently (69, 70).

Outer Nuclear Layer

The photoreceptor cell bodies ("outer nuclear layer"—ONL) lie internal to the plane of the external limiting membrane (Fig. 6–39). Occa-

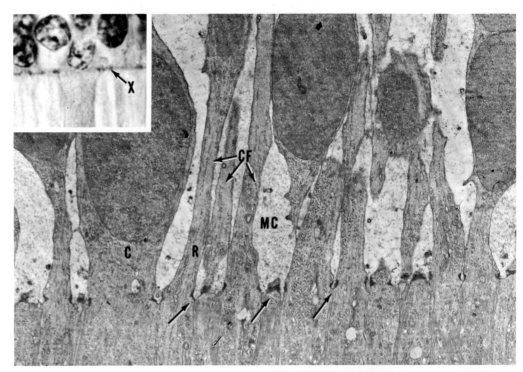

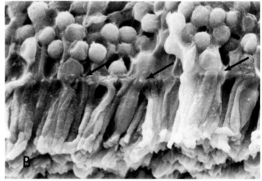

sionally a photoreceptor cell nucleus (especially of a cone because of its proximity) is found lying *external* to this membrane. The cone cell body or perikaryon is much larger than that of the rod. This difference in size is also carried over into the rod and cone inner segments and axons (Henle fibers).

The cytoplasmic connections which extend from the photoreceptor inner segments at the level of the external limiting membrane to the cell body often are referred to as the **connecting fibers** (Fig. 6–39) (79). Because most of the cone cell bodies lie nearer to the external limiting membrane than do the rod cells, these connecting fibers are necessarily short and stout for the cone cells but long and narrow for the rod cells.

Outer Plexiform Layer

The outer plexiform layer (OPL) is truly plexiform only in its inner third; its outer two-thirds is composed of the axonal extensions (Henle fibers) of the photoreceptors enveloped by the lucent outer cytoplasm of the Müller cells (Fig. 6–41, 6–42) (36). The axons contain a few segments of agranular reticulum, a small scattering

FIG. 6–39. A. External limiting membrane. Viewed by light microscopy (**inset**), membrane (**X**) appears as discontinuous series of small dots. Electron microscopy shows series of terminal bars or *zonulae adherentes* (**free arrows**), which attach Müller cells (**MC**) to photoreceptor cells (**R, C**). Nuclei of photoreceptor cells make up outer nuclear layer. **CF,** connecting fibers. (× 4500; inset, × 1500. [AFIP Neg. 61–1958]) B. Scanning electron micrograph of region traversing the external limiting membrane (**arrows**). Nuclei of photoreceptor cells are seen above; photoreceptor cell inner segments (apical cytoplasm) are seen below. (× 1200)

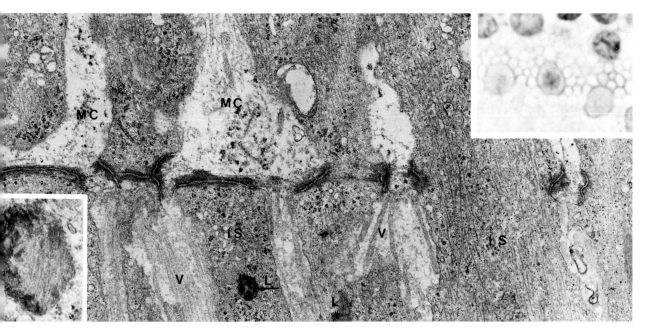

FIG. 6–40. External limiting membrane of neural retina consists of terminal bars (*zonulae adherentes* only). Portions of the *zonulae* are sectioned obliquely on the left and in cross-section on the right. **MC,** Müller cell; **IS,** inner segments; **V,** Müller cell villi; **L,** lipoidal bodies. Lower inset (× 38,000). Lipoidal material is superimposed on filamentous substructure. (× 14,500) Upper inset. Light micrograph of external limiting membrane sectioned obliquely to show more completely the "fenestrated membrane" or "zonulae." (TB, × 1100; AFIP Neg. 73-3713).

of individual (apparently glycogen, *i.e.,* TSC-positive) particles, a few elongated mitochondria, and uniform packing of microtubules (neurotubules) embedded in a moderately dense ground substance (see sections on Ganglion Cell Layer; Nerve Fiber Layer, later in this chapter).

These thick and thin axons of cone and rod photoreceptor cells together with their surrounding "packing" of Müller cells (Fig. 6–43) make up the Henle fiber layer of the outer plexiform layer.*

* The term "Henle fiber layer" has become widely used as synonymous with the oblique fibers present in the foveal (macular) region. Except for the obliquity and consequent greater length, the fibers do not differ substantially from similar photoreceptor axonal exten-

Near the dendrites of the bipolar cells (Fig. 6–44), the photoreceptor axons dilate into large *synaptic expansions.* The cone expansion is much the larger of the two and the more inwardly placed (Fig. 6–45). With the metal impregnation techniques of light microscopy, the cone expansion appears as a pedicle or foot, with small branches. The rod axon expands into a somewhat teardrop-shaped expansion termed the **rod spherule** (see Fig. 6–47) (71).

Electron microscopic examination shows that these synaptic expansions are filled with myriad small (200–300 A) vesicles called **synaptic vesicles** (21, 57). The vesicles are believed to contain acetylcholine (23), which is released at the cell surface upon appropriate stimulation.

sions elsewhere, where they are vertical in section. The latter also once were called "Henle fibers." The term "outer plexiform layer" originally referred *only* and specifically to the narrow truly plexiform layer of dendrites and axons lying closely apposed to the bipolar cell layer (inner nuclear layer) (81). Presumably some later confusion arose because the Henle fiber layer superficially may resemble the outer plexiform layer under certain conditions of tissue sectioning (Fig. 6–50). The inner plexiform layer always is plexiform in appearance regardless of the plane of section or of the level of the layer examined.

Because of general usage the term "outer plexiform layer" is retained here for the entire zone lying between the two nuclear layers. The contemporary outer plexiform layer therefore would be divisible into two parts, the outer Henle fiber portion and the inner plexiform portion.

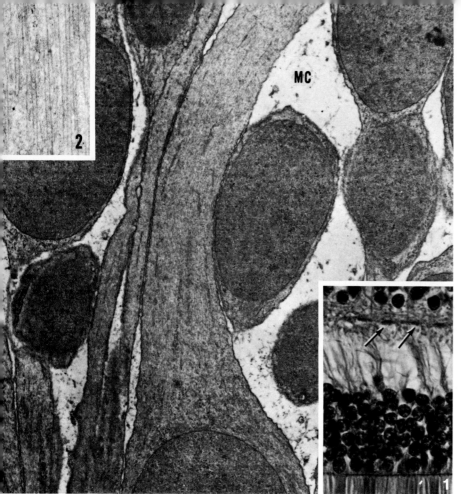

FIG. 6–41. Electron micrograph showing a number of photoreceptor cell bodies, their nuclei, and their axonal extensions (Henle fibers) surrounded by lucent cytoplasm of Müller cells (**MC**). (× 6800) Inset 1. Light micrograph showing outer plexiform layer (see footnote, Outer Plexiform Layer). Inner third is plexiform and outer two-thirds is fibrous (Henle fibers), union being marked by plane of photoreceptor synapses (**arrows**). (H&E stain, × 600) Inset 2. Electron micrograph showing cytoplasmic microtubules ("neurotubules") present within axoplasm. (Glutaraldehyde fixation, × 24,000) (Modified from Fine BS, Zimmerman LE: Invest Ophthalmol 1:304, 1962)

FIG. 6–42. Nasal retina. Section through outer nuclear layer parallel to external limiting membrane. Cross-sections of large-diameter cone axons (**C**) small-diameter rod axons (**R**), and cell bodies are enveloped by lucent Müller cell cytoplasm (**MC**). (× 12,000)

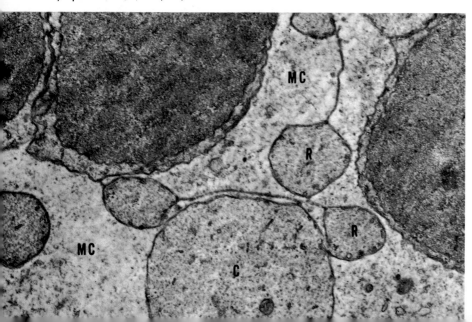

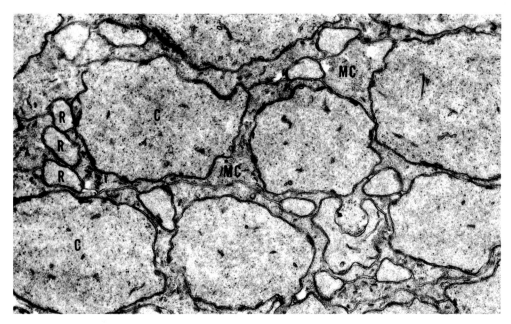

FIG. 6–43. Henle fiber layer, consisting of packed photoreceptor axons (**C, R**) surrounded by Müller cell cytoplasm (**MC**). (× 16,000)

FIG. 6–45. Cone pedicle or foot. Basilar plasma membranes are invaginated by bipolar or horizontal cell processes. Mitochondria (**M**), region of synaptic vesicles (**SV**), and synaptic ribbons (lamellas) (**SL**) are present within pedicle. **RS,** adjacent rod spherule is located along a plane external to that of cone pedicles. (× 6000)

FIG. 6–44. Light micrograph showing plane of photoreceptor synapses (**arrows**) in zone of middle limiting membrane. (H&E stain, × 305)

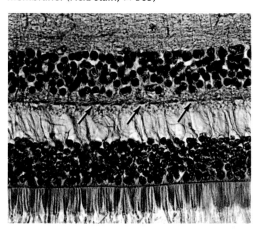

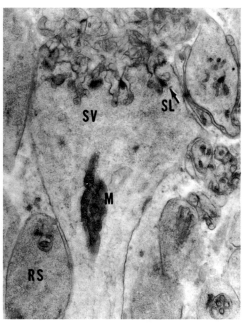

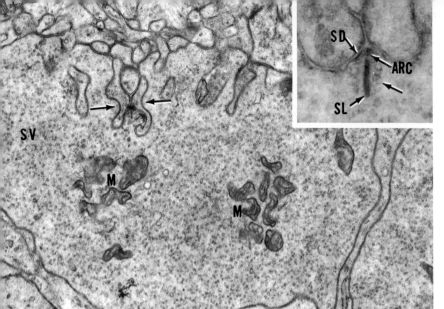

FIG. 6–46. Cone pedicle. Synaptic vesicles (**SV**) and mitochondria (**M**) are evident. Invaginating two neurites of horizontal cell (**arrows**) and adjacent bipolar cell envelop a portion of cone foot containing a synaptic lamella. The three parts form a triad. (× 16,000) Inset. Arrangement of synaptic lamella (**SL**), special halo of synaptic vesicles (**free arrow**), arciform density (**ARC**), and density of adjacent membranes. Modified punctum adherens or synaptic density, **SD.** (× 66,000)

FIG. 6–47. Rod spherule with its synaptic ribbon or lamella (**arrow**) in cleavage plane formed by invaginating neurites of adjacent bipolar and horizonal cells. **SV,** synaptic vesicles; **MC,** Müller cell. (× 22,860) (Fine BS: J Neuropathol Exp Neurol 22:255, 1963) Inset. Almost complete longitudinal section of single ribbon or lamella, illustrating its three-dimensional ribbon-like appearance. Special vesicle halo and adjacent arciform density (**arrow**) are also recognizable. (× 32,800) (Fine BS: In McPherson A (ed): New and Controversial Aspects of Retinal Detachment. New York, Hoeber, 1968)

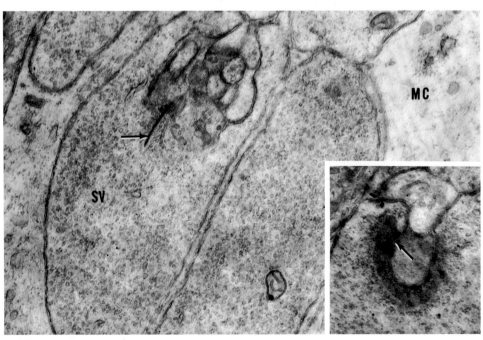

Many TSC-positive particles are also present within the cone pedicles, suggesting a small content of glycogen.

The many infoldings at the innermost cell surface of the synaptic expansions of both rod and cone cells are produced by the "plugged-in" blind endings of adjacent bipolar cell dendrites (Fig. 6–46) as well as by both dendrites and axons of such lateral interconnecting neurons as the *horizontal cells*. Dense attachment foci (**synaptic densities** [53, 75] or modified puncta adherentes* are present along this surface. Frequently, within the synaptic expansion and the cleavage formed by two adjacent impinging neurites, short dense strips are seen, the synaptic **lamellas** (32, 52, 57, 60) or **ribbons** (86),† around which a peculiar "halo" of synaptic vesicles is arranged. The ribbons or lamellas are multiple in the cone foot,‡ but generally single within a rod spherule; occasionally, however, two lamellas are present in a spherule. In both varieties of synaptic expansions the lamellas are separated from the surface plasma membrane by a dense band of material known as the **arciform density** (52) (Fig. 6–46, 6–47). The two lucent invaginating cell processes in a cone pedicle lying on either side of the synaptic ribbon (lamella) lying within the *synaptic ridge* generally are considered to represent dendrites of the horizontal cell (28, 75). The axial process beneath the synaptic ridge is considered to belong to an *invaginating midget bipolar cell*, the three invaginations producing a triad. Superficial contacts or synapses made lateral to the bipolar and horizontal cell invaginations are made by *flat bipolar cells* (see Fig. 6–49). The axial invagi-

nating process in a rod spherule is that of a rod bipolar cell. The bipolar cells possess ribbon synapses at their axonal ends. The horizontal cell differs by making conventional (*i.e.*, lacking a ribbon or lamella) synaptic contacts onto bipolar dendrites and/or other horizontal cell processes.

Mitochondria, although few in number, are also present within the synaptic expansions.

The arrangements within the photoreceptor synaptic expansions are repeated "in miniature" for the smaller synaptic expansions of the ribbon bipolar cells in the *inner plexiform layer* (28, 32, 46, 57, 76) (Fig. 6–53, 6–54).

Similar arrangements are present in all synaptic expansions of the central nervous system except for the lack of synaptic ribbons (lamellas) and arciform densities. The latter structures are peculiar to the retina, the hair cells of the cochlea of the inner ear (91), the photoreceptor-like cells in the pineal gland of amphibia (45), and specialized sensory cells of certain fish (5). Although their peculiar localization is clear, their significance is not. Embryologically (90), the ribbon synapses appear almost simultaneously in the inner and outer plexiform layers, before photoreceptor outer segments appear. Cone synaptogenesis precedes that of the rods.

Occasionally, lateral projections of the photoreceptor expansions may be seen abutting against an adjacent expansion. These abutments are sometimes interpreted to function as lateral communicating channels (16, 18, 62).

Inner Nuclear Layer

The inner nuclear layer (INL) contains the nuclei of the bipolar, the Müller, the horizontal, and the amacrine cells.

Bipolar Cells. Bipolar cells possess typical dendrites which make up most of the narrow, truly plexiform portion of the so-called outer plexiform layer (Fig. 6–48). The dendritic stalks (Fig. 6–49) are filled with a considerable number of poorly oriented mitochondria (Fig. 6–51),* segments of agranular reticulum, and especially with glutaraldehyde fixation, large numbers of neurotubule-like structures or microtubules.

The many branches of the dendritic stalk are interwoven with other dendrites and with the

---

* Although morphologists generally tend to equate the site of synaptic density with the physiologic event of transmission of the nerve impulse, such equation remains uncertain. Originally, Sherrington (84) defined a synapse as a *postulated* anatomic site (which he had inadequate means at the time to observe directly) for the physiologic event of transmission of the nerve impulse.

Synaptic vesicles congregated along a synaptic density or punctum adherens are generally considered to represent a chemical synapse, while similar vesicles clustered near a gap junction or macula communicans are considered to represent an electrical synapse.

† Although the structure is ribbon-like in three dimensions (hence the name "synaptic ribbon"), it is recognizable in most sections as a cross section of the ribbon (hence the name "synaptic lamella").

‡ Up to 25 lamellas, as determined by serial reconstruction of a single cone synaptic pedicle (60).

* Disarray of mitochondria is a useful electron microscopic criterion for identifying a dendrite in a tissue section.

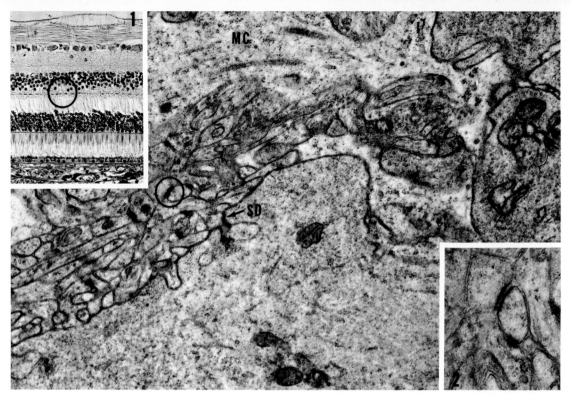

axons of laterally communicating cells such as the horizontal cells. This basket-weave arrangement of dendrites and axons forms a layer the strength of which is augmented by many desmosome-like attachment plates (36, 74) or puncta adherentes* (Fig. 6–48). The zone of desmosome-like attachments of the photoreceptor synaptic expansions (**synaptic densities or modified puncta adherentes**) can be seen by light microscopy as a series of dashes in the innermost part of the outer plexiform layer (inset, Fig. 6–48) and is termed the **middle limiting membrane** (MLM) (36). This membrane has considerable strength and restraining ability, much like that of the external limiting membrane. Its strength is explained by three morphologic observations: 1) the interweaving of the neurites, 2) the desmosome-like attachment plaques (or puncta adherentes), and 3) the synaptic densities (which possess the adhering property of desmosomes).

In pathologic tissues such a ''membrane'' may act as a temporary internal barrier to exudates that may accumulate between the photoreceptor axons (Henle fiber layer or outer plexiform layer). Since

* These are distinguished from chemical synapses by their lack of associated synaptic vesicles.

FIG. 6–48. Electron micrograph showing cone pedicle indented by horizontal and bipolar dendrites. Desmosome-like densities or *puncta adherentes* (**circle**) are present, attaching adjacent neurites to one another within plexiform zone. **MC,** Müller cell; **SD,** synaptic density. (× 18,000) (Fine BS: In McPherson A (ed): New and Controversial Aspects of Retinal Detachment. New York, Hoeber, 1968) Inset 1. Light micrograph with circle indicating approximate region illustrated in electron micrograph. (H&E stain, × 130) (AFIP Neg. 61-1960) Inset 2. Enlargement of circled area in electron micrograph. (× 32,400)

this membrane also demarcates the outermost capillary reach of the normal retinal vasculature, it may serve to direct neovascularization inward at least in the early stages of this pathologic form of endothelial proliferation.

The middle limiting membrane is observed easily in properly oriented conventional H&E-stained sections (Fig. 6–41, 6–44, 6–48) and resembles the external limiting membrane (terminal bars) more closely than the internal limiting membrane (basement membrane). These relations and differences are augmented by special staining techniques such as iron hematoxylin, which accentuates terminal bars and desmosomes, but not basement membranes.

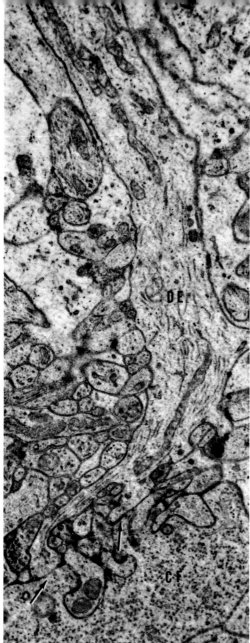

FIG. 6–49. Branches of flat bipolar dendrite (**DE**) in contact (**arrows**) with cone foot pedicle (**CF**). (× 14,000)

The bipolar cell perikaryon (Fig. 6–50, 6–51) is generally scanty, and the axonal extension is quickly lost in the complexity of the inner plexiform layer. The axons, however, are easily recognized by the axial arrangement of their cytoplasmic components (like photoreceptor axons), particularly when their highly oriented microtubules are accentuated by initial glutaraldehyde fixation.

Accessory Neurons. Many forms of bipolar cells have been described on the basis of their varying morphology as determined by metal impregnation or coating techniques (11, 71), as well as by correlative techniques of electron microscopy. Their various functional significances, however, are generally unclear. The nuclei of the Müller (glial) cells may lie at any level of the bipolar layer. Two special cells that often are considered to act as laterally communicating neurons are also present in this zone (11). One, the horizontal cell, lies just anterior to the middle limiting membrane; the other, the amacrine cell, an analogous cell, lies near the innermost bipolar cell bodies (Fig. 6–25).

The horizontal cell is generally identified in the *human* retina by the presence of a

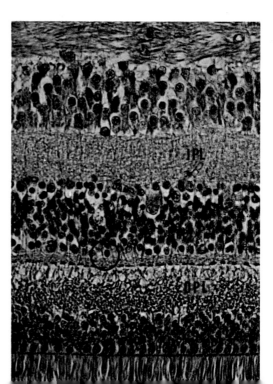

FIG. 6–50. Light micrograph with **circle** indicating approximate region illustrated in Figure 6–51. Note that sectioning *across* Henle fibers produces an outer plexiform layer (**OPL**) that only *superficially* resembles the inner plexiform layer (**IPL**). (H&E, × 300)

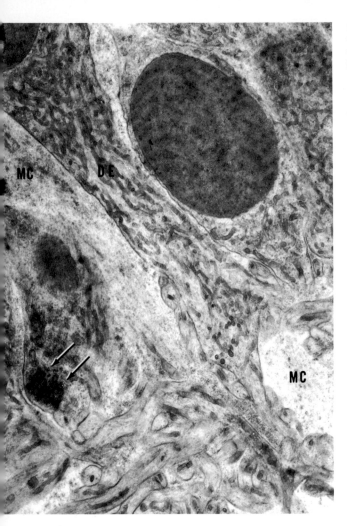

FIG. 6–51. Outer boundary of bipolar cell layer. Stout mitochondria-filled dendrites of bipolar cell (**DE**) are prominent. A cluster of large tubules (Kolmer crystalloid) is present (**arrows**) in adjacent cell lying just internal to plane of middle limiting membrane. **MC,** Müller cell. (× 7500)

analogous amacrine cell lacks such a characteristic structure but is generally identified by its lobulated nucleus (27) and its position along the innermost boundary of the bipolar cell layer.

Pathologic accumulations that may occur within the inner nuclear layer generally are localized to discrete pockets by the anteroposterior orientation of the entire bipolar cells much as they are similarly localized by the Henle fibers in the extrafoveal retina.

Inner Plexiform Layer

The inner plexiform layer (IPL) is composed of the axons of the bipolar and amacrine cells and their synapses and the dendrites of the ganglion cells. The bipolar cell synaptic expansions are most easily identified as miniature photoreceptor synaptic expansions (ribbon synapses) with mitochondria, typical synaptic vesicles, and a typical but much smaller synaptic ribbon or lamella lying generally within the cleavage of two dendrites inpouching from a ganglion cell (Fig. 6–53). The appearance of these two inpouching dendrites is known as a **dyad*** (26, 28) configuration (Fig. 6–54).

Myriad synapses occur within the inner plexiform layer (92). In sections of bird retinas this layer is clearly subdivided into three or more zones, each of which is presumably a different level for synapse. In sections of human retinas only a very slight suggestion of such layering can be seen.

peculiar body in its cytoplasm known in light microscopy as a Kolmer crystalloid (47). By electron microscopy (58, 110) (Fig. 6–51, 6–52), this structure is seen to be composed of a superimposed stack of special tubules, large in diameter, and lined by ribonucleoprotein particles (identified by specific enzyme digestion and negative for PAS by the thiosemicarbazide method). The structure only superficially resembles a stack of granular endoplasmic reticulum; its function is entirely unknown.* The

---

* Somewhat similar configurations have been observed outside the neural retina. One form devoid of ribosomes and continuous with the remainder of the smooth endoplasmic reticulum was found in the pigment epithelium of naturally hibernating bats (49). The others were observed in some examples of corneal endothelial cells from a variety of corneas with patho-

logic changes (44). Another peculiar cylindrical structure described as a "crystal" (98) or "cylinder organelle" (19), seen only by electron microscopy in the region of synaptic related processes of the horizontal cell has been observed. Apparently separate and unrelated to the Kolmer crystalloid, its composition and function are unknown.

* These terms are useful only in proper context because the same terms, dyad and triad, are also used for specialized regions of agranular endoplasmic reticulum (sarcoplasm) of striated muscle cells (78).

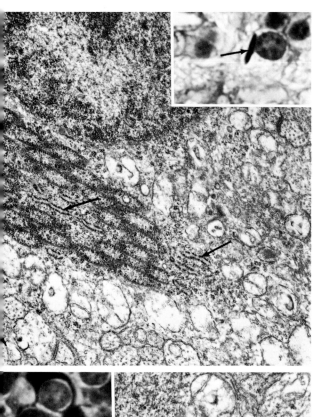

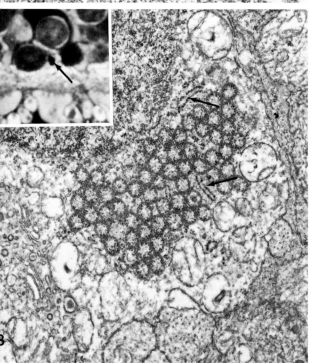

FIG. 6–52. Kolmer crystalloid. A. Longitudinal section of crystalloid (**arrow**) lying alongside nucleus of the cell. Temporal fovea (× 1040) (AFIP Neg. 72-6761) The larger figure is an oblique section of the ribosome-lined, superimposed large tubules. Note interwoven segments of more conventional rough or granular endoplasmic reticulum (**arrows**). (× 12,500) B. Cross-section of crystalloid (**arrow**) lying adjacent to cell nucleus. Temporal fovea. (TB, × 1040) (AFIP Neg. 72-6763). The TEM shows a cross-section of characteristic ribosome-lined large tubules of the crystalloid. Segments of conventional rough or granular endoplasmic reticulum are present within the crystalloid (**arrows**). (× 14,000)

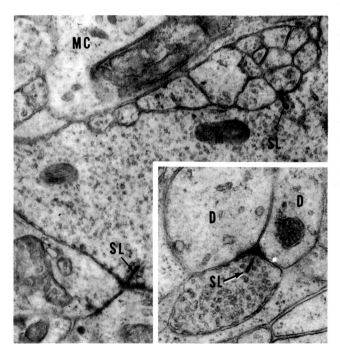

FIG. 6–53. Bipolar ribbon synapse within inner plexiform layer. Miniature synaptic ribbons or lamellas (**SL**) as well as synaptic densities and vesicles are present. **MC,** Müller cell; **M,** mitochondrion. (× 21,800) Inset shows dyad arrangement of bipolar synapse with its ribbon or lamella (**SL**) and two adjacent dendrites (**D**). (× 35,200). (Fine BS: J Neuropathol Exp Neurol 22:255, 1963)

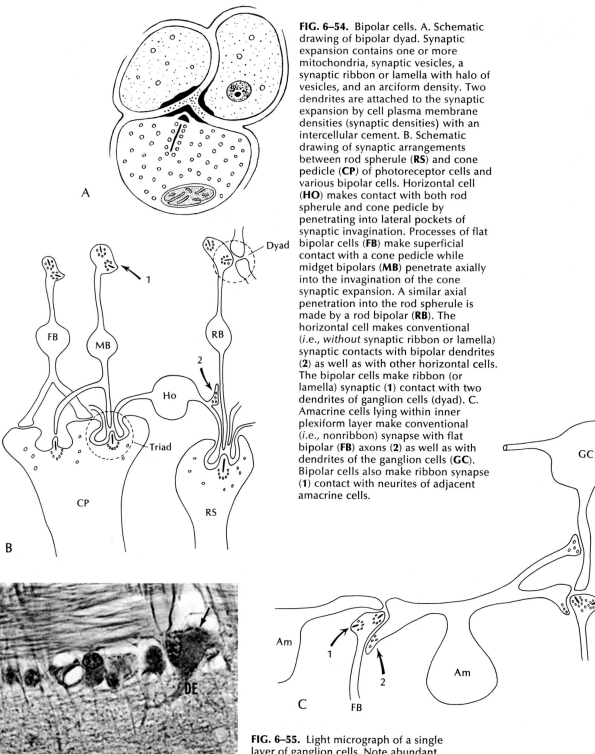

FIG. 6–54. Bipolar cells. A. Schematic drawing of bipolar dyad. Synaptic expansion contains one or more mitochondria, synaptic vesicles, a synaptic ribbon or lamella with halo of vesicles, and an arciform density. Two dendrites are attached to the synaptic expansion by cell plasma membrane densities (synaptic densities) with an intercellular cement. B. Schematic drawing of synaptic arrangements between rod spherule (**RS**) and cone pedicle (**CP**) of photoreceptor cells and various bipolar cells. Horizontal cell (**HO**) makes contact with both rod spherule and cone pedicle by penetrating into lateral pockets of synaptic invagination. Processes of flat bipolar cells (**FB**) make superficial contact with a cone pedicle while midget bipolars (**MB**) penetrate axially into the invagination of the cone synaptic expansion. A similar axial penetration into the rod spherule is made by a rod bipolar (**RB**). The horizontal cell makes conventional (*i.e., without* synaptic ribbon or lamella) synaptic contacts with bipolar dendrites (**2**) as well as with other horizontal cells. The bipolar cells make ribbon (or lamella) synaptic (**1**) contact with two dendrites of ganglion cells (dyad). C. Amacrine cells lying within inner plexiform layer make conventional (*i.e., nonribbon*) synapse with flat bipolar (**FB**) axons (**2**) as well as with dendrites of the ganglion cells (**GC**). Bipolar cells also make ribbon synapse (**1**) contact with neurites of adjacent amacrine cells.

FIG. 6–55. Light micrograph of a single layer of ganglion cells. Note abundant cytoplasm, basophilic Nissl bodies (**arrow**), and a dendrite (**DE**) of one of the ganglion cells extending into plexiform layer. (H&E, ×520) (Fine BS: Arch Ophthalmol 69:83, 1963)

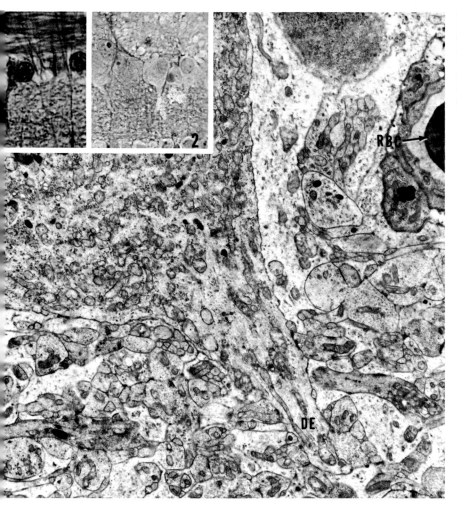

FIG. 6–56. Portion of ganglion cell dendrite (**DE**) emerging from adjacent inner plexiform layer. Small blood vessel (**RBC**) is present at right. (× 7700) Insets show comparable regions by light microscopy: **1.** Conventional 8- to 10-μ section. **2.** Plastic-embedded 1.5-μ section.

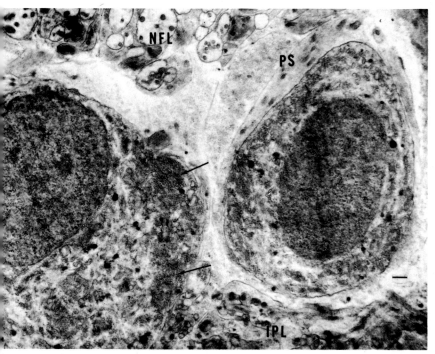

FIG. 6–57. Two ganglion cells from nasal retina lying between nerve fiber layer (**NFL**) and inner plexiform layer (**IPL**). Patches of Nissl substance (rough endoplasmic reticulum, **arrows**) are present, as are many dense cytoplasmic bodies. **PS,** nonspecific periganglion satellite cells. (× 4,500). (Fine BS: Arch Ophthalmol 69:83, 1963)

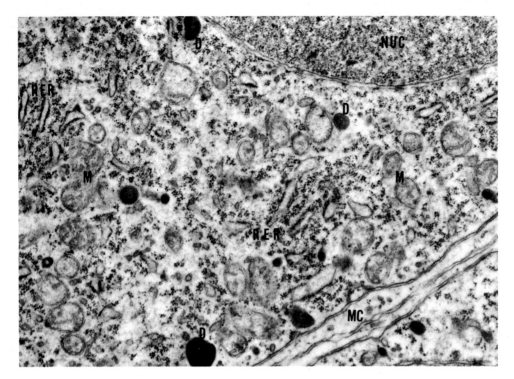

FIG. 6–58. Higher magnification of portion of ganglion cell. Basophilic Nissl granules or substance are formed of clusters of granular or rough endoplasmic reticulum (**RER**). Many dense bodies (**D**) are present throughout cytoplasm. **M,** mitochondria; **MC,** Müller cell; **NUC,** nucleus of ganglion cell. (× 24,000)

FIG. 6–59. Nerve fiber layer (**NFL**) of retina passing through arcades formed by stout columns and footplates (**arrows**) of Müller cells. **GC,** ganglion cell; **ILM,** internal limiting membrane. (Epon, PD, × 350) (AFIP Neg. 69-7570)

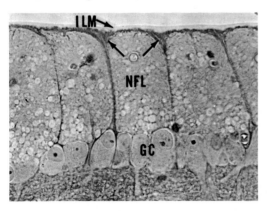

Ganglion Cell Layer

The large ganglion cell bodies form a single ganglion cell layer (GCL) throughout much of the retina (Fig. 6–55). The dendrites of the ganglion cells branch and resemble closely the dendrites of bipolar cells (Fig. 6–56). The cytoplasmic organelles of the ganglion cells differ little from those of other cells (mitochondria, Golgi complex, filaments, or tubules) except for the presence of large aggregates of granular endoplasmic reticulum (**Nissl** substance or bodies) and many small bodies of varying density (6, 31) (Fig. 6–57, 6–58). With increasing age, the small bodies increase in density. Glycogen is absent.

Dissolution of the basophilic areas of Nissl substance is an early sign of either physiologic or pathologic disturbance to the ganglion cell.

Nerve Fiber Layer

The axons of the ganglion cells are aggregated into nerve fiber bundles, which pass parallel to the retinal surface through the arcades formed by the stout columns and footplates of the Müller (glial) cells (Fig. 6–59, 6–60) to compose the nerve fiber layer (NFL) of the retina. The axons in tissues initially fixed in osmium

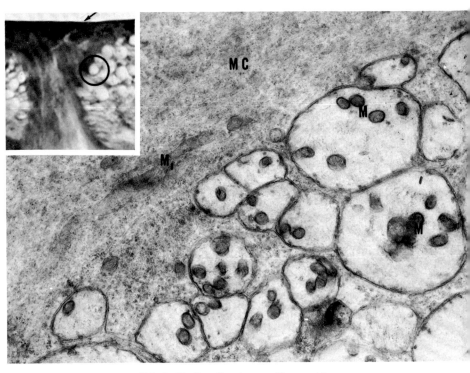

FIG. 6–60. Bundle of nerve fibers cut in cross-section. Their lucency is due to initial osmium fixation (filaments plus lucent ground substance). Adjacent Müller cell cytoplasm (**MC**) is dense, filament-filled in the columns, but relatively filament-free between axons. **M₁** Müller cell mitochondrion; **M** cross-sectioned axonal mitochondria. (× 14,000) (Fine BS, Zimmerman LE: Invest Ophthalmol 1:304, 1962) Inset. Light micrograph showing approximate region (**circle**) of electron micrograph. **Arrow** points to anterior surface of internal limiting membrane. (1.5-μ methacrylate section, PAS-hematoxylin, × 1500) (AFIP Neg. 61-2158) (Fine BS: Arch Ophthalmol 66:847, 1961)

tetroxide (Fig. 6–60) look different from those in tissues fixed initially in glutaraldehyde (33, 48) (Fig. 6–61). With the former, the axoplasm contains myriad neurofilaments (Fig. 6–60, 6–61) embedded in a very lucent ground substance. Mitochondria and some segments of agranular reticulum are present and longitudinally oriented, but the small particles (*i.e.,* glycogen-like) of the photoreceptor axons are lacking. With initial glutaraldehyde fixation, the neurofilaments are entirely replaced by *neurotubules,* and the ground substance is more prominent and more dense (Fig. 6–61). In the human retina the axons are unmyelinated because during embryonic development myelination ceases abruptly when it reaches the scleral lamina cribrosa of the optic nerve head (Fig. 12–3) after proceeding from the chiasm down the optic nerve toward the retina.

Occasionally the process of myelination continues into the retina ("skipping" the lamina cribrosa) and may be observed by the ophthalmologist as a white patch with a serrated or feathered edge radiating from the nerve head or even as an isolated patch of myelinated nerves widely separated from the nerve head (Fig. 6–62, 6–63). Virchow (99) was the first to identify the white retinal patches both grossly and histologically as myelinated nerve fibers. By electron microscopy, the absence of oligodendroglia, together with the considerable proximity of the myelinated nerves to the Müller cells, strongly suggest that the latter cells function here as oligodendrocytes in producing the myelination. Such anatomic variations are commonly brought to the attention of the student as points in differential diagnosis to prevent confusion with such pathologic changes as exudates, cottonwool spots, and retinal tumors. Since these white superficial patches are quite opaque, they produce scotomas, which can be clearly delineated on tangent screen (central field)

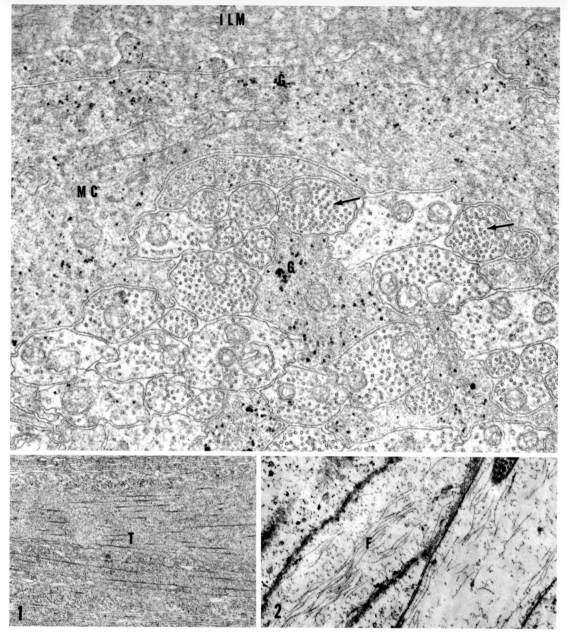

FIG. 6–61. Ganglion cell axons in tissue fixed initially in glutaraldehyde. Microtubules (**arrows**) within axons are seen here mainly in cross-section. Müller cell (**MC**) cytoplasm contains glycogen particles (**G**) and envelops many of the axons. Many axons are not separated by Müller cell cytoplasm. **ILM,** internal limiting membrane. Inset 1. Microtubules (**T**) in longitudinal section. Inset 2. Filaments (**F**) within axoplasm in tissue fixed initially in osmium tetroxide. (All × 16,800)

FIG. 6–62. A. Section of retina shows myelination localized exclusively to nerve fiber layer. (Epon, PD, × 80) (AFIP Neg. 72-10790) Inset shows myelinated nerve fibers as they appear grossly within the retina. Note the "skip" area (**arrow**) between the edge of the optic disc and the myelination. The retinal vessels are hidden by the opaque white fibers which attenuate in a "feathered" appearance above. B. Enlargement to show myelinated nerve fibers clearly outlining the nerve fiber bundles. **IPL,** inner plexiform layer. (Epon, PD, × 300) (AFIP Neg. 72-10791)

examination. Some animals (*e.g.*, the rabbit) normally possess a band of myelinated retinal nerve fibers (Fig. 6–64).

Internal Limiting Membrane

Along the posterior human retina the **internal limiting membrane** (ILM) is a thick (0.5μ or more) basement membrane (30) (Fig. 6–65). Its inner or vitreal surface is extremely flat, whereas its outer surface follows closely the uneven surface of the Müller cell basal plasma membranes. Frequently the inner surface of the Müller cell footplates is deeply pocketed and the basement membrane fills this pocket (Fig. 6–66). The inner plane of the basement membrane therefore is maintained. These basement-membrane-filled pockets are called **basement membrane facets** (34) (Fig. 6–66).

Reflections from the inner surface of the glasslike internal limiting membrane produce the retinal "sheen" that may be observed with the ophthalmoscope. Similarly, it is likely that the basement membrane facets (Fig. 6–67) are the anatomic reason for the normal glistening spots or "Gunn's dots" so frequently observed in this sheen.

Artifactitious separations of the internal limiting membrane of the retina invariably take some of the footplates of the Müller cells with them.

The *submembranous cleavage plane* is a meaningful artifact in that a number of pathologic processes involve this potential space.

Such anatomic observations may also be of some value to the clinician in differentiating ophthalmoscopically a true, otherwise uncomplicated, subvitreal hemorrhage from a submembranous (*i.e.*, superficial intraretinal) hemorrhage, for no sheen will be seen on the surface of the uncomplicated subvitreal hemorrhage, whereas it will be present over the intraretinal hemorrhage. A submembranous intraretinal hemorrhage should also be easily distinguishable from one into the deeper layer of nerve fibers (ganglion cell axons) by means of the characteristic "flame shape" of the latter. The internal limiting membranes of retinas of some animals, such as rabbit (Fig. 6–68) or frog (Fig. 6–69) are

FIG. 6–63. Electron micrograph of myelinated nerve fibers. The characteristic layers of myelin are seen clearly, as are some of the mesaxons (**arrows**). The ganglion cell axons ("nerve fibers") here contain both filaments and tubules. (× 42,000)

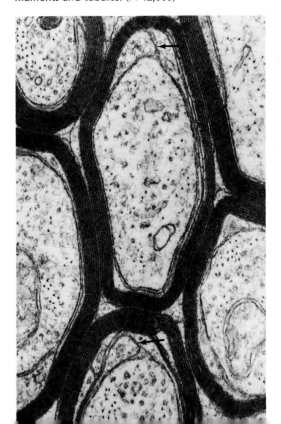

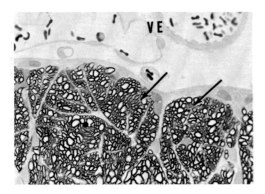

FIG. 6–64. Rabbit retina, showing band of myelinated nerve fibers (**arrows**) normally present in the species. Retinal vasculature (**VE**) in this species is preretinal. (Epon, PD, × 395) (AFIP Neg. 66-6700)

FIG. 6–65. Internal limiting membrane. A. Internal limiting membrane of posterior retina (**ILM**), a thick basement membrane closely applied to basal plasmalemmas of Müller cells (**arrows**). Inner surface of this basement membrane is smooth. **FIL,** Müller cell cytoplasmic filaments; **MC,** Müller cell. (× 11,700) B. Thick internal limiting membrane in region near temporal edge of fovea. Note areas of lucency and feltwork structure. A few cell processes also are present. (× 18,000)

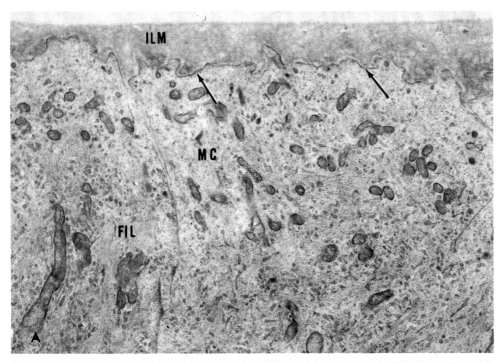

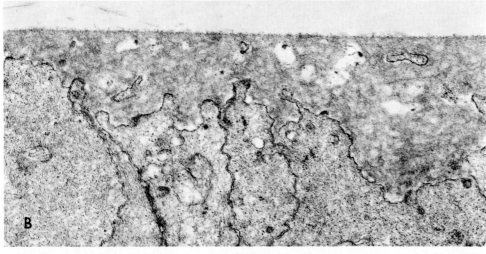

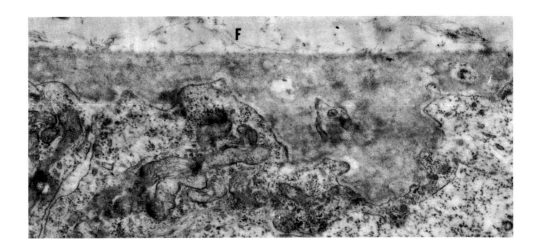

exceedingly thin and therefore produce no ophthalmoscopic sheen.

Peripherally, toward the equator of the eye (40), the thick basement membrane of the retina rather abruptly becomes thinner (Fig. 6–70 A, B). More peripherally, in the region of the vitreous base the retinal basement membrane becomes a typical thin basement membrane (Fig. 6–70 C) resembling closely the thin basement membrane present along the posterior retina in infancy (Fig. 6–71). In the region of the ora serrata the thin basement membrane frequently is interrupted with aging (Fig. 6–72). Toward the ora serrata/pars plana the basement membrane becomes multilaminar.

THE GLIAL SYSTEM

The Müller Cell

This, the largest glial cell in the retina, makes up the largest volume of glial tissue in the retina. The cell cannot be demonstrated in its entirety by conventional staining techniques, but requires special silver stains, such as those of Golgi (11). With that metal-impregnation method the cell can be seen to have at least two distinct parts: a stout inner trunk with rather small lateral branches, and a delicate honeycomb-like outer part that forms delicate sheaths of cytoplasm around the cell bodies of the photoreceptor cells in the outer nuclear layer (Figs. 6–39 A, 6–41, 6–42). Delicate apical villi, once known as the "fiber baskets of Schultze," can be seen protruding outward through the plane of the external limiting membrane (Fig.

FIG. 6–66. Deep pocket filled with internal limiting membrane, a basement membrane facet. Vitreous filaments (**F**) are present, attached to smooth inner surface of membrane. (× 22,500) (Fine BS: In McPherson A (ed): New and Controversial Aspects of Retinal Detachment. New York, Hoeber, 1968)

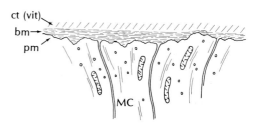

FIG. 6–67. Schematic drawing of basement membrane facet; **bm,** basement membrane; **ct** (**vit**), vitreous filaments; **MC,** Müller cell; **pm,** plasma membrane.

FIG. 6–68. Thin basement (internal limiting membrane, **arrow**) of rabbit retina. (× 16,000)

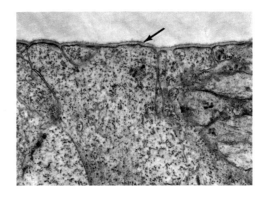

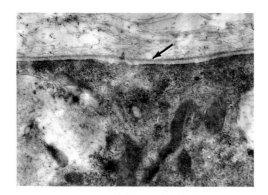

FIG. 6–69. Thin basement membrane (internal limiting membrane, **arrow**) of frog retina. (× 13,250)

FIG. 6–70. Basement membrane of 18-year-old subject, showing internal limiting membrane at various points. A. At nasal equator. **MC,** Müller cells. (× 15,000) B. At temporal equator. **MC,** Müller cells. (× 15,000) C. At retinal periphery. **f,** vitreous filaments. (× 7800)

6–40) to terminate between the inner segments of the photoreceptors.

By electron microscopic examination, the cytoplasm of the Müller cell is seen to be subdivided into three parts: the inner filamentous cytoplasm, the outer lucent cytoplasm, and the intermediate portion or transitional zone.

1. *The inner dense cytoplasm.* The inner part of the Müller cell, especially its footplates or expansions, separates the nerve fiber bundles from the internal limiting membrane (Fig. 6–61) except in a few areas where smaller glia intervene. The stout portion of the cell contains many filaments aligned along its axis. From the stout filamentous columns, delicate, almost filament-free processes, containing glycogen particles (Fig. 6–60, 6–61), pass between many of the axons in each nerve fiber bundle. The processes occupy much of the retinal space except for the typical ~150 A intercellular spaces. The intercellular spaces, although appearing small, are highly functional as a pathway for ionic and nutritional exchanges (65, 89).

2. *The outer, lucent cytoplasm.* This easily disrupted part of the cell contains clusters of mitochondria near the external limiting membrane and some filaments (*i.e.,* microtubules in tissue fixed initially with glutaraldehyde).

3. *The intermediate portion or transition zone.* This zone of the Müller cell lies apical to the nucleus (Fig. 6–73) and contains the Golgi complex as well as a few segments of granular endoplasmic reticulum. Individual particles of glycogen are widely dispersed within the lucent cytoplasm.

Presumably, the intracellular filaments are partly the reason why, in Formalin-fixed retinas (Fig. 6–23), the stout inner columns of the Müller cells are seen

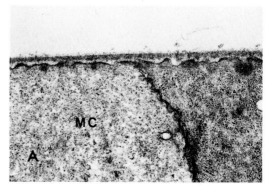

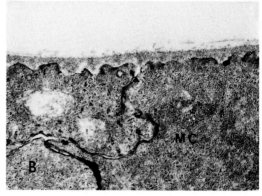

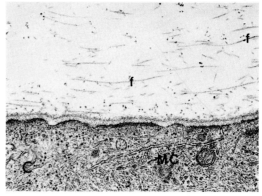

easily and thus called Müller fibers. The inner segments of the cells also appear more "fibrous" when the nerve fiber bundles are cross-sectioned (Fig. 6–59). The outer segments or cytoplasmic leaflets lack the large number of filaments and dense ground substance, so they are almost impossible to detect in convention H&E-stained sections except perhaps by their absence or "negative" staining. Small hemorrhages can track easily along the axons within the nerve fiber layers because the delicate Müller cell cytoplasmic filament-free processes offer little resistance. The distribution of blood in the nerve fiber layer produces the "feathered-edge" hemorrhage observed by the clinician, an observation which identifies for him the retinal layer involved.

Accessory Glia

The smaller glia, fibrous and protoplasmic astrocytes, and oligodendrocyte-like cells, normally are found only in the nerve fiber, ganglion cell, and inner plexiform layers. As their names imply, they are roughly identified by the concentration of their cytoplasmic filaments. The small astrocytes (Fig. 6–74) probably are responsible for much of the retinal gliosis in pathologic conditions.

Some of the smaller glia (mostly astrocytes, fibrous or protoplasmic), which lie beneath the ILM of the retina migrate from the retina through the thick basement membrane (109) onto its surface, where they proliferate. The sheet of preretinal glial cells so formed often produces distortions ("cellophane macula") of the ILM, most noticeable in the region of the fovea (macula). There is some evidence that the Müller cell also may participate in the formation of this preretinal gliosis. Traction by detachment of the vitreous body may be one of the stimuli to initiate the migration.

The astrocytes may also undergo a form of degeneration that produces small intracytoplasmic bodies known as **corpora amylacea** found in the inner retinal layers (34, 73) (Fig. 6–75). The properties of the oligodendrocyte-like cells in the retina* are not clear because in the retina

* The presence of true oligodendroglia in the retina has long been disputed by those who seek to identify them by metal-impregnation techniques (71). Some investigators say that the Müller cells function in the retina as oligodendroglia (see section on Nerve Fiber Layer earlier in this chapter). By current electron microscopic cytologic criteria, however, a few cells are present that possess a number of characteristics of oligodendroglia. Some of these latter cells may also represent "resting" microglia. They may also be another source for preretinal gliosis (i.e., in addition to fibrous astrocytes).

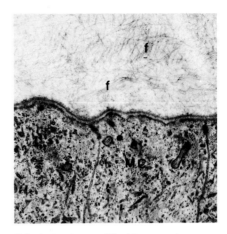

FIG. 6–71. Internal limiting membrane, posterior retina, 5-month-old infant. **f,** vitreous filaments; **MC,** Müller cells. (× 12,000)

FIG. 6–72. Rupture of thin internal limiting membrane (**arrow**) at retinal periphery. (× 9300)

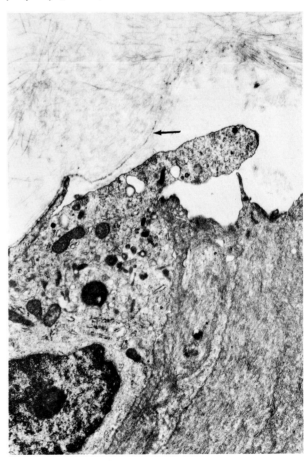

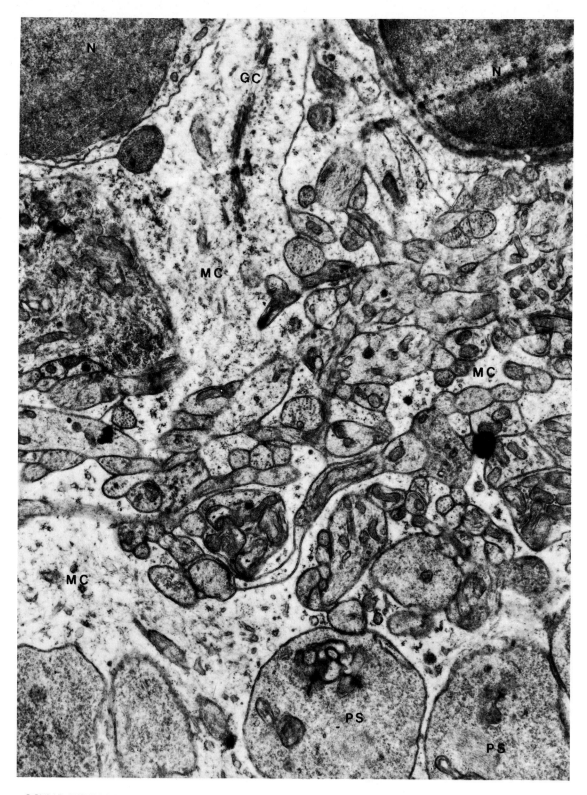

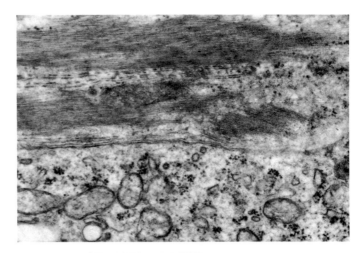

FIG. 6–73. Intermediate zone of Müller cell lying just apical to its nucleus. Golgi complex (**GC**) is present in this region. Lucent cytoplasm (**MC**) of Müller cell permeates plexiform layer as well as all levels occupied by photoreceptor cells internal to external limiting membrane. **N,** nuclei of bipolar cells; **PS,** photoreceptor synaptic expansions. (× 15,000) (Fine BS, Zimmerman LE: Invest Ophthalmol 1:304, 1962)

FIG. 6–74. Fibrous astrocytes, recognizable by their cytoplasmic content of filaments. Fovea. (× 24,000)

the cells do not produce myelin as they do in the central nervous system. Other cells are found which lack some of the clear-cut criteria for astrocytes, but because of their close association with ganglion cells they have been called, in a nonspecific way, periganglion cells (like perineuronal cells of the central nervous system).

Microglia, the central nervous system counterpart of the histiocytes or macrophages found elsewhere, are difficult to identify in normal tissue. In fact, they generally are identified only when they have become macrophagic (have actually ingested material). Many of the macrophagic cells observed in pathologic tissues probably originate from the bloodstream.

Various "nourishing" and "structural" functions frequently are attributed to these glial cells. Some evidence for their nutritional function is their high glycogen content (50) (Müller cells) (Fig. 6–61) and their uptake of necrotic materials (Müller cells and newly arrived macrophages). Evidence for their structural function is the aggregation of cytoplasmic filaments (inner ends of Müller cells, fibrous astrocytes).

THE VASCULAR SYSTEM

The human retina is vascularized in its inner layers outward to the level of the middle limiting membrane.* The choriocapillaris of the choroid mostly is responsible for nourishing the photoreceptor and enveloping Müller cell

* The zone where, in the terminology of the older anatomists (79), the "neuroepithelial layers meet the cerebral layers," *i.e.,* where the cerebral layers are vascularized.

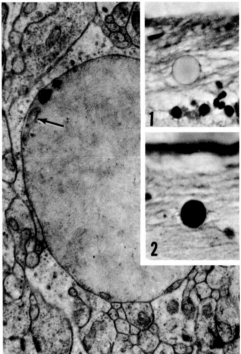

FIG. 6–75. Corpora amylacea formed from fibrous astrocytes. Electron micrograph, showing single body lying within a cell membrane and containing a few dense bodies as well as a mitochondrion (**arrow**). The main mass consists of short, needle-like filaments in disarray. (× 12,000) (Fine BS: In McPherson A (ed): New and Controversial Aspects of Retinal Detachment. New York, Hoeber, 1968) Inset 1. Single body in nerve fiber layer. (H&E stain, × 395) (AFIP Neg. 70-3670) Inset 2. Similar body stained with PAS. (× 530) (AFIP Neg. 70-3846)

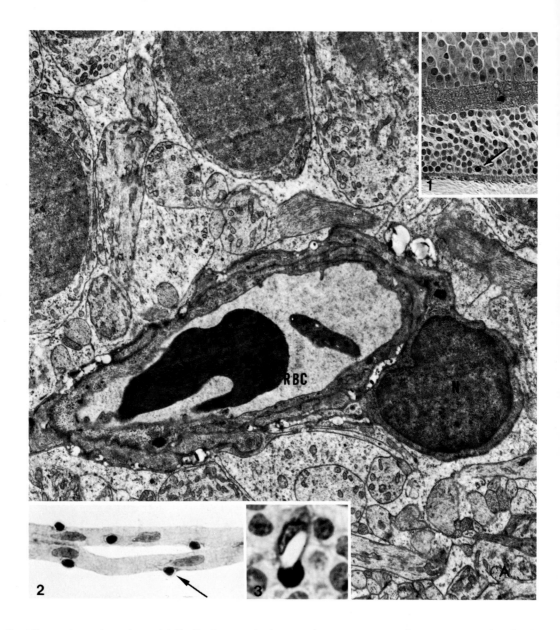

cytoplasm that lies external to the middle limiting membrane.

The retina has no real arteries or veins except possibly just adjacent to the optic disc. The largest vessels are arterioles and venules; the smallest are capillaries.

The capillaries are easily identified by their single endothelial lining and basement membrane (34, 59) (Fig. 6–76). Outside the endothelial basement membrane is an interrupted layer of cells. These cells, pericytes (periendothelial or "mural" [51] cells), are also surrounded by

their own basement membrane material, which fuses with that of the capillary endothelium, giving an appearance of a cell "embedded in basement membrane." With aging, some of the basement membrane degenerates, producing dense bodies and a vacuolated appearance.

The observation of preferential loss of pericytes in relation to endothelial cells from the retinal capillaries is considered to be highly characteristic of diabetes mellitus (108).

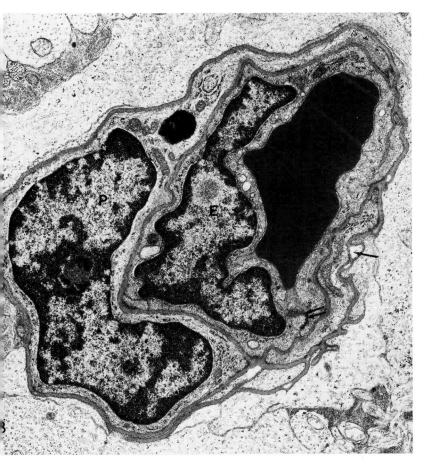

FIG. 6–76. A. (opposite page) Retinal capillaries. 1) Outermost capillary layer lying just anterior to middle limiting membrane (**arrow**). (PD, × 210) (AFIP Neg. 63-6895) 2) Segments of retinal capillaries following retinal digestion with trypsin. Large axial pale-staining nuclei of endothelial cells are easily distinguished from denser rounded nuclei of pericytes. A thin "shell" of PAS-positive basement membrane can be seen around the pericyte present in profile. (PAS, ×440) (AFIP Neg. 64-7004) 3) Section of capillary. Nucleus of endothelial cell stains lightly while that of surrounding pericyte stains darkly. (TB, × 1040) (AFIP Neg. 73-3714) B. Nasal retina, rhesus monkey. Pericyte (**P**) and endothelial cell (**E**) of retinal capillary. Small lumen is occupied completely by distorted erythrocyte. Endothelial cell has a basement membrane as does the pericyte. The basement membranes fuse where they meet. A few foci of basement membrane vacuolation or rarefaction are present (**arrows**). Endothelial cell *zonula adherens* is identifiable (**double arrows**). (× 12,000)

To the pericyte basement membrane are attached glial cells (generally Müller cells) or, in the larger vessels, collagenous connective tissue.

Capillary endothelial cells are attached to one another by terminal bars (Fig. 6–77). Most of the terminal bar attachment is formed by a zonula adherens (easily recognized by the adjacent cytoplasmic densities, whether cut normally or obliquely). A very short zonula occludens is present on the luminal side of the adherens (83).

The very short occludens is difficult to demonstrate. It is best detected physiologically by the use of horseradish peroxidase. Intravascular peroxidase is barred from the intercellular space near the lumen. Extravascularly placed peroxidase passes readily along the entire zonula adherens to stop abruptly near the capillary lumen. One part of the blood–retina barrier, therefore, lies here. Another part of the blood–retina barrier lies at the level of the zonula occludens in the retinal pigment epithelium (see section on pigment epithelium earlier in this chapter).

Near the attachments the endothelial cells frequently project into the lumen in the form of villi or flaps, which may, on occasion, be so marked as to produce bizarre configurations.

The capillary endothelial cells also possess micropinocytotic vesicles, as do cerebral capillaries and capillaries elsewhere. Considerable argument has taken place over the functional significance of the vesicles that are present under the best conditions of fixation and that can be demonstrated to transport particles in either direction.

Physiologists have long been concerned with the transport of nutrient and waste materials across the endothelial lining of capillaries (103). Experimental

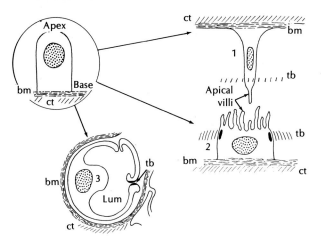

FIG. 6–77. Schematic drawing showing arrangement of retinal cells to form 1) Müller cells, 2) pigment epithelial cells, and 3) vascular endothelium. All cells possess apical attachments and basement membranes (**bm**), connective tissue (**ct**), and terminal bars (**tb**). (Fine BS: In McPherson A (ed): New and Controversial Aspects of Retinal Detachment. New York, Hoeber, 1968)

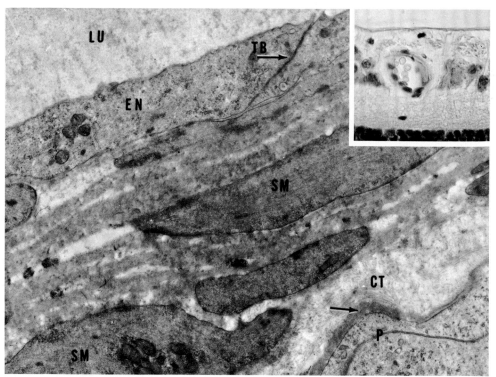

FIG. 6–78. Arteriole. Lumen (**LU**), endothelial lining (**EN**), zonula adherens of terminal bar (**TB**), and wall of smooth muscle cells (**SM**), all surrounded by layers of basement membrane. Parenchymal cells (**P**) are separated from outermost smooth muscle cells by basement membrane (**free arrow**) and layer of connective tissue (**CT**). (× 16,000) Inset. Light micrograph showing comparable retinal arteriole near internal limiting membrane. (H&E, × 300)

FIG. 6–79. A. Topography of major retinal vessels and their relation to adjacent nerve fiber. B. Superior edge of area centralis. Note several layers of capillaries throughout inner retinal layers. Inner plexiform layer is attenuated in vicinity of superior temporal arteriole. Henle fibers are oblique (**arrow**). (PD, × 90) (AFIP Neg. 75-12995) C. Inferior edge of area centralis. Temporal retinal arteriole (**a**) and venule (**v**) are present. Note attenuation of inner plexiform and bipolar cell layers in region of major vessels. Henle fibers are oblique (**arrow**). (TB, × 90) (AFIP Neg. 75-12997)

observations combined with theoretical considerations have indicated that there are at least two sizes of "apertures" or "pores" across a capillary lining, a hypothetic "large pore system" ~400–700 A diameter, and a hypothetical "small pore system" ~40 A diameter. Because no static apertures of such dimension are seen in electron micrographs, it has been assumed by many investigators that the typical intercellular space of ~150 A width represents the small-pore system (54), and that the endothelial cell micropinocytotic vesicles (see Ch. 11) the large-pore system. For example, intravascular injection of horseradish peroxidase, a small protein molecule (40,000 molecular weight, ~25–30 A diameter) (Fig. 6–15A; see also Fig. 1–14, 10–47, 10–48, 10–50) was shown to pass readily through the intercellular spaces of some muscle capillary endothelia. Ferritin, a larger molecule (500,000 molecular weight, ~90–110 A diameter) was found to enter the micropinocytotic vesicles but did not pass between the endothelial cells. Basement membranes are all highly permeable to both tracers. The functions of a "pore" system may of course be modified by additional factors (e.g., presence of a zonula occludens).

An arteriole is easily differentiated from a venule by its thicker wall, which takes a darker stain in flat preparations, and by its more circular cross section. The arteriole lacks an internal elastic lamina and a continuous layer of smooth muscle cells. Smooth muscle cells are typical of those found elsewhere in the body and are separated by their own basement membranes (Fig. 6–78). The outermost muscle cells are generally separated by a layer of collagen fibrils or filaments ("adventitia") from the adjacent parenchymal cells.

The major retinal vessels (Fig. 6–79) arise as branches of their corresponding central retinal vessel in the optic nerve head. The central retinal artery lies on the nasal side of the central retinal vein. As they enter the retina, the artery and the vein divide into four main branches: the upper and lower nasal and the upper and lower temporal. The arterioles are slightly smaller in diameter than the corresponding venules. Generally mirroring the pattern of contiguous nerve fibers, these major vessels lie near the internal limiting membrane or not far beneath it.

Where the vessels approach the surface, the internal limiting membrane may be extremely attenuated (Fig. 6–80) thereby causing a "weakness" in this basement membrane analogous to that in the regions of the optic disk and fovea (Fig. 6–91, 12–4).

By both light and electron microscopy the internal limiting membrane becomes attenuated wherever the cytoplasmic footplates of the Müller cells become attenuated (Fig. 6–80, 6–81). A thin internal limiting membrane (Fig. 6–82, 6–83, 6–84) is therefore sporadically pres-

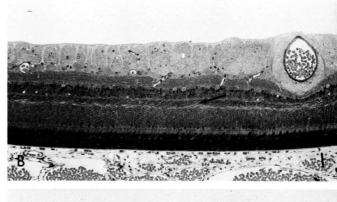

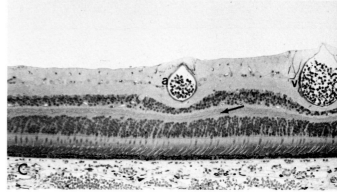

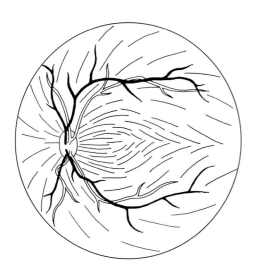

A

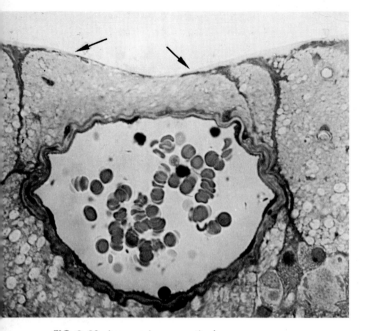

FIG. 6–80. Large vein near retinal surface. Internal limiting membrane is attenuated (**arrows**), mirroring attenuation of adjacent Müller cell cytoplasm. (Epon, PD, × 485) (AFIP Neg. 69-7567)

FIG. 6–81. Large vessel near retinal surface. Internal limiting membrane (**arrow**) remains thick, mirroring thick underlying layers of Müller cell cytoplasm. (Epon PD, × 485) (AFIP Neg. 69-7566)

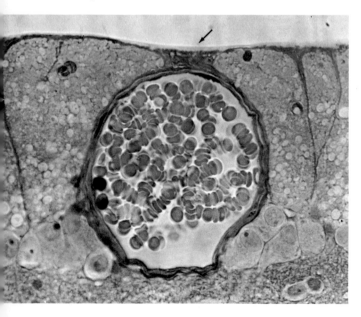

FIG. 6–82. Thin internal limiting membrane (**ILM**) overlying thin cytoplasmic leaflets of Müller and superficial glial cells (**GL**). The latter cells are perivascular astrocytes, as determined by their cytoplasmic content of filaments and glycogen. Cells are also associated with a basement membrane. Edge of large retinal vessel (**V**) is present just external to small glial cell. **NFL,** nerve fiber layer. (× 16,500)

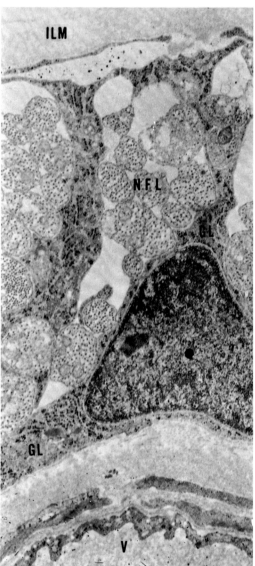

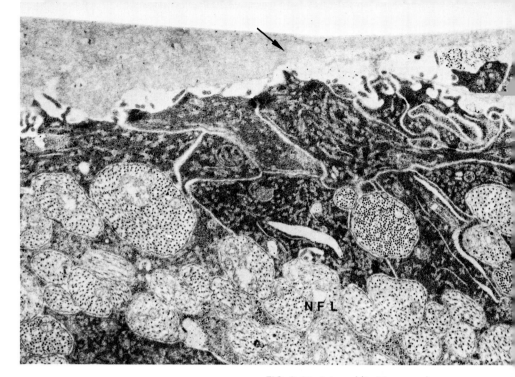

FIG. 6–83. Internal limiting membrane peripheral to that in Figure 6–82, overlying large retinal blood vessel. Transition of a thick to a thin internal limiting membrane can be seen at arrow. Dense cytoplasm underlying membrane is that of Müller cell. Axons of nerve fiber layer (NFL) are clearly seen, mostly cut in cross-section. (× 16,500)

FIG. 6–84. Internal limiting membrane, thinnest where underlying glial cell cytoplasm is minimal. These regions of membrane thinning suggest regions of weakness. Note "loose" spaces occupied by basement membrane (arrows) along retinal surface in close relation to its vasculature. GL, perivascular astrocyte; NFL, nerve fiber layer. (× 16,000)

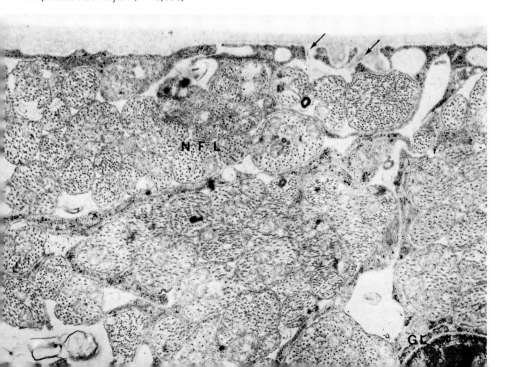

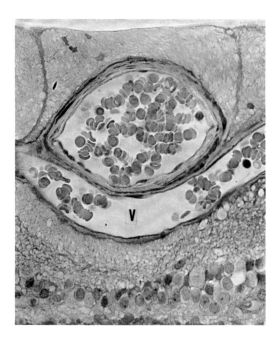

FIG. 6–85. Arteriovenous crossing. Arteriole generally crosses internal to venule (**V**). Adventitia of the two vessels is here in continuity. (Epon, PD, × 350) (AFIP Neg. 69-7564)

FIG. 6–86. Venule draining lower temporal retina appears to pass directly into choroidal vasculature at temporal edge of optic disc (**arrow**). Inset. Fluorescein angiography in the early venous phase shows clearly venous drainage into region of choroidal vasculature. (Courtesy of Dr. John J. Weiter)

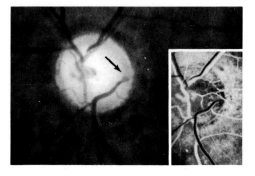

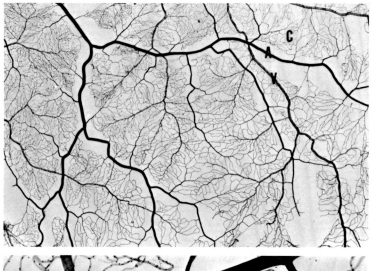

FIG. 6–87. Trypsin-digested specimen of retina, showing distribution of vasculature. **A,** arterioles; **C,** capillaries; **V,** venules. (PAS, × 8) (AFIP Neg. 64-7007)

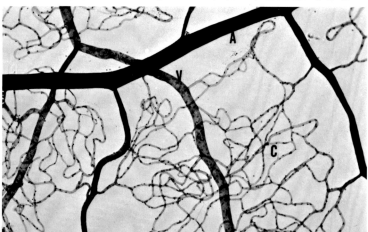

FIG. 6–88. Trypsin-digested specimen of retina. Large dark-staining vessel has a thick wall, indicating it is an arteriole (**A**). Relatively capillary-free zone is present alongside arterioles. Cellular large vessel represents a small venule (**V**). **C,** capillaries. (PAS, ×50) (AFIP Neg. 64-7002-B)

ent along the distribution of the major retinal vessels. The foci of thin basement membrane may indicate sites of "weakness," through which early changes of preretinal disease processes (e.g., preretinal gliosis, early neovascularization) may gain access to the vitreous compartment. (Compare with the basement membrane lining the optic cup of the optic nerve head, Figure 12–4.)

The arteriole generally overlies (lies internal to) the corresponding venule (Fig. 6–85). Because both vessel walls normally are transparent, the clinician sees one column of lighter colored blood (oxygenated in the arteriole) overlying a column of slightly darker blood (deoxygenated in the venule). With aging or with disease processes that accelerate aging (e.g., diabetes, hypertension), the arterial wall may thicken (arteriolar sclerosis) and hide from view a small segment of the underlying venular blood column ("arteriolar-venous nicking").

In approximately 25% of the population a retinal vessel arises directly from the choroidal vasculature at the temporal edge of the optic disk (the **cilioretinal artery**) to nourish much of the macula and the papillomacular bundle. Smaller, less significant cilioretinal vessels can be found in as much as 50% of the population.

Central retinal artery occlusion occurring in a person having a cilioretinal artery may have little effect on his central visual acuity. Conversely, embolization of such a cilioretinal vessel (a rare event) may severely damage central acuity, leaving the peripheral vision intact. An accompanying vein is rare. Even more rarely, a major portion (e.g., lower temporal retina (Fig. 6–86) of the retina is drained by a vessel directly into the choroidal vasculature (3, 4).

A relatively wide capillary-free zone lies adjacent to the arterioles (Fig. 6–87, 6–88). A similar but much less prominent capillary-free zone accompanies the venules.

The retinal vasculature at the posterior pole terminates in the fovea as a capillary net or ring (see Foveola), producing the retinal avascular zone of the fovea (macula) (Fig. 6–89). At the retinal periphery the vasculature terminates in delicate arcades ~1 mm short of the ora serrata; the arterioles are therefore often called **"end arteries."**

TOPOGRAPHIC VARIATIONS

Area Centralis

Temporal to the optic disc is a region of posterior fundus much larger than the optic disc and roughly demarcated by the arcuate temporal retinal vessels (Fig. 6–90). The region, approximately 6 mm in diameter (approximately 15° of field) is known historically as the **area centralis** (71), a region wherein histologically more than one layer of ganglion cells can be found (see section on the macula lutea later in this chapter). The remainder of the retina is generally termed peripheral retina (i.e., temporal periphery, nasal periphery, upper, lower, etc.).

Fovea (Centralis)

Approximately in the center of the area centralis lies a pit or depression slightly oval in shape, the fovea (centralis), the horizontal diameter of which, in the human, mirrors that of the optic disc, ~1.5 mm (approximately 5° of field) (Fig. 6–91).

In the smaller eye of the rhesus monkey the more circular fovea centralis has a smaller diameter, averaging approximately 1 mm (Fig. 6–92 and 6–93) and in this species also mirrors the horizontal diameter of the corresponding optic disc.

The thick basement membrane present on the surface of the retina posterior to the equator (Fig. 6–91 a) which reflects light as the retinal sheen, is attenuated along the slopes or **clivus** of the fovea (Fig. 6–91 b to d). The attenuation of the thick basement membrane along the clivus closely approximates thinning of the underlying ganglion cell layer, at the termination of which (Fig. 6–91 e) it continues across the floor as a thin basement membrane (105) (Fig. 6–91 f). The floor of the fovea, therefore, is covered entirely by a thin basement membrane, which follows the contours of the smooth curve produced by the underlying flaps or sheets of Müller glial cells and a few presumably isolated smaller glia, as indicated by the few nuclei present in the region.

The transition of basement membrane from thick to thin also closely approximates the level of transi-

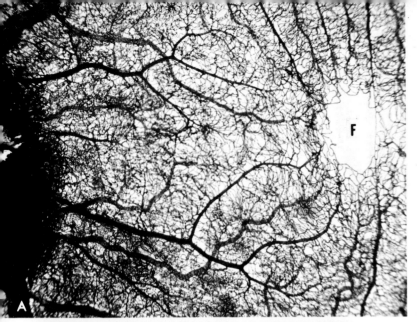

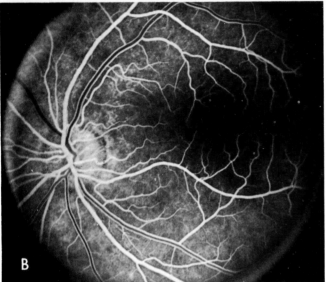

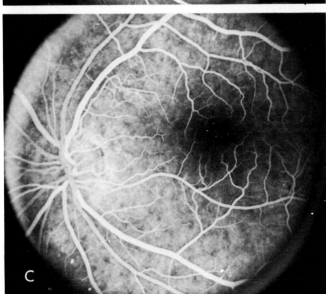

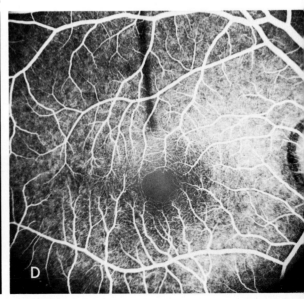

FIG. 6–89. Retinal vasculature. A. Trypsin-digested specimen of retina showing vasculature in region between optic disc on left and avascular foveal region (**F**) on right. Vasculature terminates at foveal declivity as series of capillary arcades. (PAS, × 22.) (Scheie HG, Albert DM: Adler's Textbook of Ophthalmology. Philadelphia, WB Saunders, 1969) B. Fluorescein angiogram—early venous stage. Arteries are filled and venous return (laminar flow) has begun. Large area of posterior pole appears dark. (Courtesy of Dr. J. W. Berkow) C. Fluorescein angiogram—late arteriovenous phase. Both arteries and veins are filled completely with dye. Lumens of veins are larger than those of arteries. Dye in arteries has begun to fade. Note dark area of posterior pole ("macula") is now approximately the size of the optic disc. Lobular pattern of choriocapillaris still can be seen (see Fig. 10–36). (Courtesy of Dr. J. W. Berkow) D. Arteriovenous phase of angiogram reproduced with maximum contrast to show vessels of the posterior pole to best advantage. The central (foveal) capillary net and ring (see Fig. 6–90B) are clearly seen as is the central retinal avascular zone. The capillary net adjacent to the avascular zone is two-dimensional (see Fig. 6–96), and therefore stands out sharply since it is not superimposed on other retinal vessels. (Berkow JW, Kelley JS, Orth DH: Manual of American Academy of Ophthalmology and Otolaryngology. Rochester, MN, 1977)

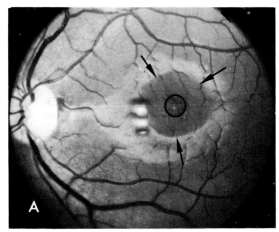

FIG. 6–90. Fundus of human eye. A. Area centralis occupies region of posterior pole between the arcuate temporal vessels. Ring reflex (**arrows**) indicates edge of retinal pit or fovea centralis. The small circle outlines the small red disc of the foveola or foveal floor. B. Schematic drawing superimposing anatomic terminology on fundus topography. The central capillary ring also is called the perifoveolar capillary ring. (Modified from Orth DH *et al.*: Trans Am Acad Ophthalmol Otolaryngol 83:OP506–OP514, 1977)

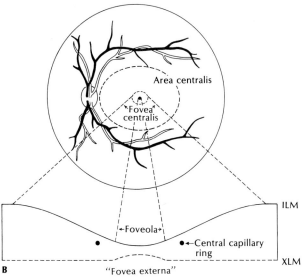

Clinically (Fig. 6–90A), the boundary of the fovea can be noted by the partial or complete annular or foveal (ring) reflex, a reflection of light from the thick basement membrane that passes over the rim of the depression where it begins to attenuate (67). By moving the ophthalmoscope back and forth, a corresponding attenuation of the annular reflex toward the floor of the fovea may be observed. Not infrequently, and especially in the young, the attenuated reflex can be observed all the way to the plane of the retinal vasculature (*i.e.*, to the plane of transition of basement membrane from thick to thin—see preceding paragraph). The deepmost penetration of the foveal pit by the ophthalmoscopic reflex also outlines the outer edge of the *foveola* (Fig. 6–90A), a deeper red disc-shaped area comprising the foveal floor.

The tiny reflex commonly observed in the center of the fovea, *i.e.*, the **foveolar reflex (central foveal reflex)** (see following section) apparently results from the geometry of the foveolar area (Fig. 6–94) and is unrelated directly to the presence of a thin basement membrane. Apparently the geometry may vary from a saucer shape to that of a concave circular mirror to that of a parabola. The variation in curvature would help to explain the clinical observation of an absent reflex, a reflex that forms a small arc (the caustic of a concave circular mirror with large aperture) or a pinpoint reflex (the focal point of a parabolic mirror). The image can be observed clinically to be smaller than, and to lie actually suspended anterior to, the foveolar disc.

tion from vascular to avascular (relatively anoxic) retina in the fovea. The two observations suggest an anatomic basis for some of the mysterious proliferations that occur in this region, proliferations that distort or wrinkle the foveomacular region to such an extent that visual acuity may be severely impaired. In accordance with other observations (see retinal vessels, equatorial retina, and optic nerve head) basement membrane transition from thick to thin is generally accompanied by an increase in strength of vitreous body attachment. Traction through such an attachment may be one stimulus initiating migrations and proliferations of glial cells. Glial proliferations (apparently of Müller cell origin) can occur in this plane of relative anoxia and thin basement membrane (see Fig. 6–96) and migrate up the walls of the fovea along the smooth surface of the thick basement membrane as the small glial cells do over posterior retina or from the optic nerve head (Fig. 12–6).

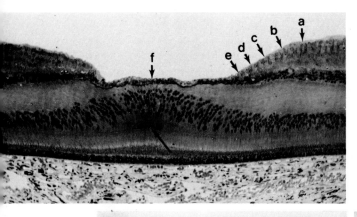

FIG. 6–91. Fovea of 18-year-old subject. Note somewhat flattened foveal floor (foveola). Outer nuclear layer is thicker and more anteriorly placed in the foveola. The connecting fibers are longer and there is a fovea externa (**arrow**). Variations of thickness of the retinal internal limiting membrane (ILM) are sampled from **a** to **f** and illustrated in the accompanying figures. (TB, × 90) (AFIP Neg. 75-13002). (**a**) Posterior pole ILM near edge of fovea. (**b**) The ILM in early foveal declivity. (**c**) The ILM midfoveal declivity. (**d**) The ILM deep in foveal declivity. (**e**) The ILM passing onto floor of fovea. Note last ganglion cell (**GC**) on right. (**f**) The ILM at center of foveal floor or foveola. (**a–f,** × 15,000)

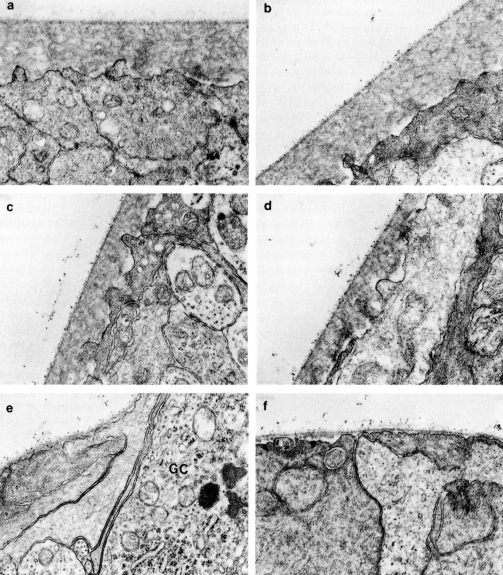

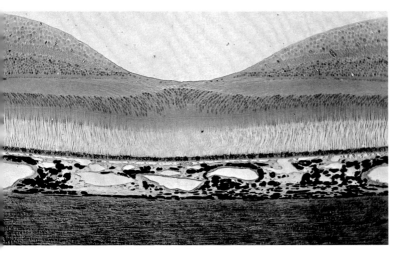

FIG. 6–92. Rhesus monkey fovea. A. Section through center of fovea. Ganglion cell layer is five to seven cell layers thick at periphery. At foveal floor all layers, except internal limiting membrane and entire length of photoreceptor cells, and their associated pigment epithelial cells, are absent. (Epon, PD, × 90) (AFIP Neg. 66-8920) B. Horizontal diameter of fovea approximates that of disc in same eye. The human fovea is more ovoid than that of the rhesus monkey.

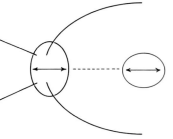

Human 1500μ diameter
(1.5mm)

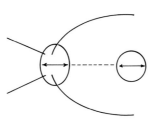

Rhesus monkey 1000μ diameter
(1.0mm)

FIG. 6–93. The foveola. A. Exact center of rhesus monkey foveola. Only internal limiting membrane (see Fig. 6–91, f), a few glial cells and processes, part of the photoreceptor cell length, and pigment epithelium remain of the thickness of the same layers elsewhere in retina. Photoreceptor nuclei (**ONL**) appear piled up, there is a slight anterior bowing of external limiting membrane ("external fovea"), and photoreceptor outer and inner segments are delicate cylinders closely packed together. Choriocapillaris here is at its greatest concentration of aperture versus area. Retinal capillary closest to fovea is seen at **arrow**. (Epon, PD, × 200) (AFIP Neg. 66-8921) B and C. Two sections through floor of rhesus foveola showing approximate center (**B**), indicated by presence of a few cross-sectioned photoreceptor axons (Henle fibers, **arrow**), and exact center (**C**), where no cross-sectioned photoreceptor axons are present (**arrow**). (Epon, PD. **B,** × 395 [AFIP Neg. 66-8923]; **C,** × 395 [AFIP Neg. 66-8922])

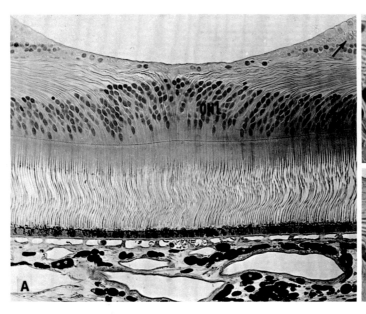

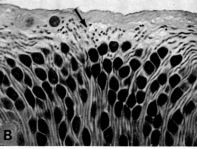

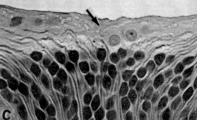

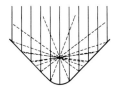 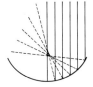 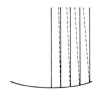

FIG. 6–94. Schematic drawing illustrating proposed mechanisms that produce the various foveal reflexes observed clinically. (Orth DH *et al.*: Trans Am Acad Ophthalmol Otolaryngol 83:OP 506, 1977)

Foveola

For practical correlation of clinical and anatomic viewpoints, the area of retina underlying the observed central foveal reflex may be designated the **foveola.**

The area of the underlying foveola can be clinically seen as much larger than the well-focused light reflex. The area generally appears as a small disc of deeper red color than the adjacent vascularized retinal layers of the fovea (see preceding discussion). It is this area that produces the relative "cherry-red spot" in such pathologic conditions as Tay-Sachs' disease, wherein the ganglion cells accumulate lipids producing a clouding of adjacent retina.

Histologically, this area would approximate that portion of the fovea that is wholly rod-free, correlating well with the physiologic property of being the area of highest visual acuity (approximately 350μ in diameter or slightly more than $1°$ of field). Histologically, the same region can be estimated by measuring the extent of the **fovea externa,** the small central region of inward bowing of the external limiting membrane of the retina, produced by the extra long cylindrical central cones or by the line of anterior displacement of the outer nuclear layer from the external limiting membrane.

Although the fovea may be defined as twice the distance from the center to the first recognizable rods, such measurements are difficult to make on histologic sections but are made with less difficulty on flat preparations. Other measurements can be made on a suitable histologic section which may provide useful criteria, *viz.,* from the last ganglion cell on one side to a similar cell on the opposite side, a similar measure in the plane of the bipolar cells or identification of a zone in which discrete photoreceptors cannot be easily visualized up to $400 \times$ to $500 \times$ magnification (Fig. 6–95). In the latter case the zone measures roughly the region of the foveolar cones and is roughly equal to the extent of the fovea externa.

The foveal terminal capillary arcade of the

FIG. 6–95. Schematic representation of histologic section through fovea of rhesus monkey. Various measurements are indicated, giving a variety of criteria for measurement of *fovea centralis* and foveola from such a preparation. ▶

retinal vasculature, a single plane of capillaries, approaches the clivus of the fovea approximately one-third of the distance between the plane of the retinal surface and the pigment epithelium (Fig. 6–96). The vasculature, therefore, falls short of the critical foveola, the retinal avascular zone measuring approximately $500–600\mu$ in diameter in the human retina.*

The lack of vasculature in the foveola is a necessary specialization to permit light to pass unobstructed into this region of highest visual acuity (102).

The foveola lacks several of the inner retinal layers (Fig. 6–91, 6–92) namely, the nerve fiber layer, the ganglion cell layer, the bipolar cell layer, and the middle limiting membrane. The retinal vasculature is also absent (Fig. 6–93, 6–96).

The ratio of cones to rods increases toward the fovea until the population becomes exclusively cones in the foveola. Although foveolar cones resemble rods superficially (Fig. 6–97, 6–98), they possess all the cytologic characteristics of cones elsewhere (Figs. 6–97 to 6–99), except for their shape. Their inner segments here, however, contain greater numbers of

* To avoid confusion between widely used clinical terminology and anatomic terminology, a simple equation has been proposed (67, 109) so that when speaking clinically, clinical terms are used, and when speaking anatomically, anatomic terms are used, *viz.,*

Anatomic	Clinical
Area centralis ("Histologic macula")	Posterior pole
Fovea centralis	Macula
Foveola	Fovea
Central (perifoveolar) capillary net and ring	Perifoveal capillary net and ring

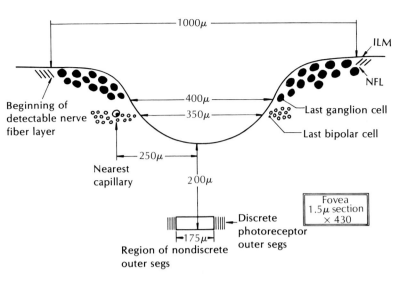

1000μ

ILM

NFL

Beginning of
detectable nerve
fiber layer

400μ

350μ

Last ganglion cell

Last bipolar cell

Nearest
capillary

250μ

200μ

175μ

Region of nondiscrete
outer segs

Fovea
1.5μ section
× 430

Discrete
photoreceptor
outer segs

FIG. 6–96. Inset shows section of central (perifoveolar) capillary ring (**double arrows**). Termination of ganglion cell layer and transition from foveal clivus to foveola is indicated by the **single arrow.** (TB, × 220) (AFIP Neg. 75-13004.) The large figure shows the central capillary, its pericytes (**P**) separated from the endothelial cells by slightly vacuolated basement membranes. The outermost basement membrane layer is covered by processes of the Müller cells. (× 18,000)

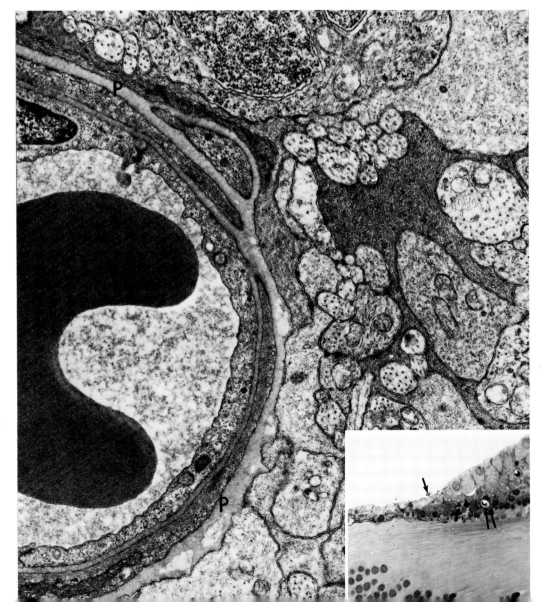

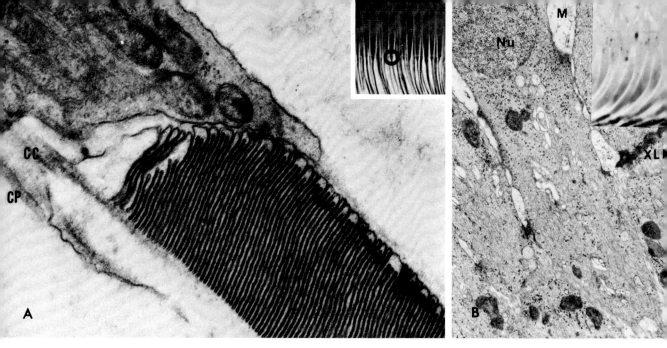

lipoidal bodies (Figs. 6–40, 6–97B). These striated lipid bodies may represent here the equivalent of oil droplets (often yellow in color) present in ellipsoids of lower animals. The outer segments are cylindrical and elongated like rods but possess lamellas that are typical of cones. The lamellas are of the "tight" or closely apposed type, with direct connections to the surface plasma membrane. Longitudinal furrows are absent. The calyces differ slightly in being elongated into villous-like extensions around the inner portion of the outer segment (Fig. 6–97, 6–98). Their synaptic expansions are all typical broad cone "feet" or pedicles containing the characteristic multiple synaptic ribbons (lamellas). The foveolar cones' relation to the pigment epithelium here resembles that of rods elsewhere (*i.e.*, they reach to the surface of the pigment cell and are enveloped by extremely delicate apical villi of the pigment epithelial cells [Fig. 6–99]).

Macula Lutea

An oval zone of yellow coloration seems to permeate most of the retinal layers in and near the fovea but is present in greatest concentration in the outer plexiform layer. The coloration is most intense along the clivus, disappearing from view in the region of the foveola, as well as peripherally toward the edge of the fovea.

FIG. 6–97. A. Junction between outer and inner segments of parafoveolar cone from rhesus monkey (**circled area** in inset). Connecting cilium (**CC**) is only slightly sectioned and calyceal processes (**CP**) are better appreciated in cross-sectional views (Fig. 6–98) (Main figure, × 29,000; inset, PD, × 300) B. Numerous lipoidal bodies are present in foveal cone inner segments. The bodies consist of linear deposits of lipid upon a striated or filamentous support (see Fig. 6–40). **M,** Müller cell; **XLM,** external limiting membrane; **Nu,** nucleus of cone cell. (Main figure, × 5400; inset, Epon PD, × 600)

FIG. 6–98. Parafoveolar receptors from rhesus monkey. A. Light micrograph. Circles **1, 2,** and **3** indicate approximately parts of photoreceptors illustrated in **B, C,** and **D.** (Epon, PD, × 300) (AFIP Neg. 66-8679) B. Oblique section of photoreceptor near its junction of inner and outer parts. Note long calyceal processes (**CP**) that extend for some distance along outer segment. (× 29,000) C. Cross-sectioned cone is characterized by its "fingerprint-like" appearance. Outer segment is ringed by long calyceal processes (**CP**). (× 17,000) D. Distal to termination of calyceal processes, long villi of pigment epithelial cells (**V**) envelop photoreceptor outer segments. Fingerprint-like outer segment cross-sections are cones; cross-sectioned outer segments with scalloped periphery are rods. Mixture of rods and cones indicates the parafoveolar location of this section. **MP,** interreceptor mucopolysaccharides. (× 17,000)

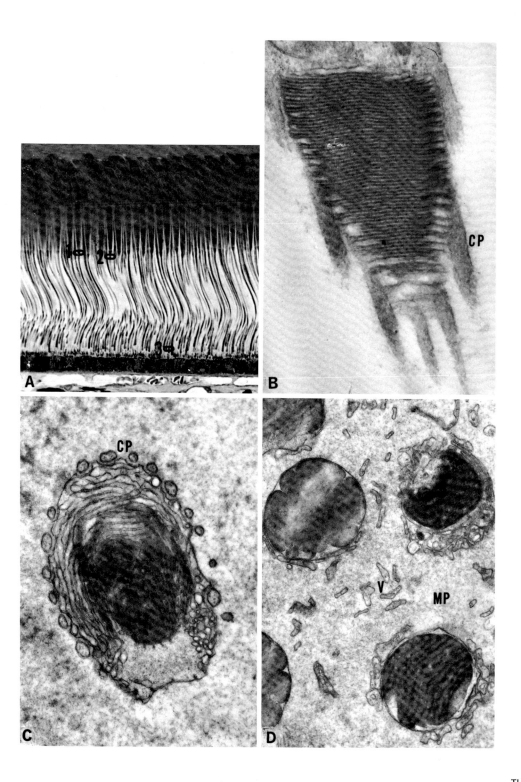

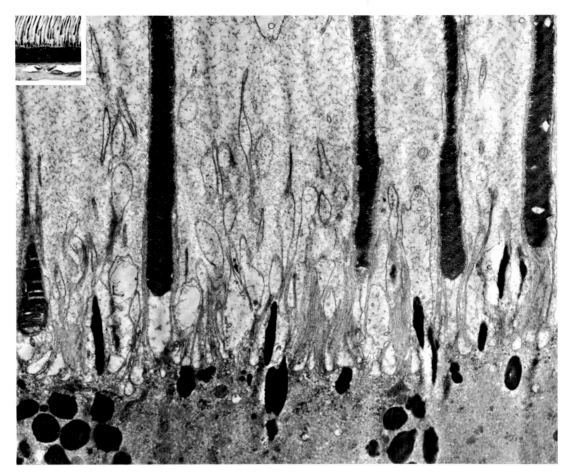

FIG. 6–99. Junction of foveolar cones with pigment epithelium. Inset is a light micrograph of junction region in rhesus monkey. (Epon, PD, × 300) (AFIP Neg. 66–8679) Main figure is an electron micrograph of similar region. Cylindrical cones make contact with many delicate villous processes of pigment epithelial cells. (× 7200)

Thus, the extent of the macula lutea falls short of the area of the fovea (~1.5 mm diameter), and the term macula is thus frequently used clinically to refer to the area of the anatomic fovea.

The context in which each term is used clinically should alert the reader to the appropriate meaning. Therefore, when *macula** is used for the

* The term **macula** when used alone, without the adjective "lutea," is a purely clinical one. The area of the posterior pole so designated has, to our knowledge, never been universally agreed upon so that it may vary in usage from clinician to clinician. Some will consider

area encompassed by the *annular reflex*, the term fovea will refer to the region underlying the foveolar reflex.

The ganglion cells in the area are somewhat smaller than elsewhere in the retina, and may reach five to seven layers in thickness at the edge of the fovea centralis (Fig. 6–91, 6–92). Two layers of ganglion cells may frequently be

the *apparent* avascular area surrounding the ophthalmoscopic foveal reflex as the macula, while others may accept an area of as much as 2–3 disc diameters of the posterior pole as the macula. Because of this broad range of imprecision, together with a current and pressing need for a uniform terminology, we have proposed that the area encircled by the ring reflex, about one disc diameter in size and sometimes known as the macular ring reflex, be used as the definition for the clinical macula. This area obviously outlines precisely the anatomic fovea. Such equation has been noted by others in the past and should provide a more useful topographic marker in addition to that of the retinal avascular zone.

present at the temporal edge of the optic disc. The cytoplasmic organelles and inclusions of the ganglion cells are identical to those elsewhere in the retina (Fig. 6–100).

The presence of two or more layers of ganglion cells temporal to the optic disc and occupying most of the region between superior and inferior temporal ascuate vessels generally defines the region of the area centralis, a region widely used and defined as the extent of the *histologic* macula (synonymous with area centralis).

The histologic macula is additionally recognized in tissue sections by the presence of the oblique and elongated Henle fibers (photoreceptor axons) in the

FIG. 6–100. Electron micrograph showing sampling of multiple ganglion cell layers. Except for being slightly smaller in size, ganglion cells appear identical to others throughout retina. **Arrows,** granular endoplasmic reticulum (Nissl body or substance); **D,** dense (?lysosome) bodies; **IPL,** inner plexiform layer; **MC,** Müller cell cytoplasmic leaflets. (× 3,700) (AFIP Neg. 61-1959) (Fine BS: Arch Ophthalmol 69:83, 1963) Inset. Light micrograph showing multiple ganglion cell layers present in parafoveal region. Note thick internal limiting membrane and nerve fiber layer. (H&E, × 350)

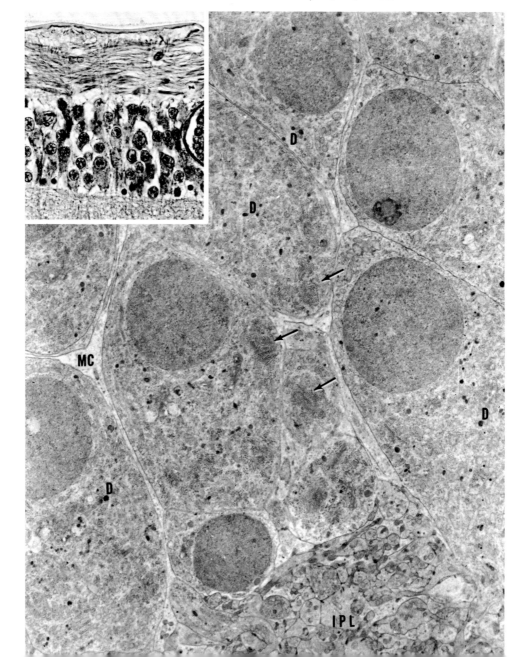

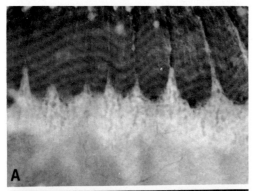

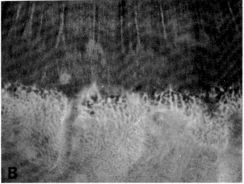

FIG. 6–101. Gross appearance of *ora serrata*. Toothlike configuration is much more prominent on nasal side of eye (**A**) than on temporal side (**B**). Cystoid changes within peripheral retina are more pronounced on temporal side.

FIG. 6–102. *Ora serrata* and anterior subretinal cul-de-sac. Sensory retina is continuous with nonpigmented ciliary epithelium (**NPE**). External limiting membrane unites with fenestrated membrane of pigment epithelium (**arrow**). Photoreceptors (**P**), mostly short malformed cones, disappear. (Epon, PD, × 485) (AFIP Neg. 70-3848)

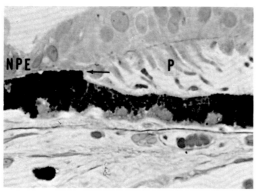

outer plexiform layer, and by the relatively high concentration of cones among the photoreceptors.

The dense cytoplasmic inclusions (31) (?lysosomes) closely resemble the dense or yellow-orange colored cytoplasmic inclusions common to neurons in the central nervous system.

The yellow substance of the macula lutea is somewhat labile as it is soluble in ether or discolored by alcohol or acetone. Additionally, in the enucleated eye the yellow color fades with time. Wald identified the substance as xanthophyll, a carotenoid. Although the substance may permeate more than one layer of the retina, the layer most prominently and likely involved is that of the Henle fibers in which no discrete pigment can be seen at the electron microscopic level. The region of the foveola may also contain some of the yellow pigment, but it is not obvious grossly and, if present, is extremely attenuated, as are the Henle fibers in this same region. The yellow pigment is most intense where the Henle fiber layer is most thick.

The yellow filter present in the fovea would account for the phenomenon of the "Haidinger brushes" by absorbing the incident blue light. The filter also would assist in improving central visual acuity by removing more of the chromatic aberration present in the human eye.

The Henle fibers (outer plexiform layer) in the foveomacula are arranged obliquely and are longer than elsewhere in the retina. They represent the axonal extensions of the photoreceptors. As elsewhere, they are enveloped by the lucent cytoplasm of the Müller cell. The oblique arrangement of the Henle fibers in the foveomacula allows greater ease of anteroposterior separation of the retinal layers in the foveomacula compared with only slight lateral separation in the more peripheral regions of the retina. Accumulations of pathologic materials (hemorrhages, exudates) therefore follow these natural tangential cleavage planes and appear to the ophthalmologist either as radiating lines ("macular stars") in the foveomacula or as more localized spherical accumulations elsewhere (focal hemorrhages or exudates). A tendency of the Müller (glial) cell to disintegrate in this region during preparation of retinal tissue for study often accentuates the cleavage planes. The lucent areas of most light microscopic preparations (*i.e.,* between the presumed eosinophilic Henle fibers [Fig. 6–23]) probably represent the interaxonal, broken-down or separated glial cytoplasm.

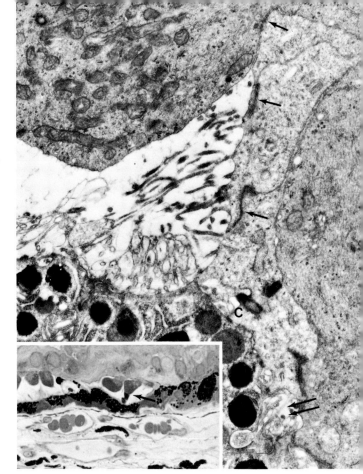

FIG. 6–103. Anterior subretinal cul-de-sac. Transmission EM, showing a bulbous cone inner segment above, joined to nearby glial cells and to pigment epithelium by apical junctional complexes (**arrows**). **C,** apical cilium; **double arrows,** villous-lined pocket between early nonpigmented ciliary epithelium above, and pigment epithelium below. (× 9000) Inset. Poorly formed cones (**arrow**) near union of external limiting membrane of retina with terminal bars of pigment epithelium. (Epon, PD, × 400) (AFIP Neg. 76-5494)

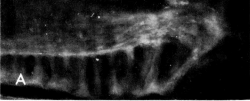

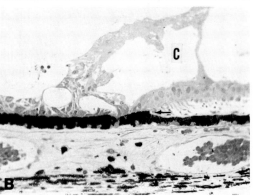

FIG. 6–104. A. Gross photo of cut edge of peripheral cystoid degeneration of retina. Note glial-neuronal columns which connect outer to inner retinal layers. B. Cystoid spaces (**C**) in peripheral retina. **Arrow,** union of external limiting membrane to pigment epithelium. (Epon, PD, × 165)

FIG. 6–105. Posterior or circumpapillary subretinal cul-de-sac of rhesus monkey. Photoreceptors terminate as a few malformed cones. External limiting membrane continues with comparable attachment girdles near free surface of pigment epithelial cells. (× 300) (AFIP Neg. 66-8674)

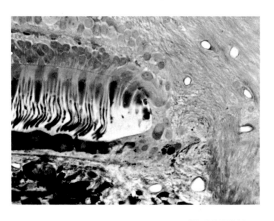

The tripartite arrangement of the Müller cell cytoplasm (see section on the Müller cell earlier in this chapter) is not nearly so pronounced in the foveomacula. Here the Müller cell cytoplasm is more uniformly lucent.

The anatomic observation that the Müller cell cytoplasm is more uniformly lucent in the foveomacula than elsewhere may be related to the well-known observation that both edema and cystoid spacing can occur as easily in both outer and inner layers in this region as they can in outer layers of the more peripheral retina.

The Subretinal Space

The subretinal space* ends blindly in two circumferential cul-de-sacs. The anterior and larger circumferential cul-de-sac occurs at the ora serrata; the smaller, posterior or circumpapillary cul-de-sac encircles the intraocular portion (i.e., retinal layer) of the optic nerve head.

Ora Serrata and Anterior Subretinal Cul-de-Sac. The peripheral neural retina thins abruptly anteriorly and becomes continuous with the nonpigmented epithelium of the ciliary body. Grossly (Fig. 6–101), the transition occurs circumferentially in a serrated fashion, the serrations, or teeth, being most prominent on the nasal side of the globe. Deep to the neural retina (Fig. 6–102), within the anterior cul-de-sac of the subretinal space, the photoreceptor outer and inner segments (mainly cones) become malformed and disappear as the external limiting membrane unites with the fenestrated membrane (terminal bars) of the pigment epithelium to form the attachments (Fig. 6–103) that continue anteriorly between the two layers of ciliary epithelium. This union produces the large circumferential anterior cul-de-sac of the subretinal space.

* Although this space lies embryonically *between* the two layers of neuroepithelium, it is convenient to continue to use the well-established clinical term of subretinal.

The strong adhesion of the nonpigmented cell layer to the pigmented cell layer prevents, except in most unusual circumstances, extension of a retinal detachment or accumulating subretinal fluids into the epithelium of the pars plana.

Within the peripheral neural retina the cells become separated by an accumulating watery material as the retina ages (Fig. 6–104). The *cystoid degeneration* of the peripheral retina is more prominent on the temporal side of the retina and is accentuated by aging or by many disease processes (109). The separation of cells within the neural retina occasionally traverses the ora serrata to appear within the adjacent nonpigmented epithelium of the ciliary body. When exaggerated, the latter fluid-filled pockets are called **cysts of the pars plana.**

Posterior Subretinal Cul-de-Sac. Posteriorly, the subretinal space ends blindly as a smaller circumferential cul-de-sac around the retinal layer of the intraocular portion of the optic nerve head (Fig. 6–105). The photoreceptor inner and outer segments cease, and the external limiting membrane of the neural retina is continuous with comparable attachment girdles (terminal bars) near the apexes of the pigment epithelial cells via terminal-bar-like attachments between a number of intervening large glial cells. This union produces the smaller, posterior or **circumpapillary cul-de-sac** of the subretinal space.

Experiments by Zauberman and Berman (115) point up the importance of the concept of an anatomically "sealed" subretinal space. From these experiments Zauberman (114) postulated that the forces which maintain apposition of the neural retina to the pigment epithelium *in vivo* may be in part related to a *negative pressure*, an explanation which we believe is the most useful concept to date and one that is well supported by the anatomic evidence. The presence of the watery interreceptor mucoid would, in all probability, serve to improve this adhesion. More recently (116), the vitality of the cell layers on either side of the subretinal space is considered to be of importance.

REFERENCES

1. Angelucci A: Histologische Untersuchungen über das retinale Pigmentepithel der Wirbelthiere. Arch Physiol (Leipzig), Physiol Abt Jahrg, 1878, p 353–386
2. Arey LB: Retina, choroid and sclera. In Cowdry EV (ed): Special Cytology, 2nd ed., vol 3. New York, Hoeber, 1932
3. Awan KJ: Anomalies of the retinal veins and their incidence. J Pediat Ophthalmol 13:353, 1976
4. Awan KJ: Arterial vascular anomalies of the retina. Arch Ophthalmol 95:1197, 1977
5. Barets A, Szabo T: Appareil synaptique des cellules sensorielles de l'ampoule de Lorenzini chez la torpille, Torpedo marmorata. J Micro 1:47:1962
6. Beams HW, Tahmisian TN, Anderson E, Devine R: Studies on the fine structure of ultracentrifuged spinal ganglion cells. J Biophys Biochem Cytol 8:793, 1960
7. Berkow JW, Kelley JS, Orth DH: Fluorescein angiography: a guide to the interpretation of fluorescein angiograms. Manual of American Academy of Ophthalmology and Otolaryngology, Rochester, MN, 1977
8. Berman ER, Bach G: The acid mucopolysaccharides of cattle retina. Biochem J 108:75, 1968
9. Breathnach AS, Wyllie LMA: Ultrastructure of retinal pigment epithelium of the human fetus. J Ultrastruct Res 16:584, 1966
10. Burnside B, Laties AM: Actin filaments in apical projections of the primate pigmented epithelial cell. Invest Ophthalmol 15:570, 1976
11. Cajal SR: Studies on Vertebrate Neurogenesis. Guth L (trans). Springfield, IL, CC Thomas, 1960
12. Cohen AI: The ultrastructure of the rods of the mouse retina. Am J Anat 107:23, 1960
13. Cohen AI: The fine structure of the extrafoveal receptors of the rhesus monkey. Exp Eye Res 1:128, 1961
14. Cohen AI: A possible cytological basis for the "R" membrane in the vertebrate eye. Nature 205:1222, 1965
15. Cohen AI: New details of the ultrastructure of the outer segments and ciliary connectives of the rods of human and macaque retinas. Anat Rec 152:63, 1965
16. Cohen AI: Some electron microscopic observations on interreceptor contacts in the human and macaque retina. J Anat 99:595, 1965
17. Cohen AI: New evidence supporting the linkage to extracellular space of outer segment saccules of frog cones but not rods. J Cell Biol 37:424, 1968
18. Cohen AI: Rods and cones and the problem of visual excitation. In Straatsma BR, Hall MO, Allen RA, Crescitelli F (eds): The Retina: Morphology, Function and Clinical Characteristics. UCLA Forum in Medical Sciences No. 8. Berkeley, University of California Press, 1969
19. Craft J, Albert DM, Reid TW: Ultrastructural description of a "cylinder organelle" in the outer plexiform layer of human retinas. Invest Ophthalmol 14:923, 1975
20. DeRobertis E: Electron microscopic observations on the submicroscopic organization of the retinal rods. J Biophys Biochem Cytol 2:319, 1956
21. DeRobertis E: Submicroscopic morphology of the synapse. Int Rev Cytol 8:61, 1959
22. DeRobertis E: Some observations on the ultrastructure and morphogenesis of photoreceptors. J Gen Physiol 43 (Suppl 1), 1960
23. DeRobertis E, Delraldi AP, Rodriguez G, Gomez CJ: On the isolation of nerve endings and synaptic vesicles. J Biophys Biochem Cytol 9:229, 1961
24. DeRobertis E, Lasansky A: Submicroscopic organization of retinal cones of the rabbit. J Biophys Biochem Cytol 4:743, 1958
25. DeRobertis E, Lasansky A: Ultrastructure and chemical organization of photoreceptors. In Smelser GK (ed): The Structure of the Eye. New York, Academic Press, 1961, p 29
26. Dowling JE: Organization of vertebrate retinas. Invest Ophthalmol 9:655, 1970
27. Dowling JE, Boycott BB: Neural connections of the primate retina. In Rohen JW (ed): The Structure of the Eye. Stuttgart, Schattauer, 1965, p 55
28. Dowling JE, Boycott BB: Organization of the primate retina: electron microscopy. Proc R Soc Lond [Biol] 166:80, 1966
29. Fernandez-Moran H: Fine structure of the light receptors in the compound eyes of insects. Exp Cell Res 5 (Suppl):586, 1958
30. Fine BS: Limiting membranes of the sensory retina and pigment epithelium: an electron microscopic study. Arch Ophthalmol 66:847, 1961
31. Fine BS: Ganglion cells in the human retina, with particular reference to the macula lutea: an electron microscopic study. Arch Ophthalmol 69:83, 1963
32. Fine BS: Synaptic lamellas in human retina: an electron microscopic study. J Neuropathol Exp Neurol 22:255, 1963
33. Fine BS: Observations on the axoplasm of neural elements in the human retina. In Titlbach M (ed): Proceedings, Third European Regional Conference on Electron Microscopy. Prague, Czechoslovak Academy of Sciences, 1964, p 319
34. Fine BS: Retinal structure: light- and electron-microscopic observations. In McPherson A (ed): New and Controversial Aspects of Retinal Detachment. New York, Hoeber, 1968, p 16
35. Fine BS, Geeraets WJ: Membranes and ground substance in photic injury to the retina. In Uyeda R (ed): Proceedings Sixth International Congress for Electron Microscopy. Kyoto, Japan, 1966, p 503
36. Fine BS, Zimmerman LE: Müller's cells and the "middle limiting membrane" of the human retina. Invest Ophthalmol 1:304, 1962
37. Fine BS, Zimmerman LE: Observations on the rod and cone layer of the human retina. Invest Ophthalmol 5:446, 1963
38. Fitzpatrick TB, Miyamoto M, Ishikawa K: The evolution of concepts of melanin biology. Arch Dermatol 96:305, 1967
39. Font RL, Zimmerman LE, Armaly MF: The nature of the orange pigment over a choroidal melanoma. Arch Ophthalmol 91:359, 1974
40. Foos RY: Vitreoretinal juncture: topographic variations. Invest Ophthalmol 11:801, 1972
41. Hsieh RC, Fine BS, Lyons JS: Patterned dystrophies

of the retinal pigment epithelium. Arch Ophthalmol 95:429, 1977

42. Hudspeth AJ, Yee AG: The intercellular junctional complexes of retinal pigment epithelia. Invest Ophthalmol 12:354, 1973

43. Ishikawa T, Pei YF: Intramitochondrial glycogen particles in rat retinal receptor cells. J Cell Biol 25:402, 1965

44. Jensen OA, Hogan MJ, Wood I: Observation of Kolmer's crystalloid outside the retina: presence in the corneal endothelium in various conditions. Acta Ophthalmol (Kbh) 53:197, 1975

45. Kelley DE: Ultrastructure and development of amphibian pineal organs. Prog Brain Res 10:270, 1965

46. Kidd M: Electron microscopy of the inner plexiform layer of the retina in the cat and the pigeon, J Anat 96:2, 1962

47. Kolmer W: Uber Kristalloïden in Nervenzellen der Menschlichen Netzhaut. Anat Anz 51:314, 1918

48. Kuwabara T: Microtubules in the retina. In Rohen JW (ed): The Structure of the Eye. Stuttgart, Schattauer, 1965, p 69

49. Kuwabara T: Cytologic changes of the retina and pigment epithelium during hibernation. Invest Ophthalmol 14:457, 1975

50. Kuwabara T, Cogan DG: Retinal glycogen. Arch Ophthalmol 66:680, 1961

51. Kuwabara T, Cogan D: Retinal vascular patterns. VI. Mural cells of retinal capillaries. Arch Ophthalmol 69:492, 1963

52. Ladman AJ: The fine structure of the rod-bipolar cell synapse in the retina of the albino rat. J Biophys Biochem Cytol 4:459, 1958

53. Lasansky A: Cell junctions at the outer synaptic layer of the retina. Invest Ophthalmol 11:265, 1972

54. Lord BAP, DiBona DR: Role of the septate junction in the regulation of paracellular transepithelial flow. J Cell Biol 71:967, 1976

55. Mann I: The Development of the Human Eye, 3rd ed. New York, Grune & Stratton, 1969

56. Missotten ML: Étude des batonnets de la rétine humaine au microscope élèctronique. Ophthalmologica 140:200, 1960

57. Missotten ML: Étude des synapses de la rétine humaine au microscope élèctronique. In Houwink AL, Spit BJ (eds): Proceedings European Regional Conference on Electron Microscopy. Delft, Nederlandse Vereniging voor Electronenmicroscopie, 1960

58. Missotten ML: L'ultra-structure des cellules horizontales externes de la rétine humaine. Bull Soc Belge Ophthalmol 128:207, 1961

59. Missotten ML: Étude des capillaires de la rétine et de la choriocapillaire au microscope élèctronique. Ophthalmologica 144:1, 1962

60. Missotten ML: The synapses in the human retina. In Rohen JW (ed): The Structure of the Eye. Stuttgart, Schattauer, 1965, p 17

61. Missotten ML: The Ultrastructure of the Human Retina. Arsica Uitgaven, Brussels, 1965

62. Missotten ML, Van Den Dooren E: L'ultrastructure de la rétine humaine les contacts lateraux des pedoncules des cone de la fovea. Bull Soc Belge Ophthalmol 144:800, 1966

63. Moyer FH: Genetic effects on melanosome fine structure and ontogeny in normal and malignant cells. Ann NY Acad Sci 100:584, 1963

64. Mund ML, Rodrigues MM, Fine BS: Light and electron microscopic observations on the pigmented layers of the developing human eye. Am J Ophthalmol 73:168, 1972

65. Nicholls JG, Kuffler SW: Extracellular space as a pathway for exchange between blood and neurons in the central nervous system of the leech: ionic composition of glial cells and neurons. J Neurophysiol 27:645, 1964

66. Nilsson SEG: Receptor cell outer segment development and ultrastructure of the disc membranes in the retina of the tadpole. J Ultrastruct Res 11:581, 1964

67. Orth DH, Fine BS, Fagman W, Quirk TC: Clarification of foveomacular nomenclature and grid for quantitation of macular disorders. Trans Am Acad Ophthalmol Otolaryngol 83: 1977, p OP506–OP514

68. Parsons H: The Pathology of the Eye, vol 2. Histology, part I. London, Hodder, 1905, p 445

69. Peyman GA, Bok D: Peroxidase diffusion in the normal and laser-coagulated primate retina. Invest Ophthalmol 11:35, 1972

70. Peyman GA, Spitznas M, Straatsma BR: Peroxidase diffusion in the normal and photocoagulated retina. Invest Ophthalmol 10:181, 1971

71. Polyak SL: The Vertebrate Visual System. Chicago, University of Chicago Press, 1957

72. Porter KR, Yamada E: Studies on the endoplasmic reticulum. V. Its form and differentiation in pigment epithelial cells of the frog retina. J Biophys Biochem Cytol 8:181, 1960

73. Ramsey HJ: Ultrastructure of corpora amylacea. J Neuropathol Exp Neurol 24:25, 1965

74. Raviola E: Intercellular junctions in the outer plexiform layer of the retina. Invest Ophthalmol 15:881, 1976

75. Raviola E, Gilula NB: Intra membrane organization of specialized contacts in the outer plexiform layer of the retina. J Cell Biol 65:192, 1975

76. Raviola G, Raviola E: Light and electron microscopic observations on the inner plexiform layer of the rabbit retina. Am J Anat 120:403, 1967

77. Robison WG Jr, Kuwabara T: Microperoxisomes in retinal pigment epithelium. Invest Ophthalmol 14: 866, 1975

78. Rosenbluth J: Ultrastructure of dyads in muscle fibers of Ascaris lumbricoides. J Cell Biol 42:817, 1969

79. Salzmann M: The Anatomy and Histology of the Human Eyeball in the Normal State: Its Development and Senescence. Brown EVL (trans). Chicago, University of Chicago Press, 1912

80. Scheie HG, Albert DM: Adler's Textbook of Ophthalmology, 9th ed. Philadelphia, WB Saunders, 1977

81. Schieck-Würzburg F: Netzhaut-normale anatomie. In Henke F, Lubarsch O (eds): Handbuch der Speziellen Pathologischen Anatomie und Histologie. Berlin, Verlag von Julius Springer, 1928, p 578

82. Seiji M: Formation of mammalian melanin. Jpn J Dermatol 73:4, 1963

83. Shakib M, Cunha-Vaz JG: Studies on the permeability of the blood-retinal barrier. IV. Junctional complexes of the retinal vessels and their role in

the permeability of the blood-retinal barrier. Exp Eye Res 5:229, 1966

84. Sherrington C: The Integrative Action of the Nervous System. New Haven, Yale University Press, 1961, p 17

85. Sjöstrand FS: The ultrastructure of the outer segments of rods and cones of the eye as revealed by the electron microscope. J Cell Physiol 42:15, 1953

86. Sjöstrand FS: Ultrastructure of retinal rod synapses of the guinea pig eye as revealed by three dimensional reconstruction from serial sections. J Ultrastruct Res 2:122, 1958

87. Sjöstrand FS: The ultrastructure of the retinal receptors of the vertebrate eye. Ergeb Biol 21:128, 1959

88. Sjöstrand FS: Electron microscopy of the retina. In Smelser GK (ed): The Structure of the Eye. New York, Academic Press, 1961, p 1

89. Smelser GK, Ishikawa T, Pei YF: Electron microscopic studies of intraretinal spaces: diffusion of particulate materials. In Rohen JW (ed): The Structure of the Eye. Stuttgart, Schattauer, 1965, p 109

90. Smelser GK, Ozanics V, Rayborn M, Sagun D: Retinal synaptogenesis in the primate. Invest Ophthalmol 13:340, 1974

91. Smith C, Sjöstrand FS: A synaptic structure in the hair cells of the guinea pig cochlea. J Ultrastruct Res 5:184, 1961

92. Spira AW, Hollenberg MJ: Human retinal development: ultrastructure of the inner retinal layers. Dev Biol 31:1, 1973

93. Spitznas M, Hogan MJ: Outer segments of photoreceptors and the retinal pigment epithelium: interrelationship in the human eye. Arch Ophthalmol 84:810, 1970

94. Spitznas M, Reale E: Fracture faces of fenestrations and junctions of endothelial cells in human choroidal vessels. Invest Ophthalmol 14:98, 1975

95. Steinberg RH, Wood I, Hogan MJ: Pigment epithelial ensheathment and phagocytosis of extrafoveal cones in human retina. Philos Trans R Soc Lond [Biol] 277:459, 1977

96. Takei Y, Ozanics V: Origin and development of Bruch's membrane in monkey fetuses: an electron microscopic study. Invest Ophthalmol 14:903, 1975

97. Ts'o MOM, Fine BS, Zimmerman LE: The nature of retinoblastoma. II. Photoreceptor differentiation: an electron microscopic study. Am J Ophthalmol 69:350, 1970

98. Uga S, Ikui H: Crystal bodies in the outer plexiform layer of the human retina. Jpn J Electron Microscopy 19:278, 1970

99. Virchow R: Cellular Pathology. Chance F (trans). Philadelphia, JB Lippincott, 1863. Reprinted Dover Publications, New York, 1971, p 268

100. Wallow IHL, Fine BS, Tso MOM: Morphologic changes in photoreceptor outer segments following photic injury. Ophthalmol Res 5:10, 1973

101. Walls GL: The Vertebrate Eye and Its Adaptive Radiation. Bloomfield, MI, Cranbrook Institute of Science, 1942. Reprinted Hafner Publishing Co, New York, 1963

102. Weale RA: Fovea in human retina: theory for existence. Nature 212:255, 1966

103. Williams MC, Wissig SL: The permeability of muscle capillaries to horseradish peroxidase. J Cell Biol 66:531, 1975

104. Yamada E: Observations on the fine structure of photoreceptive elements in the vertebrate eye. J Electron Micr (Chiba) 9:1, 1960

105. Yamada E: Some structural features of the fovea centralis in the human retina. Arch Ophthalmol 82:151, 1969

106. Yamada E, Tokuyasu K, Iwaki S: The fine structure of retina studied with electron microscope. II. Pigment epithelium and capillary of the choriocapillary layer. J Electron Micro (Chiba) 6:42, 1958

107. Yamada E, Tokuyasu K, Iwaki S: The fine structure of retina studied with electron microscope. III. Human retina. J Kurume Med Assoc 21:1979, 1959

108. Yanoff M: Diabetic retinopathy. N Engl J Med 274:1344, 1966

109. Yanoff M, Fine BS: Ocular Pathology: A Text and Atlas. Hagerstown, Harper & Row, 1975

110. Yoshida M: The fine structure of the so-called crystalloid body of the human retina as observed with the electron microscope. Jpn J Electron Microsc 14:285, 1965

111. Young RW: Visual cells and the concept of renewal. Invest Ophthalmol 15:700, 1976

112. Young RW, Bok D: Participation of the retinal pigment epithelium in the rod outer segment renewal process. J Cell Biol 42:392, 1969

113. Young RW, Bok D: Autoradiographic studies on the metabolism of the retinal pigment epithelium. Invest Ophthalmol 9:524, 1970

114. Zauberman H: Personal communication, 1970

115. Zauberman H, Berman ER: Measurement of adhesive forces between the sensory retina and the pigment epithelium. Exp Eye Res 8:276, 1969

116. Zauberman H, DeGuillebon H: Retinal traction in vivo and postmortem. Arch Ophthalmol 87:549, 1972

117. Zimmerman LE, Eastham AB: Acid mucopolysaccharide in the retinal pigment epithelium and visual cell layer of developing mouse eye. Am J Ophthalmol 47:488, 1959

chapter 7

THE VITREOUS BODY

EMBRYOLOGY   131
COMPONENTS   131
  FIBROUS COMPONENT   132
  MUCINOUS COMPONENT   134
BOUNDARIES   134
ATTACHMENTS   134
  POSTERIOR ATTACHMENTS   134
  LATERAL ATTACHMENTS   138
  ANTERIOR ATTACHMENTS   138
ZONES   140
MODIFICATIONS   141

The vitreous body is an example of a tissue composed predominantly of extracellular materials. It completely fills the large posterior (vitreous) compartment of the eye (Fig. 7–1). The vitreous body thus accounts for most of the volume of the eye (Fig. 7–2); it is a very delicate transparent connective tissue—probably the most delicate of all the connective tissues in the body.

EMBRYOLOGY

The vitreous body develops in three stages (1, 11). In the first stage the cavity of the optic cup is filled with a mass of ectodermal and mesodermal filaments from which the primary vitreous forms. The ectodermal components originate mostly from the cells of the retina, and the mesodermal elements, including the hyaloid vessels, enter into the vitreous space through the fetal fissure inferiorly. The primary vitreous is thus vascularized by the hyaloid vascular system.

In the second stage, which occurs after the embryo reaches a size of 13 mm, new vitreous (secondary vitreous) is formed by the cells of the inner layer of the optic cup when the hyaloid vascular channels in the primary vitreous stop growing and begin to atrophy. Eventually the secondary vitreous surrounds the primary vitreous, which then becomes limited to a cone-shaped region running through the vitreous compartment (see Fig. 7–7). Because the primary and secondary vitreous bodies differ in optical density, a line of demarcation (the wall of Cloquet's canal) can be detected at their interface. The hyaloid artery courses within Cloquet's canal to supply the vascular network surrounding the lens.

In the third stage, the tertiary vitreous or zonular fibers develop. This begins at about the 65-mm stage, when the primitive nonpigmented ciliary epithelium is in contact with the

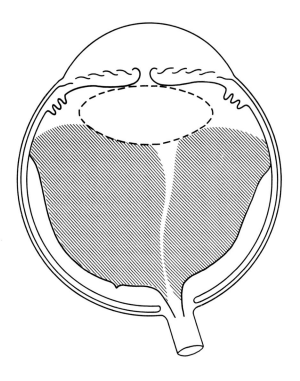

FIG. 7–1. Schematic drawing of vitreous body (shaded area) occupying larger or posterior compartment of the eye (vitreous compartment).

lens capsule (see Fig. 8–4). As the eye grows anteriorly, the epithelium is displaced posteriorly, "spinning out" the vitreous-like collagen of the zonular fibers until, by the 110-mm stage, they are well visualized.

COMPONENTS

The vitreous body is readily separable into two component parts: the *fibrous* (5, 7–9, 13, 14) and the *mucinous* (12, 19). Each part is most easily observed by mechanical separation of the

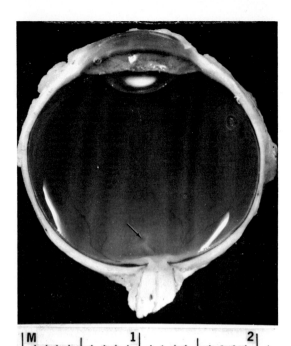

FIG. 7–2. Gross appearance of vitreous body. This delicate, transparent tissue occupies most of the volume of eye, extending from back of lens anteriorly to retinal surface posteriorly. Major temporal vessels of retina can be seen below, encircling slightly edematous fovea (macula), characteristic of fixed opened eyes. Foveola (**arrow**) lies in center of fovea. (AFIP Neg. 66-257-4)

FIG. 7–3. Filaments isolated by mechanical separation from rhesus monkey vitreous body. White, irregular-shaped particles represent debris. (U-shad, × 15,000)

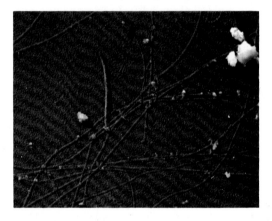

components and subsequent examination by electron microscopy.

FIBROUS COMPONENT

The fibrous component (Fig. 7–3) is composed of a delicate (~150–200 A diameter) *filament* with an apparent periodicity (~220 A) (5). In aggregates, these filaments form the substructure for the small and large sheetlike arrangements (5, 7) that, in total, make up the structural framework of the vitreous body (Fig. 7–4, 7–5). The filaments appear morphologically alike, whether in the anterior or posterior vitreous (5), and closely resemble, in both diameter and periodicity, the delicate filaments observed commonly in fetal tissues and in young cultures of fibroblasts (16). By chemical assay, this structural material (14, 15) has been shown to contain a significant amount of hydroxyproline. The foregoing criteria identify the filaments as a **collagen.**

The somewhat peculiar delicacy of this structural collagenous framework in the adult eye has stimulated much controversy regarding its true nature. If one considers that, for all practical purposes, the filamentous material is produced in the eye mainly during its growth period (2), the "fetal" or infantile

appearance of the filaments is not surprising. "Formed vitreous" (*i.e.,* that which possesses a modicum of rigidity or a clinically detectable structure) has long been known clinically never to reform in the mature eye to any significant degree, once it has been removed or lost from the eye. When the producing neuroepithelial cells have matured, they gradually (and perhaps even sequentially) lose their ability to elaborate collagen (2), but they may be called upon later to synthesize the delicate filaments, as well as mucopolysaccharides, in various pathologic processes (18).

The structural or fibrillar component of the vitreous body once was called the **residual protein.** The names **vitrein** (7, 9) or **vitrosin** (8) also have been suggested for this structural protein, but it is classified currently as a type II collagen (17) (see Ch. 4). More recently, an insoluble structural glycoprotein has been observed to be part of the composition of both lens capsule and zonules (3), and closely related to an insoluble glycoprotein that can be extracted from the vitreous body after degradation of the hyaluronic acid.

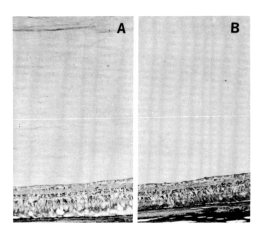

FIG. 7–4. Chemical composition of vitreous body. A. In untreated tissue, colloidal iron stains acid mucopolysaccharides. B. No staining occurs when tissue is first treated with hyaluronidase. Vitreous body contains hyaluronic acid. (Colloidal iron stain with and without hyaluronidase, × 70) (AFIP Neg. 57-1284)

FIG. 7–5. Posterior vitreous body. Shadow-cast section showing interweaving of filaments of uniform dimension to form sheetlike arrangement. (U-shad, × 20,000) (Fine BS, Tousimis AJ: Arch Ophthalmol 65:95, 1961) Inset 1. Filaments at high magnification, which emphasizes their apparent periodicity. (× 47,400) Inset 2. Similar filaments in thin section with "fluffy" adherent material representing mucinous component of vitreous, better observed as drying patterns in shadow-cast material (inset 3). (Inset 2, × 33,000; Inset 3, U-shad, × 20,000)

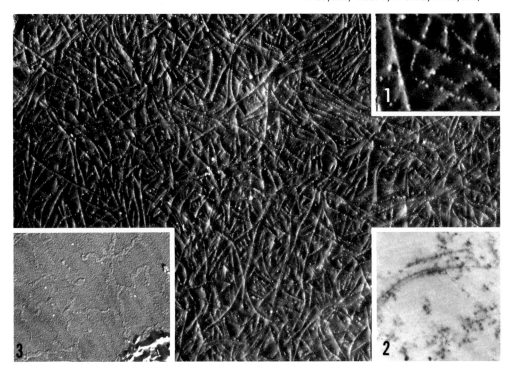

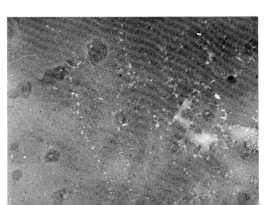

FIG. 7–6. Drying patterns of vitreous supernatant, mechanically separated from fibrous component illustrated in Figure 7–3. Drying patterns represent acid mucopolysaccharides and are similar to patterns observed in shadow-cast tissue sections (inset 3, Fig. 7–5). (U-shad, × 14,000)

MUCINOUS COMPONENT

The mucinous component, accounting for by far the larger volume of the vitreous body, can be observed morphologically by either light or electron microscopy (Fig. 7–4 through 7–6). In thin-section electron micrographs, this mucinous material can be observed as a rather "fluffy" debris, irregularly adherent to the filaments of the vitreous framework (*inset 2*, Fig. 7–5). In shadow-cast preparations of either the mechanically separated components (Fig. 7–6) or the relatively *in-situ* components of tissue sections (*inset 3*, Fig. 7–5), the mucinous material appears as flattened, irregularly distributed macromolecules ("drying patterns") of a nonfibrous material, from which the water and various ions have been removed.

BOUNDARIES

The vitreous body is bounded posteriorly by the internal surface of the retina (internal limiting membrane), axially by the surface condensations that extend in tubular fashion from the periphery of the optic disc to the posterior surface of the lens (canal of Cloquet), laterally at the ora serrata by the internal limiting membrane of the retina and of the posterior pars plana, and anteriorly by the posterior surface of the lens (Fig. 7–7). The depression formed by the posterior surface of the lens is called the **patellar fossa.**

ATTACHMENTS

POSTERIOR ATTACHMENTS

The vitreous framework is rather uniformly and tenuously attached to the thick basement membrane of the posterior retina (Fig. 7–8, 7–9) except for stronger attachments in the regions of the optic nerve head, the equator, the ora serrata, over some regions of the larger retinal vessels, and probably in the fovea centralis.

The delicate attachment along the internal limiting membrane of the posterior retina is easily disrupted. This ease of separation is accounted for by two electron microscopic observations: 1) The number of filamentous attachments per unit area of basement membrane is rather low in comparison with regions of known stronger attachment, and 2) the internal surface of the posterior retinal basement membrane is smooth, whereas the surface near the ora serrata is multilaminar (see Fig. 7–18).

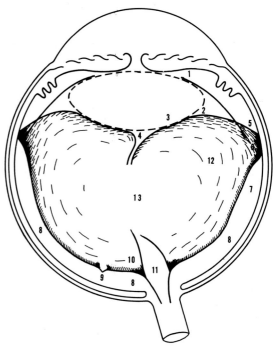

FIG. 7–7. Schematic outline of major vitreous body attachments and relations: attachment of orbiculo-anterior zonular fibers to lens (**1**); attachment of orbiculoposterior zonular fibers to lens (**2**); attachment of anterior vitreous face to posterior lens capsule (**3**); anterior extremity of canal of Cloquet (**4**); anteriormost attachment of vitreous base to mid pars plana (origin of vitreous face) (**5**); region of vitreous "base" (**6**); region of diminishing adherence of vitreous base to retinal surface (**7**); vitreous-retinal attachments (**8**); vitreous-retinal attachment in fovea centralis (**9**); attachment of posterior vitreous around optic disc, (**10**); posterior extremity of canal of Cloquet (area Martegiani) (**11**); cortical vitreous (**12**); and central vitreous (**13**). Density of lines indicates approximate relative degrees of strength of attachment.

The filaments in the preretinal or *cortical* zone of the vitreous body are arranged in aggregates (Fig. 7–10) that interconnect in a somewhat honeycomb arrangement. These delicate sheetlike aggregations, observed by electron microscopy, lie beyond the resolution of biomicroscopic examination.

The sample micrographs of vitreous structure used for illustrative purposes here are to be understood as just samples in time as well as in location

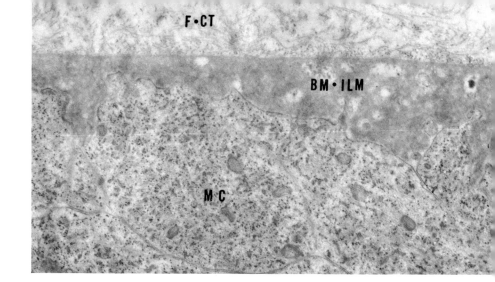

FIG. 7–8. Delicate vitreous filaments (**F·CT**) attached to smooth inner surface of thick basement membrane of posterior retina (**BM·ILM**). **MC,** Müller cell. (× 16,000)

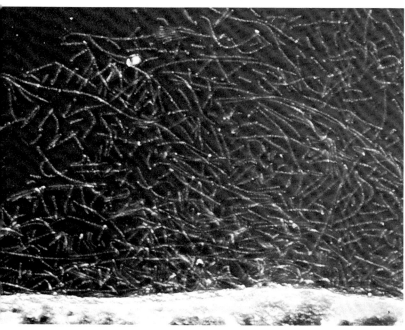

FIG. 7–9. Shadow-cast section of tissue similar to that seen in thin section in Figure 7–8. Vitreous filaments stand out clearly, but retinal detail is lost. (× 22,500)

FIG. 7–10. Shadow-cast section showing vitreous filaments forming exceedingly delicate aggregates near posterior retinal surface. Drying patterns (**arrows**) of mucinous part of vitreous body are clearly seen between filamentous aggregates. **ILM,** internal limiting membrane of retina. (U-shad, × 13,200)

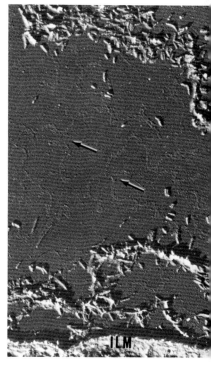

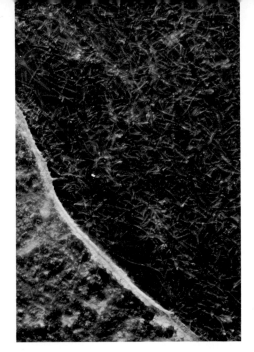

FIG. 7–11. Shadow-cast section of posterior vitreous near retinal surface. Filaments are numerous and in this minute sample do not appear aggregated. (U-shad, × 11,000) (Fine BS: In McPherson A (ed): New and Controversial Aspects of Retinal Detachment. New York, Hoeber, 1968)

FIG. 7–12. Cortical vitreous of infant eye. Note laminated (*i.e.,* aggregated) appearance near retinal surface (**arrow**) and irregularly arranged (*i.e.,* less aggregated) appearance toward central region. (Wilder reticulum stain, × 115) (AFIP Neg. 60-4411)

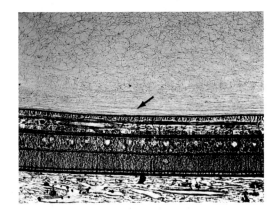

(Fig. 7–11). The vitreous body framework continually changes its arrangement throughout life,* beginning in infancy as a rather diffuse structure (*diminished relucency*), in which there are only small aggregations in the peripheral cortex (Fig. 7–12). As with collagen elsewhere, the tendency is for larger "sheets" of filaments or fibrils eventually to form (Fig. 7–13). The largest can be observed, especially anteriorly, by clinical methods. Further aggregation of collagen in connective tissue produces collapse of the "sheets" into "bands" or "strands," because aggregation of collagen with aging is associated with shrinkage or contraction. Retraction of the vitreous framework, particularly from its loose attachment to the posterior retinal surface, produces a new boundary—the newly formed "posterior hyaloid," which is detectable both clinically and histologically (Fig. 7–14). Spaces are formed between the hyaloid membrane (condensed vitreous framework, Figure 7–15) and the internal limiting membrane of the retina (Fig. 7–16). The spaces are occupied by the watery mucinous component of the vitreous body. When the vitreous body contracts (posterior vitreous detachment), if the component is more watery than mucinous, it can pass through the hyaloid membrane directly. If it is more mucinous, however, a break in the hyaloid membrane is presumed. When the vitreous framework contracts, any vitreoretinal adhesion can cause retinal tears. Both the retinal

FIG. 7–13. Scanning electron micrograph of sheet of vitreous. **ILM,** internal limiting membrane of retina (× 650) Inset. Higher power SEM of the edge of the "sheet" (× 13,000)

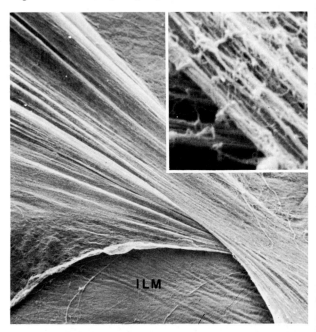

* Although the vitreous body may vary considerably *between* individuals, the lamellar structures differ very little between the two eyes of a single person if there has been no pathologic interference.

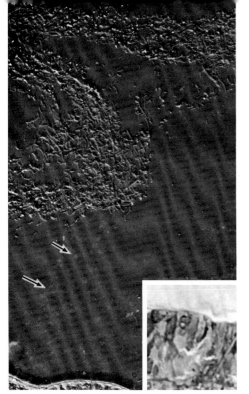

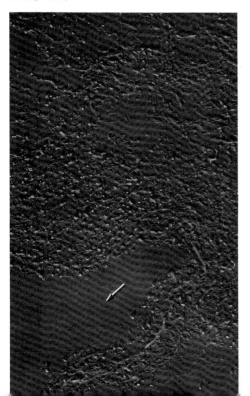

FIG. 7–14. Artifactitiously retracted posterior vitreous. Electron micrograph shows retinal surface below and retracted vitreous framework above. Newly formed posterior boundary consists of aggregated vitreous filaments. Drying patterns (**arrows**) of mucinous component are present between retracted vitreous framework and retinal surface. (× 6900) (Fine BS, Tousimis AJ: Arch Ophthalmol 65:95, 1961) Inset is light micrograph of similar area. (PAS, × 575) (AFIP Neg. 60-961) (Fine BS: In McPherson A (ed): New and Controversial Aspects of Retinal Detachment. New York, Hoeber, 1968)

FIG. 7–15. Posterior boundary ("posterior hyaloid") of retracted vitreous framework further removed from retinal surface but adjacent to section shown in Figure 7–14. Arrow points to subvitreal space. (× 7900) (Fine BS, Tousimis AJ: Arch Ophthalmol 65:95, 1961)

basement membrane (internal limiting membrane) and the retracted vitreous framework ("posterior hyaloid") stain equally with eosin or with the PAS technique, a situation which may cause some confusion in interpretation (18). If two smooth layers are present, one in continuity with the retina, the inner one is the posterior hyaloid (*inset A*, Fig. 7–16). Separation of the internal limiting membrane is generally accompanied by tags or footplates of Müller cells, which can be observed attached to the outer surface of the retinal internal limiting membrane (*inset B*, Fig. 7–16). By electron microscopy (Fig. 7–16) the distinction is easily made.

The vitreous framework has a firm attachment to the basement membrane at the edge of the optic nerve head (or disc). Where the thick basement membrane of the retina thins over the nerve head, the vitreous face turns anteriorly to form the lining walls of the canal of Cloquet. The floor of the canal is called the *area Martegiani* and is lined by a thin basement membrane covering the astrocytic glia of the nerve head (internal glial limiting membrane and central supporting tissue meniscus, see Ch. 12 and Fig. 12–4).

Retraction and separation of posterior vitreous body from the region of the nerve head often is accompanied by tearing of the glial tissue from around the optic disc to such a degree that the suspended ring of separated material is sometimes referred to clinically as the vitreous "peephole," a most appropriate term when the ring is complete.

Temporal to the optic disc, in the region of the fovea centralis, the vitreous framework has an attachment to the basement membrane that is slightly stronger than elsewhere over the posterior retina. Where the foveal declivity begins, the basement membrane changes gradually from thick to thin (Fig. 6–91). The floor of the fovea is lined by thin basement membrane (Fig. 6–91 f), and there is a paucity of vitreous filaments here. There is a transition of basement membrane from thick to thin along the clivus, such that the surface anatomic relations are somewhat analogous to those described for the nerve head. Thus a slightly firmer attachment of vitreous to retina should occur somewhere between Fig. 6–91d and Fig. 6–91e.

LATERAL ATTACHMENTS

The vitreous framework is condensed into sheets (5, 7), forming a somewhat compressed honeycomb arrangement in the cortical zone (Fig. 7–17). The sheets are coarse in contrast to the extremely delicate ones over the posterior retinal surface.

FIG. 7–16. Electron micrograph showing detached thick internal limiting membrane (**ILM**) of posterior retina and a few fragments of adhering Müller cells (**MC**). (× 11,000) Inset A. Two PAS-positive membranes near inner surface of retina. Posterior hyaloid (**HY**) is smoother and inner of the two. (PAS, × 530) (AFIP Neg. 70-3850) Inset B. Detached PAS-positive internal limiting membrane with a few outer irregularities (**arrows**) to which fragments of Müller cells frequently remain adherent. (PAS, × 270) (AFIP Neg. 67-4572)

An attachment zone of increasing strength begins at the inner surface of the peripheral retina a few millimeters behind the ora serrata. It extends anteriorly across the ora serrata and along the free surface of the ciliary nonpigmented epithelial cells, and ceases rather abruptly in the mid pars plana of the ciliary body. The zone of strong attachment is called the **base** of the vitreous body. Three structural modifications occur in this region that account for this strong attachment (Fig. 7–18): 1) The basement membrane (internal limiting membrane) becomes multilaminar and only a thin layer is applied to the basal plasmalemmas of the surface cells; 2) the basilar surfaces of the cells project into the multilaminar basement membrane and are interwoven with it; 3) large aggregates of vitreous framework filaments also are interwoven with this multilaminar basement membrane. This interweaving of the three structures is most pronounced over the region of the posterior pars plana.

ANTERIOR ATTACHMENTS

Approximately midway along the surface of the pars plana, the now condensed vitreous framework separates from the nonpigmented epithelial cells as a free surface, the face of the vitreous body (Fig. 7–19). Histologically, the

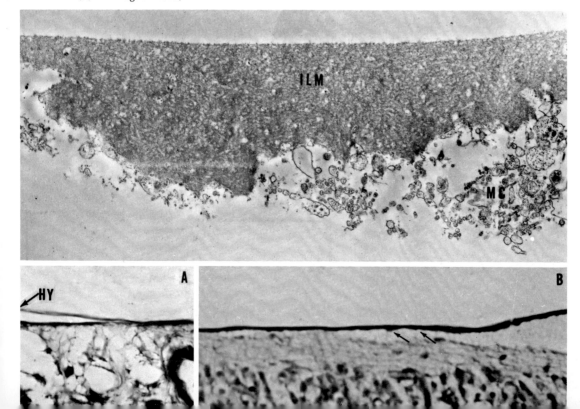

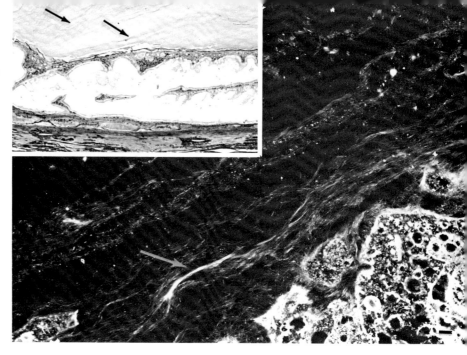

FIG. 7–17. Vitreous framework over region of *ora serrata*. Light micrograph (**inset**) shows condensation of framework into numerous sheets (**arrows**). (Wilder reticulum stain, × 70) (AFIP Neg. 60-1425) (Modified from Fine BS, Tousimis AJ: Arch Ophthalmol 65:95, 1961) Electron micrograph from similar region shows configuration produced by dense aggregates of vitreous filaments. Arrow points to a more than usually dense aggregate, which may represent a fragment of zonule. **N,** nucleus of nonpigmented epithelial cell pars plana. (× 3,440)

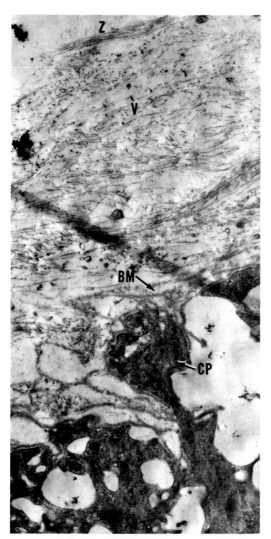

FIG. 7–18. Base of vitreous body in region of ora serrata. **BM,** multilaminar basement membrane; **CP,** cell processes; **V,** vitreous filaments; **Z,** fragment of zonular fiber. (× 8,000) (Fine BS, Zimmerman LE: Invest Ophthalmol 2:105, 1963)

FIG. 7–19. Anterior vitreous face (**arrows**) free of anterior pars plana epithelium. Fragments of zonular fibers lie within posterior chamber. (H&E, × 80) (AFIP Neg. 62-5292)

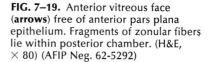

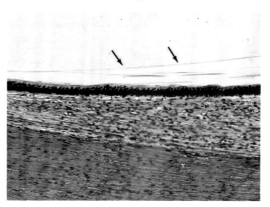

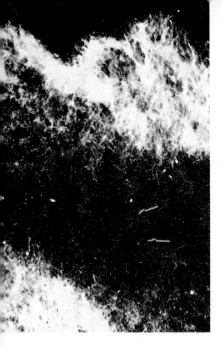

FIG. 7–20. Anterior face ("hyaloid") of vitreous body. Filament density is too great in some regions of this section to permit their individual resolution. When filaments are in lower concentration (arrows) they can be individually observed (see Fig. 7–21). (U-shad, × 2500)

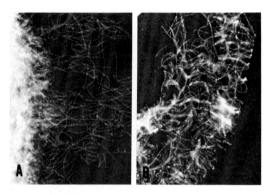

FIG. 7–21. Anterior face of vitreous body. A. Filaments are spread out on right; on left, aggregate of filaments is too dense to permit resolution of individual filaments. (U-shad, × 11,000) B. A thin "sheet" of vitreous framework is turned flat to show its filamentous composition. The two cut edges of sheet-like fragment are clearly seen. (U-shad, × 11,500)

anteriormost zone of condensed vitreous framework represents the **anterior border layer,** which is also called the **anterior hyaloid** of the vitreous body when observed clinically. The anterior border layer is composed of filaments (Fig. 7–20, 7–21) identical to those of the posterior vitreous framework and demarcates the posterior boundary of the posterior aqueous chamber. The layer attaches to the posterior lens capsule in the form of a ring ("Egger's line") ~9 mm in diameter. The strong attachment along this ring is often called the hyaloideocapsular ligament or **ligament of Wieger.** Axially, the vitreous continues more loosely attached to the posterior lens capsule until the vitreous face separates from the capsule (thick basement membrane) and turns posteriorly to form the lining border layer of the conical anterior extremity of the canal of Cloquet. A remnant of the embryonic hyaloid system may be seen on the posterior lens capsule just nasal to the visual axis and within the anterior mouth of the canal. This embryonic remnant is called the **Mittendorf dot.**

As with the posterior vitreous, the anterior vitreous face cannot be visualized optically as a distinct entity until it becomes separated from the lens capsule (i.e., detachment of the anterior hyaloid). The optically empty zone observed clinically behind the lens (except for the opening to the canal of Cloquet) in a normal eye therefore represents a zone *deep* to the vitreous face, i.e., *within* the anterior

vitreous body. This dark zone often is presumably misinterpreted as the *retrolental space of Berger*, a potential space lying between the posterior lens capsule and the vitreous face, which can be demonstrated by the injection of air between the two loosely adherent structures.

The canal of Cloquet can often be recognized *in vivo* and occasionally is seen to be occupied considerably or partially by a blood-filled vessel loop from the nerve head representing persistence of hyaloid vasculature. Less often, a small hemorrhage may be observed which may track along the canal so that it is even more clearly demarcated from adjacent, yet clear, vitreous.

ZONES

In the adult eye the vitreous body generally is divided into a condensed interweaving lamellar peripheral zone, the **cortical vitreous,** and a looser central zone, the central or medullary vitreous. The surfaces are further modified into the dense anterior border layer and the somewhat less dense boundary of the canal of Cloquet.

As mentioned previously, the loose arrangement present in fetal life constantly changes with aging, especially in the vitreous periphery, into lamellar aggregations. The loose central vitreous, therefore, represents a more watery "fetal-like arrangement" than the structurally compact cortical zone. The high concentration of acid mucopolysaccharides in the cortical zone can be attributed to their being produced by the ciliary epithelium at the "base" of the vitreous. Some observers, however, attribute their production to cells often lying freely in the posterior vitreous cortex near the retinal surface. These cells, more numerous in bovine eyes, are sometimes termed **hyalocytes** (13). It is more likely, however, that they are a variety of histiocyte or glial cell that has migrated from surrounding tissues (see retinal vessels and optic nerve head).

MODIFICATIONS

Anteriorly, in the region of the posterior pars plana or vitreous base, the densely aggregated vitreous filaments are aggregated further into "fibers." The fibers pass anteriorly and axially through the vitreous, along its face, and freely into the posterior chamber as the suspensory *ligaments* of the lens, or **zonule of Zinn** (Fig. 7–22 through 7–25).

The zonular fibers originate as myriad filaments attached to the thin basement membrane covering the markedly infolded basal plasmalemmas of the nonpigmented epithelial cells (Fig. 10–61) of the posterior pars plana or orbicularis ciliaris (6). Arranged circumferentially,

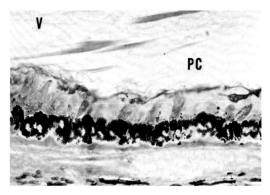

FIG. 7–22. Zonular fibers near their attachments to posterior pars plana epithelium. Zonules lie in posterior chamber (**PC**). Lens is to right and above. **V,** vitreous body. (Methacrylate section, toluidine blue stain, × 305) (AFIP Neg. 60-2490)

FIG. 7–23. Shadow-cast section of region over posterior pars plana. A zonular fiber (**Z**) is present within vitreous framework. Inset. Cross-section of filamentous zonular fiber (**FZ**) and its close relation to multilaminar basement membrane of nonpigmented ciliary epithelium (**ILM**). (Modified from Fine BS, Tousimis AJ: Arch Ophthalmol 65:95, 1961)

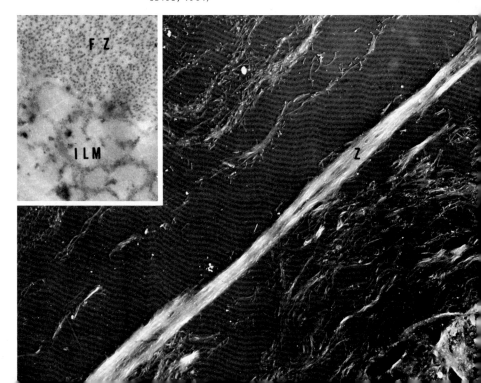

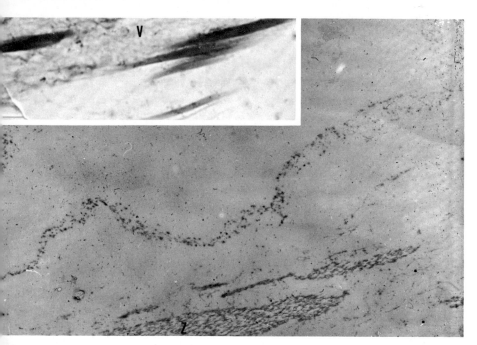

FIG. 7–24. Zonular fibers. Electron micrograph, a thin section of a region similar to that shown in inset, shows filamentous aggregates of anterior vitreous; similar filamentous aggregates form zonular (**Z**) fragments. (× 6900) Inset. Light micrograph showing zonules within vitreous body (**V**), along anterior face of vitreous body, and within posterior chamber. (Methacrylate section, toluidine blue, × 305) (AFIP Neg. 60-4101) (Fine BS, Tousimis AJ: Arch Ophthalmol 65:95, 1961)

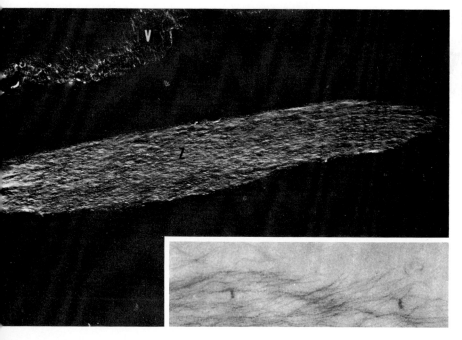

FIG. 7–25. Shadow-cast section showing fragment of an anterior vitreous "sheet" of filamentous composition (**V**) as well as large zonular fragment (**Z**). (× 2580) Inset. A thin-section electron micrograph clearly shows filamentous composition of a zonular fragment. (× 17,000) (Modified from Fine BS, Tousimis AJ: Arch Ophthalmol 65:95, 1961)

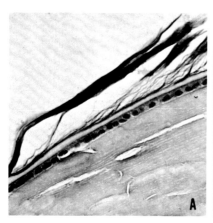
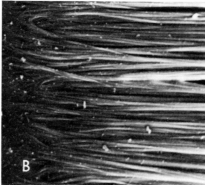

FIG. 7–26. Attachment of orbiculoanterior zonular fibers to anterior lens capsule. A. By light microscopy (Bleach-alcian blue, × 350) B. By scanning electron microscopy. (× 240)

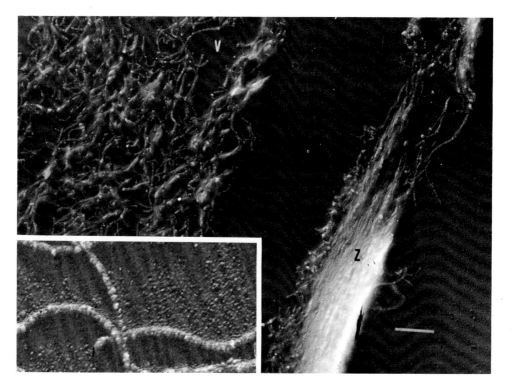

FIG. 7–27. Shadow-cast section from anterior vitreous (**V**) and adjacent anterior zonule (**Z**). Both vitreous framework and zonular fibers are composed of morphologically identical filaments. Zonular fibers are too thick at bottom of photograph for their filamentous composition to be visible. This is better appreciated above, where zonule is cut more obliquely as it passes out of plane of section. (U-shad, × 11,850) Inset. Some anterior vitreous filaments at higher magnification. (× 48,000) (Fine BS, Tousimis AJ: Arch Ophthalmol 65:95, 1961)

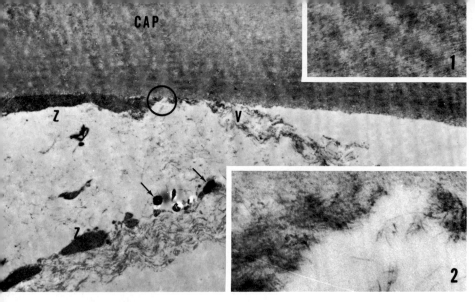

FIG. 7-28. Region of hyaloideocapsular ligament. Posterior zonular fibers (**Z**) attach to lens capsule (**CAP**) together with vitreous body face (**V**). Melanin (**arrows**) deposited here are characteristic of some adult eyes. No ease of separation of vitreous face from lens capsule. (× 3800) Inset 1. Higher magnification of lens capsule showing its filamentous composition. (× 22,8 Inset 2. Higher magnification of end zonule (circled area in main figure), showing similarity of zonular and vitreous body filaments. (× 22,800) (Fine BS: Arch Ophthalmol 67:689, 1962)

the fibers form essentially two main groups: the **orbiculoanterior** and **orbiculoposterior** zonular fibers. The former attach to the thick basement membrane or anterior lens capsule (Fig. 7-26); the latter attach to the thinner lens basement membrane or posterior lens capsule.

The orbiculoanterior zonular fibers (Fig. 7-27) attach in a ring axial to the lens equator, by spreading out over short regions of the slightly undulating capsular surface (Fig. 8-9, 8-10, 8-11). The orbiculoposterior zonular fibers attach in a ring less axial to the equator. The location of the latter ring of attachment is identical with the hyaloideocapsular ligament (Fig. 7-28, 7-29).

A true separate or discrete ligamentous component of the vitreous body in the region of the hyaloideocapsular ligament cannot be identified. The only filamentary aggregates in this zone that are observably different from those of the vitreous anterior border layer and that do not artifactitiously separate from the lens capsule are those of the orbiculoposterior zonular fibers themselves (4). Since zonular fibers are but specialized portions of the anterior peripheral vitreous framework (5), the apparent loss of a "ligament" in this region appears explicable on the basis that the hyaloideocapsular ligament is essentially synonymous with the attachment ring of the posterior zonular fibers.

Various passageways between anterior and posterior groups of zonular fibers (canal of Hanover) and between the vitreous face and some of the posterior zonular fibers (canal of Petit) have been described on the basis of injection techniques that used such methods as bubbles of air. Such methods, however, because of the surface tensions involved,

failed to point up the discrete filamentary zonular bundles which are seen by light and electron microscopy and supported by clinical observations.

Occasionally the old concept is revived that the zonular fibers are in reality parts of a continuous sheet. No strong histologic evidence exists that these are other than separate groupings of filaments. Clinically, pigment or other deposits are seen *on* but not *between* the zonular fibers.

This specialization of the vitreous framework to become the zonular fibers is in accord with the embryologic observation of a "condensation of tertiary vitreous" to form the zonules. The collagen presumably is secreted by the epithelial cells which impinge upon the lens capsule and spin out the zonular fibers as a spider its web. The fibers become longer as the cells move posteriorly with growth of the globe to come to rest as the epithelial lining of the posterior pars plana. The more anterior, or later, cells apparently lose their ability to synthesize collagen and form only irregular, vestigial, and possibly some *cilioequatorial* zonular fibers, all of which appear to be of limited functional importance. In some pathologic conditions in the adult eye, the cells may proliferate and resume their collagen-synthesizing activities; an example is the formation of new vitreous-like material by adenomatous hyperplasias of the nonpigmented ciliary epithelium (18) (see section on the Ciliary Body, Ch. 10).

REFERENCES

1. Barber AN: Embryology of the Human Eye. St. Louis, CV Mosby, 1955
2. Boyer HK, Suran AA, Hogan MJ, McEwen WK: Increase of residual protein of bovine vitreous during growth of the eye. Arch Ophthalmol 56:861, 1956
3. Dische Z, Murty VLN: An insoluble structural glyco-

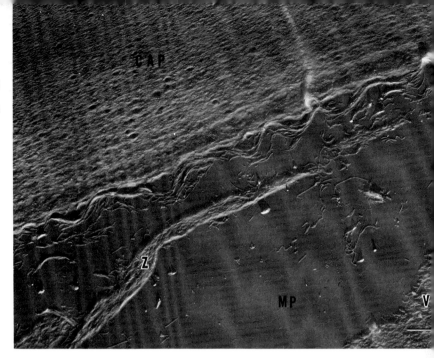

FIG. 7–29. Shadow-cast section of region similar to that in Figure 7–28. Slight undulation of capsular surface (**CAP**) is evident. Zonular filaments and filaments of vitreous body (**V**) appear identical. Mucinous drying patterns are also present (**MP**). (U-shad, × 9200) (Lerman S: Cataracts: Chemistry, Mechanisms, and Therapy. Springfield IL, CC Thomas, 1964)

protein a major constituent of the Zonula Zinni. Invest Ophthal 13:991, 1974

4. Fine BS: Correspondence. Arch Ophthalmol 67:689, 1962
5. Fine BS, Tousimis AJ: The structure of the vitreous body and the suspensory ligaments of the lens. Arch Ophthalmol 65:95, 1961
6. Fine BS, Zimmerman LE: Light and electron microscopic observations on the ciliary epithelium in man and rhesus monkey. Invest Ophthalmol 2:105, 1963
7. Friedenwald JS, Stiehler RD: Structure of the vitreous. Arch Ophthalmol 14:789, 1935
8. Gross J, Maltoltsy AG, Cohen C: Vitrosin, a member of the collagen class. Biophys Biochem Cytol 1:215, 1955
9. Krause AC: The chemistry of the vitreous humor. II. Proteolysis. Arch Ophthalmol 11:964, 1934
10. Lerman S: Cataracts: Chemistry, Mechanisms, and Therapy. Springfield, IL, CC Thomas, 1964
11. Mann I: The Development of the Human Eye, 3rd ed. New York, Grune & Stratton, 1969
12. Meyer K, Palmer JW: Polysaccharide of vitreous humor. J Biol Chem 107:629, 1934
13. Österlin S, Balazs EA: Macromolecular composition and fine structure of the vitreous in the owl monkey. Exp Eye Res 7:534, 1968
14. Pirie A, Schmidt G, Waters JW: Ox vitreous humour. I. The residual protein. Br J Ophthalmol 32:321, 1948
15. Pirie A, van Heyningen R: Biochemistry of the Eye. Springfield, IL, CC Thomas, 1956, p 234
16. Porter KR, Pappas GD: Collagen formation by fibroblasts of the chick embryo dermis. J Biophys Biochem Cytol 5:153, 1959
17. Swann DA, Constable IJ, Harper E: Vitreous structure. III. Composition of bovine vitreous collagen. Invest Ophthal 11:735, 1972
18. Yanoff M, Fine BS: Ocular Pathology: A Text and Atlas. Hagerstown, Harper & Row, 1975, p 345
19. Zimmerman LE: Demonstration of hyaluronidase-sensitive acid mucopolysaccharides: a preliminary report. Am J Ophthalmol 44:1, 1957

chapter **8**

THE LENS

EMBRYOLOGY   149
STRUCTURE   153
  CAPSULE   153
    ANTERIOR
    POSTERIOR
    EQUATORIAL
  EPITHELIUM   155
    ANTERIOR
    EQUATORIAL
  CORTEX AND NUCLEUS   156

The lens is an example of a tissue composed entirely of cells completely enveloped by the thickest basement membrane in the body.

EMBRYOLOGY

When the optic vesicle transforms into the optic cup, there is concomitant invagination of the surface ectoderm. The primordial lens separates completely from the surface layer to lie suspended within the orifice of the optic cup as a vesicle formed by epithelium, the lens vesicle (Fig. 8–1).

The delicate basement membrane associated with the surface ectoderm now encloses the vesicle in which the epithelial cells all project inward (3, 7). This basement membrane, or lens capsule, is so thin that in its early stages it cannot be appreciated by light microscopy. With further development, the posterior epithelial cells elongate to gradually occlude the lumen of the vesicle. These early, elongated lens cells ("fibers") are called the **primary lens fibers.** All subsequent lens cells ("fibers") are derived from the epithelial cell layer at the equator and are termed **secondary lens cells or fibers** (Fig. 8–2).

Presumably it is this narrow band of primary lens fibers that is seen with the slit lamp as the single, narrow, central nonrelucent zone of the lens called the *embryonic nucleus* (Fig. 8–3). The early secondary lens fibers or cells presumably form the more relucent, symmetrically paired anterior and posterior portions that "cap" this central zone. These caps, on which the Y-shaped suture is now recognizable, represent the "fetal" nucleus.

In the preequatorial zone, the lens epithelium undergoes mitotic division, and at the equator the cells elongate and rotate (apex anterior, base posterior). Further elongation occurs in the postequatorial zone (Fig. 8–2, 8–4). Successive application of these straplike cells to the underlying cells results in a layered arrangement, and where the elongated cells meet, a line or lens **suture** is formed (Fig. 8–3, 8–5).

Because all the lens cells grow equally long, and thus cannot all reach anterior and posterior points, lines of abutment—the anterior and posterior suture lines—are formed. In the human (Fig. 8–6C) the lens acquires a biconvex or flattened disc shape so that the suture lines must become quite complex. The result is a Y-shaped suture line that can be observed biomicroscopically as an inverted Y posteriorly and an upright Y anteriorly. With further addition of lens cells, suture lines increase in complexity. All these secondary cells add to the formation of the **lens cortex.**

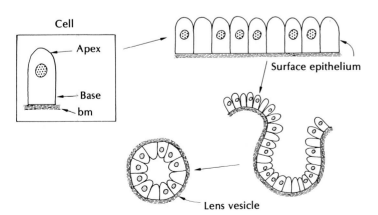

FIG. 8–1. Schematic representation of formation of lens vesicle from surface ectoderm. Polarization of epithelial cells is maintained. **bm,** basement membrane.

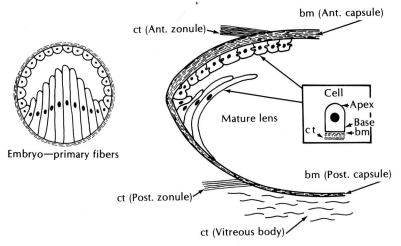

Embryo—primary fibers

Cell
Apex
Base
bm
ct

bm (Ant. capsule)
ct (Ant. zonule)

Mature lens

bm (Post. capsule)
ct (Post. zonule)
ct (Vitreous body)

FIG. 8–2. Schematic representation of maturation of primary lens fibers within lens vesicle (**left**) and final arrangement achieved in adult lens (**right**). **bm,** basement membrane; **ct,** connective tissue.

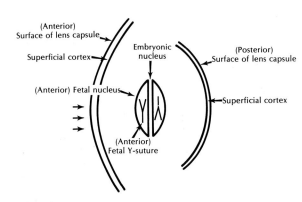

(Anterior) Surface of lens capsule
Superficial cortex
(Anterior) Fetal nucleus
Embryonic nucleus
(Posterior) Surface of lens capsule
Superficial cortex
(Anterior) Fetal Y-suture

FIG. 8–3. Slit-lamp appearance of major landmarks in lens. The three **free arrows** indicate direction of light entering eye.

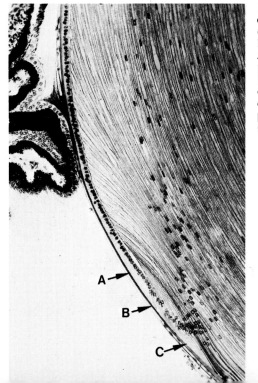

A
B
C

FIG. 8–4. Meridional section from eye of 4-month-old fetus. Preequatorial, equatorial, and postequatorial zones of lens epithelium are indicated by arrows **A, B,** and **C,** respectively. Note persistence of lens cell nuclei deep into cortex, close approximation of ciliary epithelium to lens capsule, and characteristic increased thickness of postequatorial capsule. (Masson, × 115) (AFIP Neg. 61-3077)

FIG. 8–5. Equatorial section showing formation of Y-suture where lens cells meet. (H&E, × 70) (AFIP Neg. 70-1427)

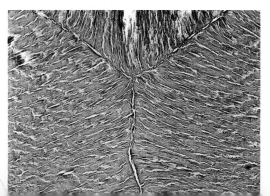

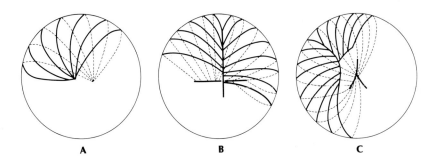

FIG. 8–6. Schematic drawing to show pole-to-pole arrangement of lens cells in early spherical arrangement (**A**). Additional cells and less spherical arrangement, e.g., rabbit (**B**) produces suture *lines* which become even more complex or Y-shaped (**C**) in the flattened human lens.

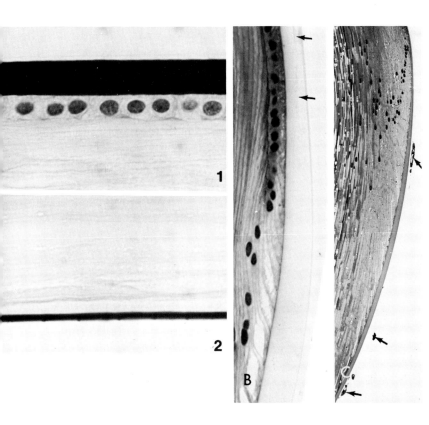

FIG. 8–7. A. Lens capsule. Thick anterior lens capsule (**1**) is applied to bases of underlying layer of epithelial cells; thinner posterior lens capsule (**2**) is applied to cortical cells only. (Both PAS, × 730) (Scheie HG, Albert DM: Adler's Textbook of Ophthalmology. Philadelphia, WB Saunders, 1969) B. The anterior lens capsule, 44-year-old subject, thickens considerably in the post-equatorial zone, altering toward a thinner posterior capsule in region of attachment of orbiculoposterior zonular fibers. Note line of division of preequatorial capsule into two parts (**arrows**) (TB × 300) (AFIP Neg. 74-1130) C. Equatorial lens capsule in 14-week fetus. Note marked thickening of post-equatorial lens capsule. **Arrows.** Segments of tunica vasculosa lentis. (TB × 90) (AFIP Neg. 74-11297)

FIG. 8–8. Surface of anterior lens capsule near periphery of pupil as seen by scanning electron microscope. Surface is remarkably smooth in this preparation at this magnification. (× 5,500)

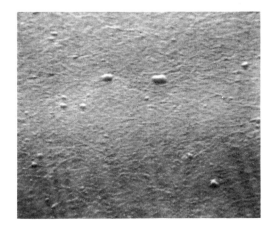

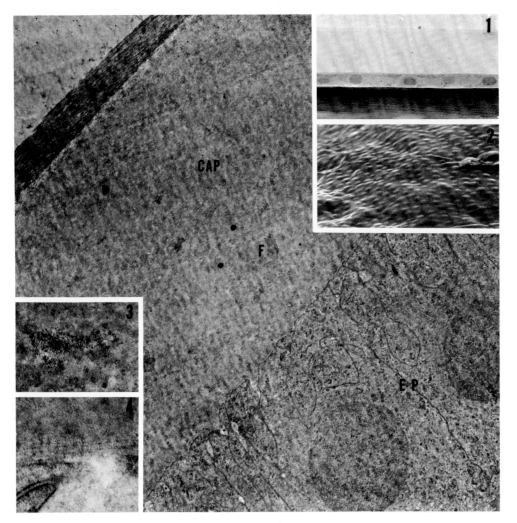

FIG. 8–9. Anterior lens capsule. Electron micrograph of anterior zonule (**Z**), lens capsule (**CAP**), fibrillogranules (**F**), and adjacent epithelium (**EP**) in area comparable to that shown in light micrograph (inset 1). (Main figure, × 5600; inset 1, Epon section, PD, × 485; AFIP Neg. 63-6905) Scanning electron micrograph (inset 2) of surface of anterior lens capsule shows nuclei of underlying epithelial cells protruding because of excessive dehydration. (× 250) Fibrillo-granular material (inset 3) is typical of anterior lens capsule. (× 15,000) Periodicity may be observed in anterior lens capsule (inset 4). (× 40,000)

FIG. 8–10. A. Anterior lens capsule to show zonules (**Z**) and fibrillogranular material (**F**) deep in lens capsule. Note faint banded appearance (~500 A) of the latter material. (× 12,000) B. Higher magnification of area of fibrillogranular material. When appropriately sectioned, a banded appearance (~500 A) can be seen (**arrows**). (× 40,000)

In more spherical lenses (e.g., dogfish, rabbit) the anterior suture is vertical and the posterior is horizontal to accommodate cells of equal length (Fig. 8–6B).

The lens epithelium remains over the anterior surface and the equatorial zone. The basement membrane or lens capsule (Fig. 8–8) continues to thicken throughout life. Because the thickening occurs mainly where epithelium is present, the posterior lens capsule remains extremely thin (Fig. 8–7A, 8–9) except in the immediate postequatorial region where the capsule is un-

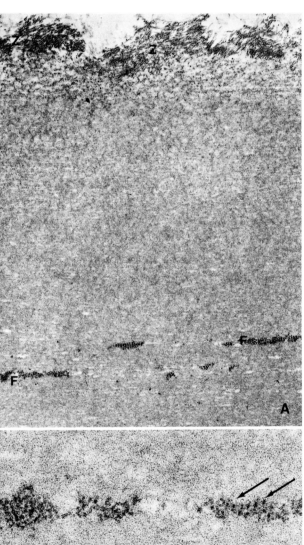

usually thick (Fig. 8–7B) a change that can be seen in the lens of a 14-week fetus (Fig. 8–7C). A similar but generally less pronounced thickening occurs in the anterior lens capsule slightly axial to the insertion of the anterior zonular fibers. The thinnest portion of the lens capsule lies always at the posterior pole.

As the cortical cells are continually layered on from the periphery, the more centrally located begin to lose their recognizable cell organelles; this is most easily noted by observing the loss of a recognizable cell nucleus toward the center of the lens. Forced deeper into the center, the cortical cells are compressed from front to back, becoming increasingly dense and folded to form a central lens mass—the **adult lens nucleus.**

STRUCTURE

After birth, the lens appears as a transparent biconvex body enclosed in a capsule, lying directly behind the pupil. The center of its anterior surface is called the anterior pole; the center of its posterior surface, the posterior pole. The radius of curvature of the anterior surface averages 10 mm, but it is subject to marked changes during accommodation. The radius of curvature of the posterior surface averages 6 mm. The lens equator is not smoothly curved, but shows, in life, numerous furrows or grooves resulting from the pull of the zonular fibers. The grooves are generally lost when the lens is removed or fixed (Fig. 8–10, 8–11).

CAPSULE

The adult lens is enclosed by the **lens capsule** (*cuticular, glass, or basement membrane*), a transparent, reflective, elastic, indigestible, PAS-positive covering.

Connective tissues are present on the outer, or nonepithelial, side of the thick basement membrane, but are modified in this special case into the anterior and posterior groups of *zonular fibers* (11) and the anterior *face* of the *vitreous body* (Fig. 8–2).

The lens capsule has a distinctly filamentous substructure (Fig. 8–9, 8–10), with the filaments aligning parallel to the surface. Numerous small patches or clusters of filaments or fibrillogranular material (inset 3, Fig. 8–9, 8–10) lying at varying levels in the equatorial and peripheral capsule differentiate the anterior lens capsule

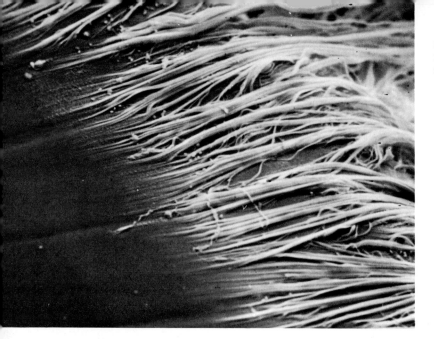

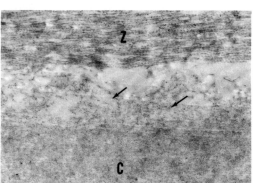

from the posterior capsule (5), where they are absent. When appropriately sectioned, the capsular basement membrane occasionally shows a periodicity (~500 A) (inset 4, Fig. 8–9), characteristic of some other banded basement membranes (13) (filamentous banded basement membrane—Ch. 4).

Exaggerations of normal structure are found in a variety of pathologic changes. Excessive fibrillation of the anterior filamentous basement membrane (capsule) may lead to (true) *exfoliation* of the lens capsule, or excessive production of the fibrillogranular banded components produces the abnormal basement membrane material in *pseudoexfoliation* of the lens capsule.

On biomicroscopic examination, the lens **shagreen** or beaten-metal-like reflex, long believed to represent a reflection from the capsular surface (known in thin optical section as the **first zone of relucency**), is observed *in vivo* to be coarser anteriorly than posteriorly. Loss of lens shagreen or surface irregularity is a sign that often alerts the surgeon to the possibility of a "weak" capsule and enables him to be more selective in his method of cataract removal. To date (Fig. 8–8, 8–11), examination of the surface of the lens capsule by scanning microscopy fails to demonstrate a gross surface irregularity. The lens shagreen, therefore, must represent optical variations *within* the lens capsule.

Although histologic studies show that a thin layer at the surface of the lens capsule can be stained differently from the remainder of the capsule, electron microscopic observations indicate that this pericapsular layer (membrane) differs mor-

phologically only in its comparative looseness from the remainder of the compact lens capsule (Fig. 8–12). That this differential staining probably is due to capsular "looseness" is supported by the observation that when the normal anterior lens capsule is split or separated mechanically into numerous layers, the loosened structure acquires similarly altered staining properties. On clinical examination, a membrane called the **zonular lamella** can be observed occasionally uniting the ends of zonular fibers that have split off from the preequatorial zone of the lens (see Fig. 8–7B). This membrane or lamella is probably composed of the looser anterior layer.

Apertures in the normal lens capsule have not yet been convincingly demonstrated, but in at least two reports on pathologic tissues (1, 2), apparent through-and-through passageways

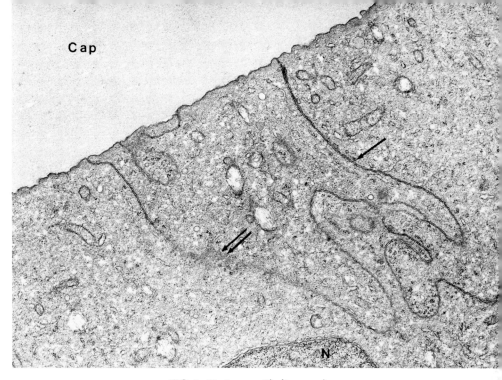

Cap

for abnormal quantities of material have been observed in the anterior peripheral capsule.

EPITHELIUM

Anteriorly, the epithelium is cuboidal, with rather flat plasma membranes applied to the equally flat basement membrane (Fig. 8–13). The cells interdigitate laterally in a fashion typical of many epithelia. The intercellular space also is typical except near the basal ends of the cells in the midperiphery, where foci of enlarged intercellular spaces may be observed (Fig. 8–14).

Some of the spaces may be artifacts; some may be physiologic, representing the histologic counterparts of the globules (*i.e.,* Vogt's "shagreen spheres") that biomicroscopists in the past have noted in the midperipheral zone; and some may represent early pathologic changes.

The organelles within the epithelial cells are not prominent, and the small Golgi complex is found in the apical cytoplasm (toward the lens cortex). The apical plasma membranes of the epithelial cells frequently are attached to one another and to the first layer of flattened cortical cells by a series of short desmosome-like densities. (Presumably, removal of lens epithelium is accompanied by a torn superficial layer of cortical cells.)

FIG. 8–13. Lens epithelium and anterior lens capsule (**Cap**). Typical intercellular space is evident where interdigitating plasmalemmas are sectioned normally (**arrow**) but is "blurred" where they are sectioned obliquely (**double arrows**). **N,** nucleus of epithelial cell. (× 12,000)

FIG. 8–14. Foci of enlarged intercellular spaces (**arrows**) filled with lucent extracellular material at anterior midperiphery. **C,** lens capsule. (× 6600) (Lerman S: Cataracts: Chemistry, Mechanisms, and Therapy. Springfield, IL, CC Thomas, 1964)

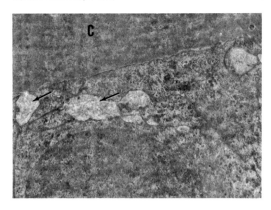

The cells undergo mitotic division in the pre-equatorial zone and elongation and rotation in the equatorial zone. The elongated cortical cells so formed are applied to the layers beneath.

CORTEX AND NUCLEUS

Because the lens nucleus is formed by increasing density of cortical cells, the cortex and nucleus are considered together. Both are made up exclusively of cells derived from the lens epithelium. The common designation of "lens fiber" for the cortical cells is a misnomer for the elongated cells of the lens substance.

Lens cortical cells ("fibers") are elongated straplike cells that appear, on cross-section, somewhat hexagonal (inset, Fig. 8–15). The cortex in this cross-section view resembles the cut surface of a honeycomb. The superficial cortical cells are relatively flat and are separated by a usual intercellular space (Fig. 8–16). Cell organelles are almost nonexistent (4, 8, 9) (Figs. 8–15 through 8–17), and the cytoplasm appears more homogeneous than that of the epithelial cells, but of comparable density (Fig. 8–18). Slightly deeper within the cortex (Fig. 8–19) the cell layers may abruptly become dense. The dense cells possess markedly irregular surfaces (Fig. 8–20) and the appearance of fusion of adjacent plasma membranes. This abrupt change in cell shape and density is interpreted as due to physiologic compression of the cells with accompanying loss of water and shrinkage.

The presence of plasmalemmal fusions in the deep cortex or nucleus is interpreted sometimes as a form of fascia occludens, together with the functional connotations that these structures carry elsewhere, where they are actively produced by adjacent cells. It is more likely, however, that, in the lens, the "fusions" are formed passively as a result of compression of the cells as they are forced inward.

The lens is but epithelium or epidermis turned inward so that the cells may no longer desquamate freely. They therefore undergo compression and loss of water, hence their increase in surface convolutions, i.e., microplicae (Fig. 8–21) and cell density. Comparable formation of microplicae and densification of the oldest cells in a stratified epithelium also is observed in the cells of the corneal epithelium (see Fig. 9–6 to 9–9).

The abrupt transition of electron microscopic density within the superficial cortex apparently represents a comparable abrupt change in optical density that can be observed in vivo and is known as the **second zone of relucency** (Fig. 8–3). A similar zone is present posteriorly, but is always more closely approximated to that of the posterior lens capsule. The difference in separation between the anterior and posterior zones of relucency is most easily explained by the combination of decreased thickness of capsule and lack of epithelium posteriorly.

In light microscopy, the transition from cortex to nucleus (Fig. 8–22) is characterized by

FIG. 8–15. Lens cells ("fibers") in cross section, showing their honeycomb-like arrangement. (× 8000) Inset. Representative light micrograph. (H&E, × 260) (AFIP Acc. 132413)

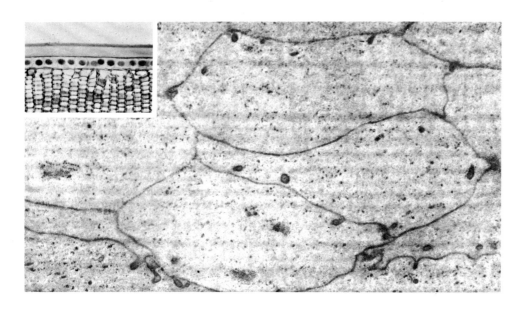

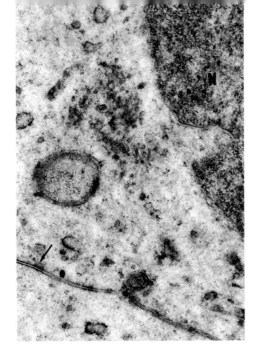

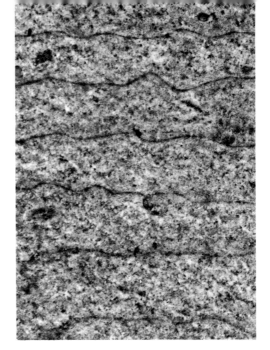

FIG. 8–16. Typical intercellular space (**arrow**) between superficial cortical cells. Cytoplasm contains few organelles. **N,** nucleus of a cortical cell. (× 27,000)

FIG. 8–17. Superficial cortical cell cytoplasm. Note its almost homogeneous appearance and the fragment of a poorly formed Golgi complex. (× 27,000)

FIG. 8–18. Adult superficial lens cortex. Cells appear homogeneous and possess relatively flat, straight boundaries. Intercellular spaces can be observed. (× 7000)

FIG. 8–19. Deep lens cortex, adult subject. Cells are dense and irregularly folded. Cell membranes are indistinct and artifactitious separations are abundant. (× 7,000)

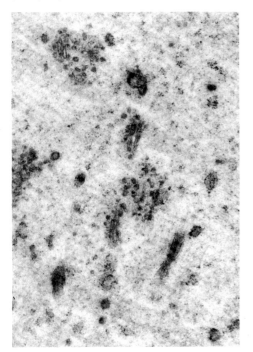

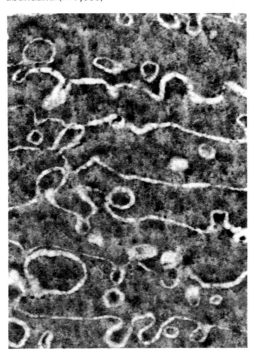

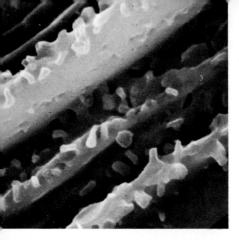

FIG. 8–20. Lens cells in superficial cortex, 28-year-old subject. Note straplike or flattened configuration. "Ball and socket" joints are present along the lateral edges of the cells. (× 7500)

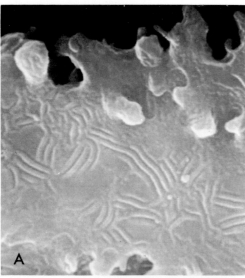

FIG. 8–21. Lens cells, infant. A. Lens cortical cell to show fingerprint pattern or microplicae along widest or flat surfaces of cell and "ball and socket" joints along the narrow lateral cell margins. (× 7000) B. Lens cell in superficial lens nucleus. Microplicae are more numerous and more densely packed along flat surface of cell. (× 9000) C. Ball-and-socket cell edge attachments can be seen separating (**arrows**) (× 3500)

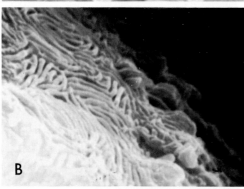

FIG. 8–22. Light micrograph showing normal transition zone (**arrows**) from cortex to nucleus in adult lens. (H&E, × 115) (AFIP Neg. 62-2043)

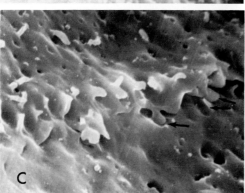

apparent loss of lamellar arrangement and increase in staining density (*i.e.,* eosinophilia). In electron microscopy, as cell density increases, so does the surface irregularity. The plasma membranes of adjacent cells become so tightly adherent to one another that intercellular spaces become impossible to distinguish and the cells may tear through the surface cytoplasm (Fig. 8–19).

These observations are compatible with the increasing density as seen by bio- and electron microscopy when deeper layers are examined. In addition, the most dense nuclear cells often show a yellow pigmentation clinically that generally increases with age. When color and density are exaggerated to a degree that encroaches upon useful vision, it is termed a nuclear *cataract.*

REFERENCES

1. Ashton N, Shakib M, Collyer R, Blach R: Electron microscopic study of pseudoexfoliation of the lens capsule. Invest Ophthalmol 4:141, 1965
2. Bertelsen TI, Drablos PA, Flood PR: The so-called senile exfoliation (pseudoexfoliation) of the anterior lens capsule: a product of the lens epithelium fibrillopathia epitheliocapsularis. Acta Ophthalmol (Kbh) 42:1096, 1964
3. Cohen AI: Electron microscopic observations on the lens of the neonatal albino mouse. Am J Anat 103:219, 1958
4. Cohen AI: The electron microscopy of the normal human lens. Invest Ophthalmol 4:433, 1965
5. Dark AJ, Streeten BW, Jones D: Accumulation of fibrillar protein in the aging human lens capsule (with special reference to the pathogenesis of pseudoexfoliative disease of the lens). Arch Ophthalmol 82:815, 1969
6. Dickson DH, Crock GW: Interlocking patterns on primate lens fibers. Invest Ophthalmol 11:809, 1972
7. Hunt HH: A study of the fine structure of the optic vesicle and lens placode of the chick embryo during induction. Dev Biol 3:175, 1961
8. Kuwabara T: Microtubules in the lens. Arch Ophthalmol 79:189, 1968
9. Kuwabara T: The maturation of the lens cell. A morphologic study. Exp Eye Res 20:427, 1975
10. Lerman S: Cataracts: Chemistry, Mechanisms, and Therapy. Springfield, IL, CC Thomas, 1964
11. McCulloch C: The zonule of Zinn: its origin, course and insertion, and its relation to neighboring structures. Trans Am Ophthalmol Soc 52:525, 1954
12. Scheie HG, Albert DM: Adler's Textbook of Ophthalmology. Philadelphia, WB Saunders, 1969
13. Yanoff M, Fine BS: Ocular Pathology: A Text and Atlas. Hagerstown, Harper & Row, 1975

chapter 9

THE CORNEA AND SCLERA

THE CORNEA   163
   TEAR FILM AND EPITHELIUM   163
   BOWMAN'S MEMBRANE (LAYER) AND
      STROMA   168
   ENDOTHELIUM AND DESCEMET'S
      MEMBRANE   171
   CENTRAL COMPARED WITH PERIPHERAL
      PORTIONS   178
THE LIMBUS   183
THE SCLERA   186
   EMISSARIA   187
   EPISCLERA   191
   STROMA   191
   LAMINA FUSCA   192

THE CORNEA

In accord with the three-tissue arrangement for describing ocular structure (Ch. 5), the cornea may be considered a tissue composed mostly of extracellular materials and covered on its anterior and posterior surfaces by a sheet of cells. The two cell layers—a multilayered epithelium anteriorly and a single-layered "endothelium" posteriorly—are apposed to their associated basement membranes and connective tissues in such manner (Fig. 9–1) as to form a three-layered sandwich. The modifications within this simplistic arrangement are described below.

Functionally, the cornea is not only a "window" to the eye but also its *major* refractive element. The corneal diameter in the adult eye averages 12 mm, with the horizontal meridian generally 1 mm longer than the vertical. When viewed from behind (as in an opened eye), the cornea appears more nearly circular. The discrepancy results from the slightly greater overlap of adjoining opaque sclera anteriorly in the vertical plane.

The cornea is ~0.5 mm thick centrally and ~1.0 mm thick peripherally.

In addition to the avascularity of the cornea, its transparency appears to be due to the relation of collagen fibrils of small and *uniform* diameter to a large bed of acid mucopolysaccharides.

The cornea may be separated into at least six layers (Fig. 9–2): 1) tear film, 2) epithelium (and its basement membrane), 3) Bowman's membrane or layer, 4) stroma, 5) Descemet's membrane, and 6) endothelium.

TEAR FILM AND EPITHELIUM

The tear film covering the corneal surface is made up of three layers: a posterior layer rich in glycoproteins derived from the conjunctival goblet cells, a middle watery layer secreted by the lacrimal tissues, and an anterior oily layer produced by the meibomian glands and the glands of Moll and Zeis in the eyelids.

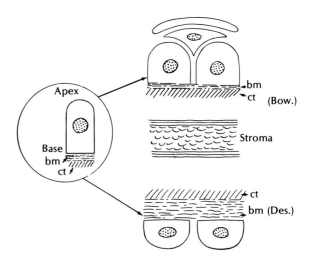

FIG. 9–1. Schematic drawing showing three-layered arrangement of cornea. **bm,** basement membrane, **ct,** connective tissue; **Bow,** Bowman's membrane (layer); **Des,** Descemet's membrane.

Although the tear film is a complex multisource secretion deposited *upon* the corneal surface and is not strictly speaking an anatomic part of the cornea, its relationship to the cornea is of such importance that it must be noted whenever the corneal epithelium is described.

The nonkeratinized squamous epithelium of the cornea consists of approximately five layers of cells that probably are more regularly arranged than any other squamous epithelium in the body. The deepest or basal layer (Fig. 9–3) is composed of columnar cells (~18μ in height), which characteristically possess a thin, irregular, occasionally diffused (i.e., slightly multilaminar) basement membrane applied to their basal plasmalemmas. Focal densities occur regularly along the basal plasma membrane. The densities appear similar to desmosomes that are attached elsewhere along the cell borders except that here they receive no reciprocity from an adjacent cell to form a complete desmosome; hence the basilar structure is termed a **hemidesmosome** (Fig. 9–4).

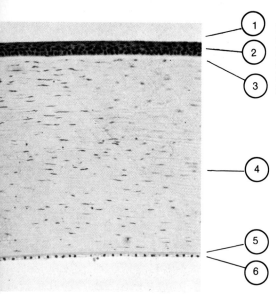

FIG. 9–2. Light micrograph of section of central cornea. Numbers indicate layers: **1**, tear film, **2**, epithelium, **3**, Bowman's membrane, **4**, stroma, **5**, Descemet's membrane, **6**, endothelium. (H&E, × 115) (AFIP Neg. 65-238)

FIG. 9–3. Basal layer of corneal epithelium. Electron micrograph shows portion of basal epithelial cells, their hemidesmosomes (**HD**), their basement membrane (**BM**), and a portion of Bowman's layer (**BL**). (× 16,000) Inset 1. Light micrograph showing Epon section of corneal epithelium, Bowman's membrane (**BM**), and adjacent corneal stroma. (Epon section, PD, × 485) (AFIP Neg. 63-6904) Inset 2. Enlargement of basal cell hemidesmosome (circled in main figure) and adjacent basement membrane (**BM**). (× 48,000) (Modified from McTigue JW: Trans Am Ophthalmol Soc 65:591, 1967)

Although they are structurally unilateral, evidence exists that hemidesmosomes accentuate focally the usual attachment of a cell to its thin basement membrane (2, 18). Experiments with tissue cultures of rabbit corneal epithelium indicate that epithelial cells may separate readily through "dissolution" of the intercellular cement substance of desmosomes. Hemidesmosomes, however, remain so adherent to their basement membrane that when migrating basal cells separate from a surface, they may leave behind small cytoplasmic pseudopodia in the region of these basal plasmalemmal densities.

The basal cells have a centrally located nucleus as well as the usual complement of mitochondria and apical Golgi complex. Their cytoplasm contains a high concentration of filaments (characteristic of a number of epithelial cells). Some of the filaments are believed to be actin filaments (7).

As the basal cells undergo mitotic division by dividing in an apicobasilar plane, the slide of adjacent basal cells forces a daughter cell outward into the next or **adbasal** cell layer. Because the daughter cells now are flattened and curved slightly in their horizontal dimension, they are called **wing** cells and the layer is known as the **wing cell layer.** Persisting in this layer are the myriad desmosomal attachments to adjacent cells (Fig. 9–5) as well as the high concentration of cytoplasmic filaments. The filamentous bundles as seen by light microscopy are called **tonofibrils** which are made up of **tonofilaments** as seen by electron microscopy.

Although difficult to demonstrate, it appears highly likely that the basal cells of the corneal epithelium are arranged topographically in a whorl-like manner, the more superficial layers being progressively less well arranged. This is reflected in normal eyes of heavily pigmented individuals by the vortexlike arrangement often seen with excessive extension of the limbal pigment onto the cornea. Similar patterns occur as a result of abnormal deposits within basal cells in such conditions as Fabry's disease (*cornea verticillata*) (31) and chloroquine keratopathy. The whorl-like arrangements in the two eyes of a single individual are generally symmetrical, the pattern being clockwise or counterclockwise or opposites in the two eyes.

Beyond this layer, the cells become more flattened and more dense (presumably because of increased dehydration), with loss of most recognizable cell organelles except for the nucleus, which persists. The broad, flattened surface cells continue to possess their surface irregularities (microvilli or microplicae (1), (Figs. 9–6 to 9–8), which are smoothed over by the tear film (Fig. 9–9), especially its mucoprotein and lipoidal components. On occasion, the dried-out remains of the tear film layer can be observed in a micrograph (Fig. 9–6).

The corneal epithelium is continuous with the epithelium of the bulbar conjunctiva at the limbus. Goblet (mucus-secreting) cells appear in the bulbar conjunctival epithelium (Fig. 9–44).

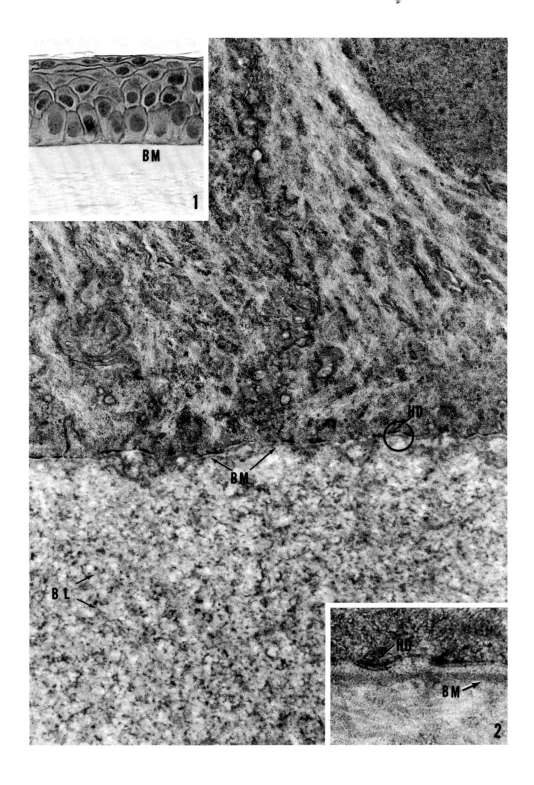

BM

1

HD

BM

BL

HD

BM

2

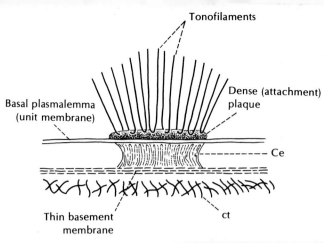

Tonofilaments

Basal plasmalemma
(unit membrane)

Dense (attachment)
plaque

Ce

Thin basement
membrane

ct

FIG. 9–4. Schematic of hemidesmosome. **Ce,** cement substance; **ct,** connective tissue.

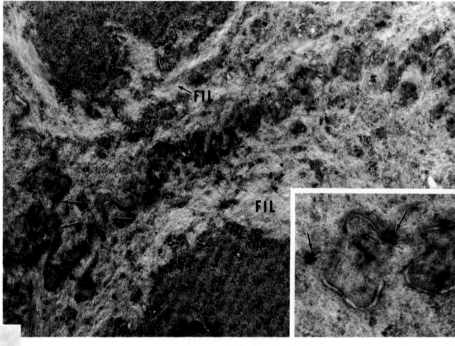

FIL

FIL

FIG. 9–5. Wing cell layer of corneal epithelium. Adjacent cells are attached by myriad desmosomes (**arrows**), shown enlarged in inset. **FIL,** intracellular filaments. (× 16,000; inset, × 80,000)

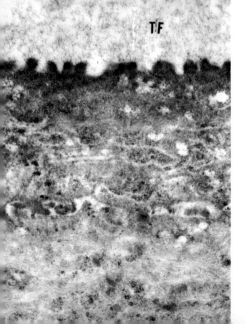

TF

FIG. 9–6. Surface cells of corneal epithelium. Anteriormost cell has its surface projections or microplicae exposed. **TF,** dried remains of tear film. (× 14,500)

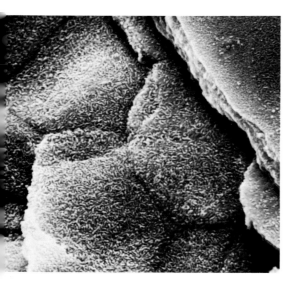

FIG. 9–7. Rabbit corneal epithelium fractured to show the surface microplicae of cells at all levels. Flattened surface cells are present in upper right. Apexes of wing and basal cells occupy most of the figure on left. (× 3600)

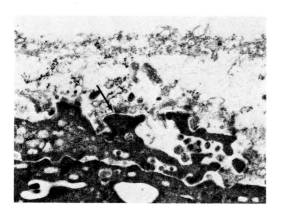

FIG. 9–8. Desquamating disintegrating superficial epithelial cell is distinguished easily from tear film by its recognizable cell fragments, e.g., filaments and particles. Note identifiable remains of a desmosome (**arrow**). (× 21,000)

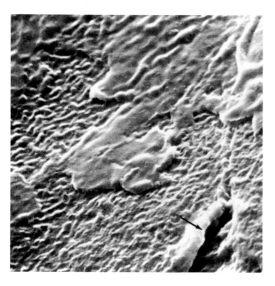

FIG. 9–9. Corneal surface as viewed by scanning electron microscope. Tear film (**above**) obscures surface microplicae that are more easily observed below. **Arrow.** Free edge of a flattened surface epithelial cell that has begun to peel away. (× 2000)

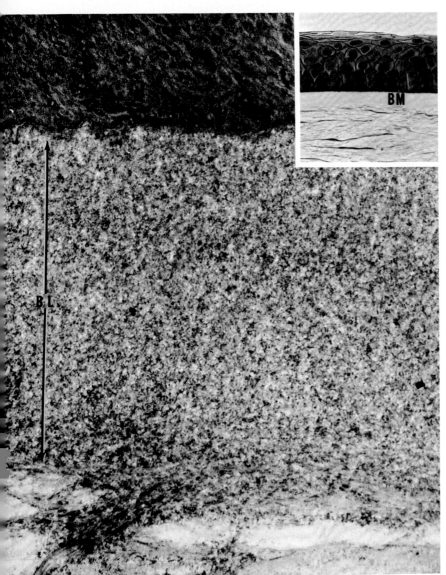

FIG. 9–10. Bowman's membrane or layer. By light microscopy (inset) structure appears as a membrane (**BM**). By electron microscopy it is a thick acellular layer of collagen fibrils in random distribution. **BL,** Bowman's layer. (× 8400) (Inset, Epon section, PD, × 300)

BM

BL

BOWMAN'S MEMBRANE (LAYER) AND STROMA

On the posterior (deep) side of the epithelial basement membrane lies the adjacent connective tissue layer. By light microscopy (inset, Fig. 9–10), this layer ~10–16μ thick is seen as a relatively homogeneous, acellular sheet known as **Bowman's membrane.** In reality, this zone, as seen by electron microscopy (11, 12, 14, 20), is a specialized layer resembling corneal stroma and not a true membrane. The layer is composed of collagen fibrils (Fig. 9–10) in random distribution, which, except for a slight difference in diameters,* are otherwise similar to those of the deeper stroma. Where it joins un-

derlying lamellar stroma, the "membrane" alters via a narrow transition zone in which the collagen fibrils aggregate into the first recognizable, obliquely arranged, collagenous lamellas of the superficial corneal stroma proper.

To avoid confusion in terminology and to specify the method used for a particular description, the term **Bowman's membrane** refers to this structure's

---

* Jakus (10) gives a range of 160–240 A diameter (peak ~190 A) for fibrils in Bowman's layer and 240–280 A diameter in the deeper stroma, with a slight increase in diameter to ~340 A near Descemet's membrane.

appearance by light microscopy, whereas **Bowman's layer** (12) refers to its appearance by electron microscopy. The transition into obliquely arranged stromal lamellas prevents the layer from being easily separated from the remainder of the stroma. The collagen of Bowman's membrane is produced prenatally by the corneal epithelium. Postnatally, therefore, if Bowman's membrane is destroyed it cannot be regenerated but rather is replaced by thickened epithelium ("epithelial facet") or by scar tissue.

The membrane or layer contains apertures inset, Fig. 9–11), pores, or canals to allow the corneal nerves to pass through to reach the epithelial cells. Groupings of these nonmyelinated neurites often are observed between adjacent basal epithelial cells (Fig. 9–11), but their canals through Bowman's layer and the appearance of their endings within the epithelium have not as yet been seen by electron microscopy.

Because the layer is normally acellular, one of the earliest pathologic alterations that may be noted is the appearance of one or more cell nuclei. Some cell migration between superficial stroma and epithelium may be aided by the presence of the normal apertures or pores that allow for passage of the corneal nerves.

The adjacent corneal stroma (approximately the anterior one-third) is arranged much like a flattened honeycomb into obliquely oriented bundles of collagen fibrils (Fig. 9–12) known as **lamellas.** Lying between the lamellas are the keratocytes (Fig. 9–12, 9–13), believed to represent fibrocytes that can become fibroblastic after appropriate stimulation (e.g., trauma [27]).

The keratocytes generally are recognized in H&E-stained sections by their very basophilic

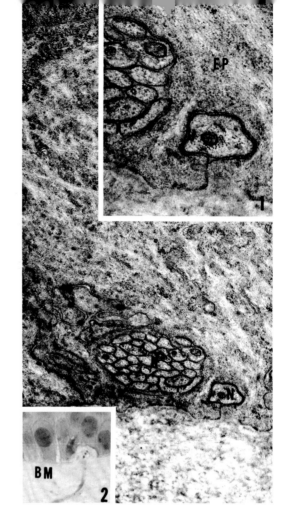

FIG. 9–11. Electron micrograph shows groups of neurites (**N**) present between adjacent epithelial cells. (× 16,000) Inset 1. Outer neurites in each group are enveloped only by adjacent epithelial cells (**EP**). (× 32,000) Inset 2. Light micrograph showing passage of presumed nerve fiber bundle through Bowman's membrane (**BM**). (Epon section, PD, × 575) (AFIP Neg. 66-6701)

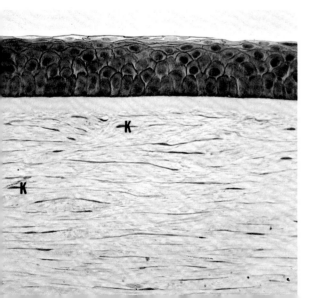

FIG. 9–12. Anterior corneal stroma composed of obliquely arranged collagenous lamellas. **K**, keratocytes. (Epon section, PD, × 300) (AFIP Neg. 67-5144).

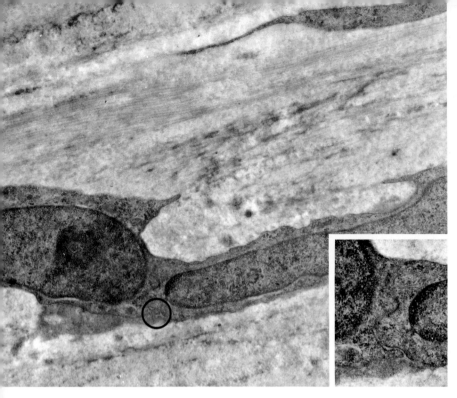

FIG. 9–13. Keratocytes lying between corneal stromal lamellas. Presence of two nuclei in main figure indicates either presence of two adjacent cells or sectioning of a bilobed or grossly folded nucleus. (× 16,000) Inset. A higher magnification of area circled in main figure shows typical intercellular space, which indicates that the two nuclei may belong to two separate but adjacent cells or a single cell folded. (× 25,000) (Modified from McTigue JS: Trans Am Ophthalmol Soc 65:591, 1967)

FIG. 9–14. Schematic representation of morphogenesis of corneal stroma. Stroma is formed by collagen-producing keratocytes, which surround themselves with collagen. This produces a flattened honeycomb-like arrangement, which is more prominent in anterior than in posterior corneal stroma.

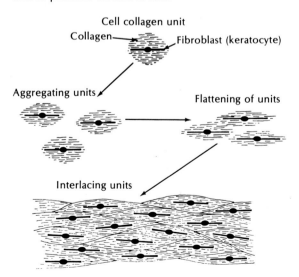

nuclei. Their cytoplasmic extensions are poorly seen by light microscopy but can be seen by electron microscopy to extend for enormous distances.

Artifactitious "clefting" of the stromal lamellas usually occurs from separation in the plane of the keratocytes. The lamellas themselves do not readily come apart. The concept of a flattened honeycomb-like arrangement (Fig. 9–14) in this region is further supported by the observation that artifactitious clefting does not extend for any great distance in any single plane. A corneal surgeon attempting a lamellar dissection or *keratectomy* at these superficial levels also appreciates this arrangement.

A single stromal lamella is made up of collagen fibrils of uniform diameter (~300 A or 30 nm)* in highly ordered array (Fig. 9–15). The various acid mucopolysaccharides, which occupy the interfibrillar spaces, are best visualized by applying to a conventional tissue section such light microscopic histochemical staining procedures as the colloidal iron (AMP) or alcian blue techniques. In electron micrographs the delicate weblike material that frequently may be observed spanning the interfibrillar spaces is

* The average diameter remains remarkably constant from 43 days of gestation (22).

interpreted as the drying patterns of these same acid mucopolysaccharides.

Patches of basement-membrane-like material are frequently observed in direct contact with the plasmalemma of keratocytes, especially in the peripheral cornea (Fig. 9–16). The material is occasionally observed to be filamentous. Close association of similar material with collagen fibrils produces a banded structure which may also be observed in the uveal meshwork (see Ch. 11).

Deeper within the stroma (at the approximate junction of the anterior one-third and posterior two-thirds) a transitional zone occurs. The lamellas become arranged more parallel to the corneal surface (Fig. 9–17), and therefore the long cytoplasmic extensions of the keratocytes can be traced with greater ease. The parallelism continues posteriorly to Descemet's membrane.

It has been generally and widely believed that the corneal layer equivalent to skin was limited to the epithelium. It appears, from the combined evidence of phylogeny (26), embryology (Fig. 9–18), histology, and biomicroscopy, that all the layers of the skin are represented in the anterior cornea. The epithelium, therefore, represents the epidermis, and the anterior third of corneal stroma, the dermis. The analogy can be carried even further, with Bowman's layer being represented by the loosely arranged (i.e., reticulin staining, collagen of the papillary layer of dermis, and the obliquely arranged lamellas of anterior corneal stroma by the densely arranged bundles of collagen that compose the "reticular" layer of the dermis. The deeper layers of corneal stroma would, therefore, represent the subcutaneous tissue. Vasculature, present in the skin, is, of course, normally absent in the cornea. The histologic difference between the arrangement of the anterior one-third and the posterior two-thirds of the corneal stroma (Fig. 9–19) is also well reflected by the normal biomicroscopic differences in relucency of these two zones (Fig. 9–20). These differences in relucency are exaggerated in early stromal edema (19), or in *congenital hereditary stromal dystrophy* (28) of the cornea. The *increase* in relucency anteriorly with swelling was apparently confusing because of experiments which indicated that swelling occurred more easily and to a greater degree in the posterior stroma. The anatomic arrangements of lamellar obliquity anteriorly and lamellar parallelism posteriorly appear to explain both the experimental and clinical observations. Corneal clouding or opacification is not synonymous with corneal edema.

ENDOTHELIUM AND DESCEMET'S MEMBRANE

Lining the posterior surface of the cornea (Fig. 9–21) and forming the anterior boundary of the anterior aqueous chamber is a single layer ($\sim$5 to 6μ thick) of flattened hexagonally arranged cells generally known as the corneal endothelium. The total number of endothelial cells lining the central cornea has been estimated *in vivo* by means of the clinical specular microscope and has been found to decrease with age (3). The cell density has been reported as 3015/sq mm in a 6-year-old central cornea and as a mean of 2776/sq mm in 40 normal corneas (range of 1547 to 4003/sq mm with ages from 74 years to 12 yrs, respectively [3]). The findings indicate that human corneal endothelial cells that are lost from the central region are replaced by spread, and thus thinning, of adjacent cells.

Proliferation of endothelial cells, however, does appear to occur when endothelium overgrows the drainage angle and the anterior border layer of the iris (31).

The "endothelium" is not a true endothelium (*i.e.,* lining a vascular or lymphatic channel), but a *mesothelium* (*i.e.,* resembling those cells that line such body cavities as peritoneum and pleural or pericardial clefts or spaces). Furthermore, cells called *mesothelia* frequently are considered to possess the property of readily undergoing alteration into fibroblasts, a property that is not widely attributed to true endothelia. If such is the case, then the concept becomes readily acceptable that this layer of cells produces connective tissue membranes, either normal or pathologic. On this basis, the peculiar changes observed in certain disease processes (Fuchs' endothelial dystrophy [15, 20] or congenital stationary hereditary dystrophy [16]) as well as the mysterious formation of *some* acellular retrocorneal fibrous membranes are more easily explained.

Like some epithelia, the endothelial cells are attached by densities to one another in a plane near the cell apex (Fig. 9–21). The attachment densities are apically located similar to terminal bars elsewhere. Here, however, they are somewhat discontinuous (Fig. 9–22) and are seen frequently in several parts, due to the overlapping flaps of adjacent endothelial cells (Fig. 9–23, 9–24). The adjacent cells, separated by intercellular spaces, are well interdigitated. No desmosomes are present. The basal plasmalemmas are quite flat, are closely applied to a thick

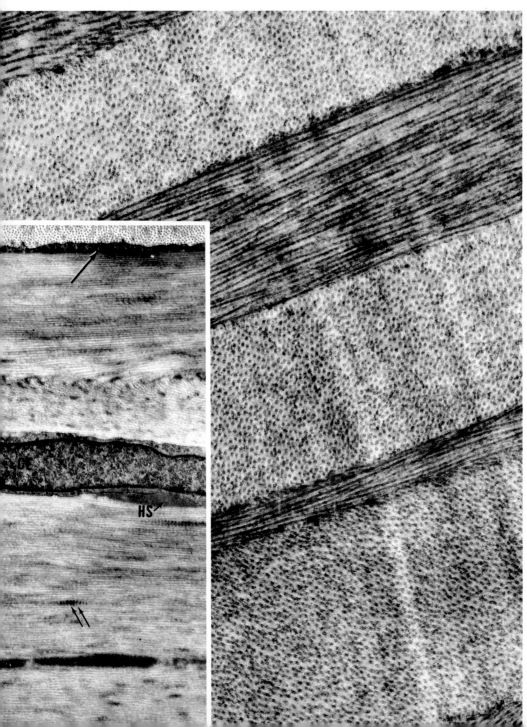

FIG. 9–15. Corneal stromal lamellas, showing arrangement of collagen fibrils. (× 18,000) Inset. Attenuated cytoplasm of a keratocyte (**single free arrow**) lies between lamellas; adjacent to a keratocyte cell body (**CE**) is a homogeneous substance (**HS**), and some collagenous aggregates (**free double arrows**) have a banded appearance. (× 11,000)

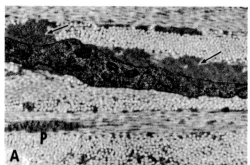
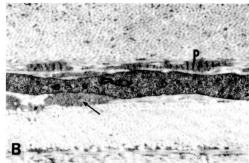

FIG. 9–16. Peripheral cornea. A. Extracellular masses of homogeneous basement-membrane-like material closely applied to keratocyte (**arrows**). Occasionally homogeneous extracellular material appears filamentous. Patches of similar material involving several collagen fibrils produce a banded pattern (**P**). (× 13,500) B. Another keratocyte with adjacent patches of basement-membrane-like material (**arrow**) and banded pattern (**P**). (× 16,000)

FIG. 9–17. Light micrograph of posterior cornea, showing more parallel arrangement of stromal lamellas. (Epon, PD, × 300) (AFIP Neg. 68-5145)

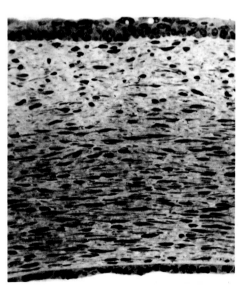

FIG. 9–18. Fetal cornea at 12 weeks' gestation. Stroma is clearly separable into anterior layer (one-third) and posterior layer (two-thirds). (Epon section, toluidine blue, × 220) (AFIP Neg. 71-876).

Mature cornea

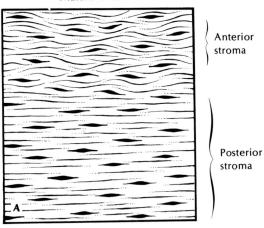

Anterior stroma

Posterior stroma

FIG. 9–19. Cornea. A. Arrangement of anterior and posterior corneal stromal lamellas. B. Scanning electron micrograph of cut surface of cornea, 28-year-old subject. Endothelium is present in lower left. Note how posterior corneal lamellas separate easily and widely from one another, compared to the compactness of the anterior stroma. (× 100)

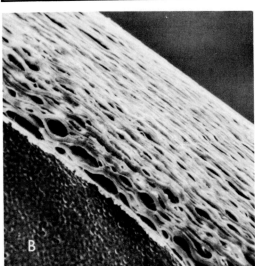

FIG. 9–20. Slit-lamp differences in zones of relucency of anterior and posterior corneal stroma.

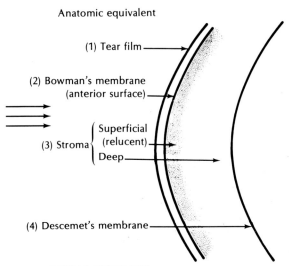

Anatomic equivalent

(1) Tear film

(2) Bowman's membrane (anterior surface)

(3) Stroma { Superficial (relucent) / Deep

(4) Descemet's membrane

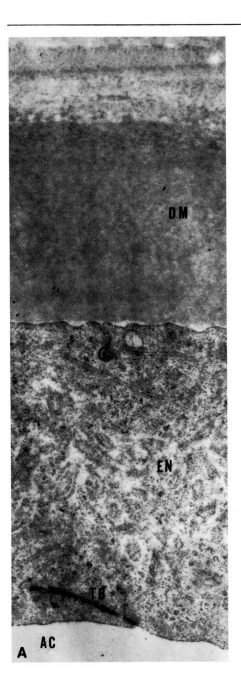

DM

EN

TB

AC

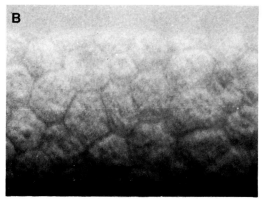

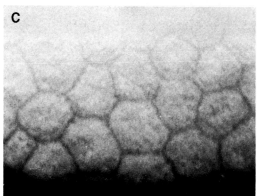

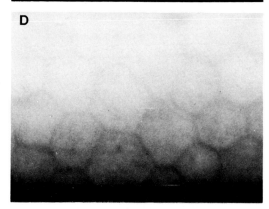

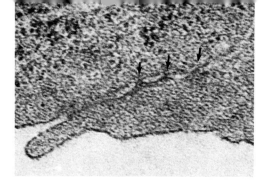

FIG. 9–22. Apexes of adjacent corneal endothelial cells. Overlapping endothelial flap of cell on right makes multiple attachments (**arrows**) to cell on left. (× 45,000)

FIG. 9–23. Scanning electron micrograph, showing overlapping flaps of adjacent corneal endothelial cells in corneal periphery of an adult. (× 18,000)

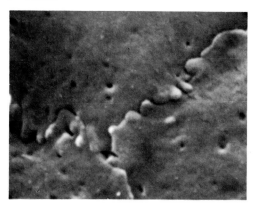

FIG. 9–24. Scanning electron micrograph, showing prominent overlapping flaps of adjacent corneal endothelial cells in corneal periphery of a newborn. (× 18,000)

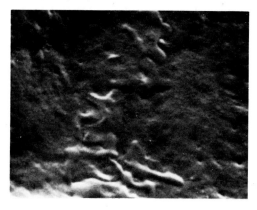

◄ **FIG. 9–21.** A. Corneal endothelium (**EN**) applied to Descemet's membrane (**DM**) and lining anterior chamber (**AC**). Endothelial cells are attached to each other by apical dense attachments (**TB**). (× 24,000) B–D. Endothelial cells as seen by clinical specular microscopy. B. 18-year-old (3400 cells/mm²). C. 69-year-old (2400 cells/ mm²). D. 83-year-old (1800 cells/mm²). (Courtesy of Dr. R. A. Laing)

basement membrane (Descemet's membrane), and are lacking in hemidesmosomes.

The only peculiarity of the cellular organelles is that of the mitochondria, which appear to possess a matrix of increased intracristal density accompanied by slight dilation of their intercristal spaces (Fig. 9–25) and so generally differ from mitochondria in other ocular tissue (except keratocytes) in their response to fixation.

Descemet's membrane, which closely resembles the lens capsule and the lamina vitrea of Bruch's membrane, has long been known as a typical ocular cuticular, glass, or PAS-positive membrane. Produced by the endothelium, the membrane is thin in infancy, increases in thickness to ~5μ in childhood, and then to ~8–10μ in adulthood (Fig. 9–26).

In the human (29), the beginnings of the thick basement membrane can be detected by the end of the second month of gestation when the mesenchymal cells have arranged themselves into a continuous sheet. By the fifth month of gestation, a multilaminar basement membrane clearly is evident. Compaction of the multilaminar membrane into a thick structure is evident by the eighth month, when the characteristic anterior banding of the adult is becoming noticeable in many areas.

Where Descemet's membrane joins the flat collagenous stromal lamellas, the deepest lamellas are slightly infiltrated by patches of basement-membrane-like material.

The anterior third or so of this thick basement membrane (the "oldest" portion and therefore the earliest to be laid down during embryonic or fetal life) possesses a peculiar structural arrangement (9). On sectioning, it presents an appearance of periodicity* that measures approximately 1000 A. Similar periodicity can be observed in other basement membranes both normal and abnormal (31) under certain conditions and planes of sectioning (Ch. 4).

The innermost (most posterior, "youngest," or latest) portion of Descemet's membrane appears quite homogeneous (except for a fine filamentous appearance that occurs under suitable conditions of fixation, sectioning, and resolution). Separation of this refractile "elastic," indigestible membrane into two or more

---

* More distinct in bovine (12) than in human eyes.

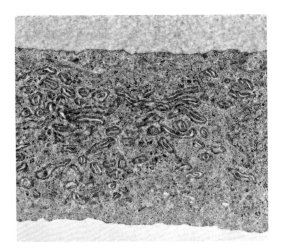

FIG. 9–25. Mitochondria of corneal endothelium with characteristically dilated, lucent intercristal spaces. (× 16,000)

layers not only is possible but also can be observed on occasion by light microscopic examination of the frayed ends of a break in it.

That Descemet's membrane is a secretory product of the endothelium is supported by the observations that a small, clean traumatic break in the membrane is bridged posteriorly by a new cuticular layer and the old cut ends are left curled slightly outward and separated (31). The location of the bridge, together with lack of interposition of another cell type (e.g., keratocyte) between it and the broken ends of the original membrane, clearly support the concept of synthesis and deposition by the overlying endothelium.

Additionally, the corneal "endothelium" can, in the adult, recreate its prenatal activities, at least in part, producing mounds of excess basement membrane, in which there also may be found foci of periodicity of ~500 A as well as ~1000 A in disarray. The mounds are considered a normal or physiologic aging change when they occur at the corneal periphery (Hassall-Henle warts, Fig. 9–35, 36) but are considered abnormal when they occur in the central or axial cornea (cornea guttata). Similar changes also can occur during the process of corneal repair following severe injury, or in certain disease processes in which proliferation of the endothelium over the adjacent drainage angle and iris stroma is often accompanied by the secretion of a new thick basement membrane layer on these surfaces ("endothelialization of the anterior chamber angle" [31]).

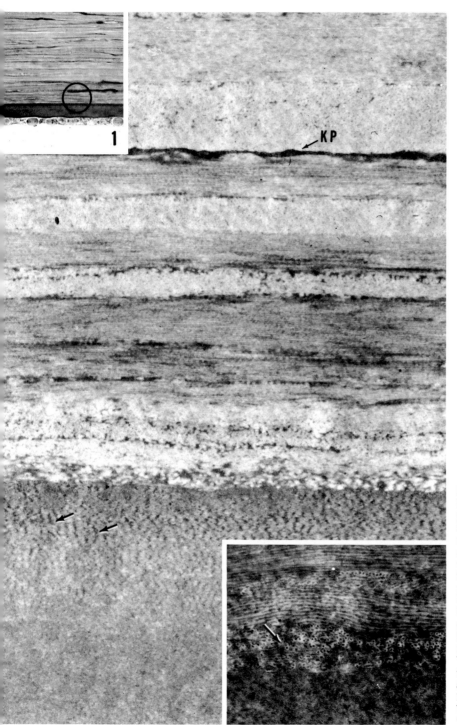

FIG. 9–26. Descemet's membrane. Electron micrograph of region comparable to that circled in inset 1. Stromal lamellas are flat and arranged relatively parallel to one another. Attenuated keratocyte processes (**KP**) extend for long distances. Characteristic periodicity (~1000 A) of anterior portion of Descemet's membrane can be seen at **free arrows.** (× 18,000) Inset 1. Light micrograph of posterior corneal stroma, Descemet's membrane, and corneal endothelium. (Epon section, PD, × 300) Inset 2. There is slight blending (**at arrow**) of this thick basement membrane with adjacent collagenous fibrils. (× 53, 700) (Modified from McTigue JW: Trans Am Ophthalmol Soc 65:591, 1967)

The preceding description has been limited for the most part to a typical example of central cornea examined from front to back. The following description is that of the cornea examined from the center to the periphery.

With age, and somewhat variable from person to person of the same age, the epithelial basement membrane increases in thickness from that of the typical thin basement membrane of the infant (Fig. 9–27) to the appearance of a multilaminar configuration with suggestive basal cell processes in the young adult (21) (Fig. 9–28). In the aged, a serrated appearance of mounds of basement membrane may appear (Fig. 9–29), or uniform masses of thickened multilaminar basement membrane containing many villous processes of the basal cells (Fig. 9–30) can often be appreciated in conventional light-microscopic sections treated with the PAS reaction (Fig. 9–31).

Peculiar banded fibrils (5, 21, 23), may be seen within the thickened basement membrane. In the skin, they often are referred to as "anchoring fibrils," but such a function for them has yet to be demonstrated. It is likely that the interweaving of the basal cell processes and their associated hemidesmosomes with the thickened multilaminar basement membrane is sufficient anatomic basis for the strong adherence of corneal epithelium to underlying Bowman's layer in this region.

The presence of foci of calcification ("spherules") within the thickened peripheral basement membrane in older, otherwise normal eyes (Fig. 9–32) suggests that the abnormal process of *calcific band keratopathy* is but an exaggeration of a normal process, an exaggeration accelerated by such other factors as chronic inflammation.

Posteriorly, proceeding from the center of the cornea to its periphery, there is again a change in the relation of cell to basement membrane (Fig. 9–33). As the corneal periphery is approached (Fig. 9–34), basil villi of the endothelial cells are seen projecting into the adjacent thick basement membrane (Descemet's membrane). The villi lack any form of "attachment" structure. The endothelial cells become slightly attenuated and the basement membrane is thicker focally. At the periphery, the foci of

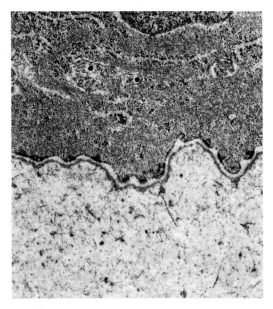

FIG. 9–27. Thin epithelial basement membrane of 4-month-old infant at periphery of cornea. (× 20,000)

FIG. 9–28. Peripheral corneal basement membrane of 28-year-old subject shows early multilaminar formation and associated basal cell processes. Note presence of hemidesmosomes.(× 14, 000)

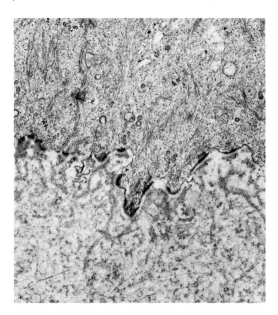

FIG. 9–29. Corneal basement membrane. A. Light micrograph, showing serrated appearance of basal cells of epithelium along periphery of Bowman's membrane (**BM**). **Arrow,** tapered end of Bowman's membrane. (Epon section, PD × 400) (AFIP Neg. 72-5647) B. Transmission electron micrograph shows thickened multilaminar basement membrane forming mounds between basal cell processes in an aged (76-year-old) eye. (× 18,500)

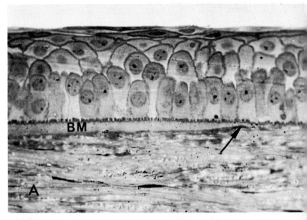

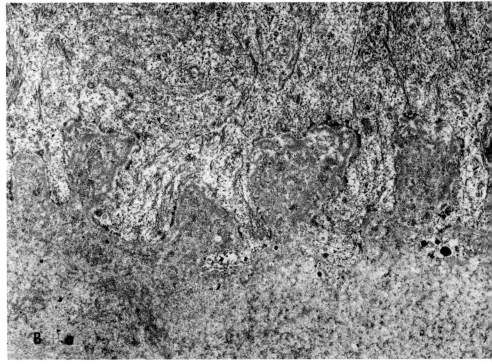

basement membrane thickening are so large (inset, Fig. 9–34) that they are easily appreciated by light microscopy as the warts of Hassall-Henle. The cell bodies containing their nuclei are located along the slopes or in the valleys between these excrescences, which are covered by an extremely attenuated endothelial cytoplasm (Fig. 9–35, 9–36). Myriad endothelial villi project into the fissures of these basement membrane accumulations (6, 12, 15, 20) (Fig. 9–35). In some instances the fissure appears to be occupied by dense globules, which are in-terpreted as degenerated fragments of pinched off cytoplasmic villi.

Exaggeration of the "physiologic" or aging process at the periphery of Descemet's membrane into the central cornea gives rise to the entity known clinically as **cornea guttata.** This condition can be identified clinically in its earliest stages by defects in the endothelial pattern noted on biomicroscopic examination (specular reflection). The defects result from displacement of the endothelium posteriorly from the plane of reflection by the enlarging foci of wartlike material. The pathologic warts or excre-

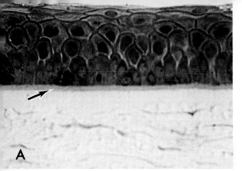

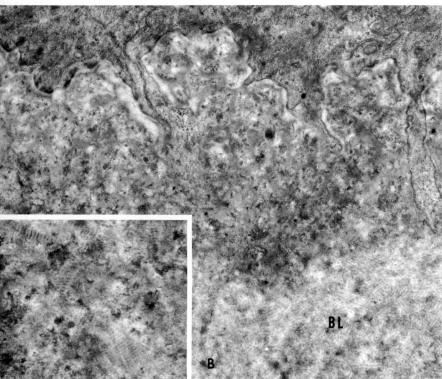

FIG. 9–30. Epithelial basement membrane, cornea. A. Light micrograph showing uniformly thick epithelial basement membrane (**arrow**) present at corneal periphery. (Epon section, PD, × 395) (AFIP Neg. 66–3320) (McTigue JW, Fine BS: In Uyeda R (ed): Proceedings, Sixth International Congress for Electron Microscopy, Kyoto, Japan, 1966, Vol. 2. Tokyo, Maruzen, 1966) B. Electron micrograph, showing long villi of basal epithelial cells projecting into thick, multilaminar, basement membrane at corneal periphery. BL, collagen fibrils of Bowman's layer. (× 16,000) Inset. Peculiar banded fibrils scattered within this basement membrane. (× 32,000)

FIG. 9–31. Variation in basement membrane (**arrows**) thickness of central cornea (**A**) compared with peripheral cornea (**B**) from same section. (PAS, × 900) (AFIP Neg. 65-12184 and 65-13102) (Modified from McTigue JW: Trans Am Ophthalmol Soc 65:591, 1967)

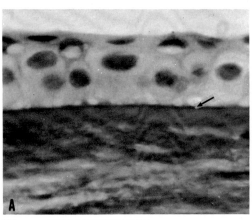

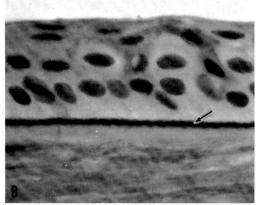

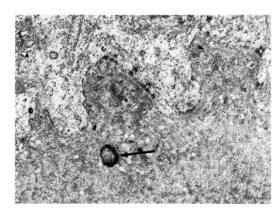

FIG. 9–32. Calcific spherule (**arrow**) present in aging multilaminar basement membrane at corneal periphery. (× 20,000)

FIG. 9–33. Typical relation of corneal endothelium to Descemet's membrane in central cornea. **D,** Descemet's membane. **N,** nucleus of endothelial cell; **TB,** terminal attachment density. Inset. Light micrograph of corneal endothelium and Descemet's membrane. (× 16,000) (Inset, H&E, × 575) (AFIP Neg. 65-237) (Modified from McTigue JW: Trans Am Ophthalmol Soc 65:591, 1967)

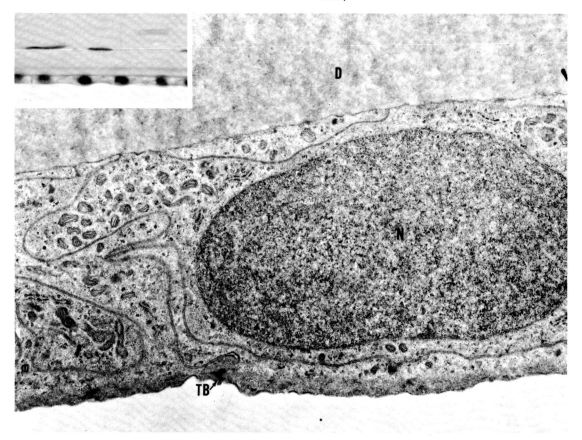

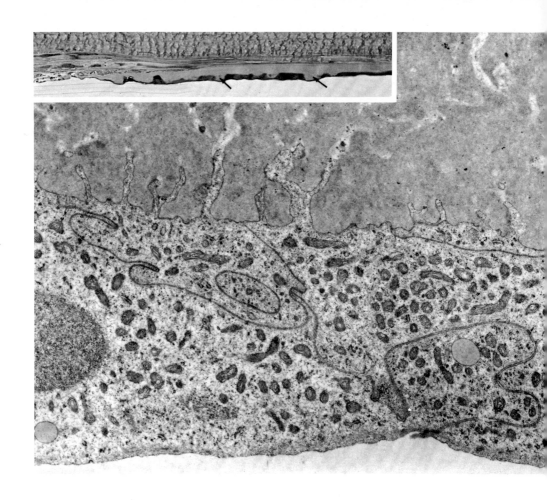

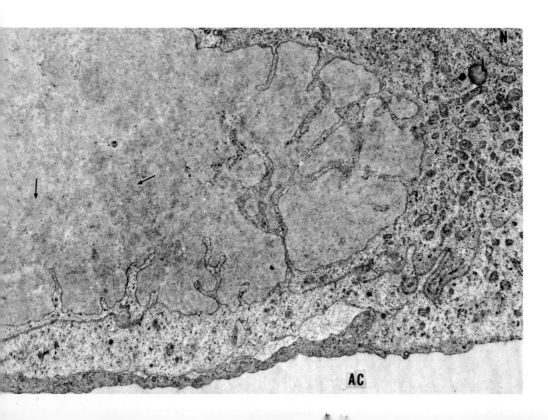

FIG. 9–34 Relations of corneal endothelium to Descemet's membrane in
peripheral cornea. Light micrograph
(**inset**) shows Descemet's membrane
with a number of excrescences, *i.e.,*
Hassall-Henle warts (**arrows**). Electron
micrograph shows fissuring of Descemet's membrane. Many processes of
endothelial cells lie within fissures.
Debris of cytoplasmic processes remain
within distal portions of fissures.
(× 10,500; inset, Epon section, PD,
× 220) (AFIP Neg. 66-1291)

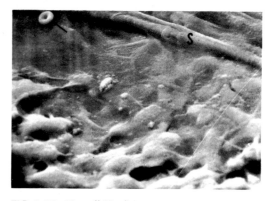

FIG. 9–36. Hassall-Henle warts as seen
by SEM. Schwalbe's line (**S**) is seen
above at extreme corneal periphery.
Arrow, isolated red blood cell lying on
corneal endothelium. (× 310)

scenses differ somewhat in morphologic composition from those normally present in the corneal
periphery. The pathologic warts contain more
prominent patches of basement membrane material
of 1000-A periodicity, a material reminiscent of the
"oldest" portions of Descemet's membrane, and
suggest a reversion of the cells to some of their
"fetal-like" activities. The combination of cornea
guttata and epithelial changes is known clinically as
Fuchs' combined dystrophy (31).

The extreme periphery of Descemet's membrane forms a ring or line, if observed in three
dimensions (*in vivo*) known as **Schwalbe's ring
(anterior border ring) or line.** Not infrequently
this line is thickened by basement membrane,
collagenous connective tissue, or a mixture of
the two (Fig. 9–37). Since endothelium (*i.e.,*
mesothelium) here has the potential to elaborate these materials, other sources need not be
strongly considered (see section on the drainage angle, Ch. 11).

A similar arrangement of mesothelium ("endothelium") basement membrane and collagenous connective tissue is carried over into the
adjacent trabecular meshwork (Fig. 9–38).

FIG. 9–35. Portion of Hassall-Henle
wart at extreme corneal periphery.
Endothelial cells are attenuated over
wart. Many endothelial cytoplasmic
processes lie within more recently
elaborated basement membrane excrescences. A suggestion of periodicity
within basement membrane is present
(**arrows**). A lipofuscin granule (**L**) is present within endothelial cell. **AC,** anterior
chamber; **N,** nucleus of endothelial cell.
(× 11,000)

THE LIMBUS

By definition the **limbus** refers to the *line* of
transition between clear cornea and opaque
sclera. The line forms an arc with a longer
radius of curvature in the vertical axis than in
the horizontal axis. The arcuate line of transition
is seen easily *in vivo* by using a gonioscopic
lens. Histologically, the line is not always so
apparent. Because many important structures
are to be found in the vicinity of the line, it is
useful to characterize a limbal *region* or *zone*
for histologic purposes. The anterior boundary
of a limbal zone or region therefore may be
defined usefully on a conventional histologic
tissue section as a straight line joining the end
of Bowman's membrane with the end of Descemet's membrane (Fig. 9–39 A). The posterior
boundary may be defined usefully as a parallel
line drawn through the posterior edge of the
scleral roll (spur). The zone, therefore, would
contain such important structures as the entire
opening to the drainage angle, the inner and
outer scleral sulci and much of the intrascleral
vascular plexus.

The description of a *surgical* limbus varies somewhat from one investigator to another.

In the region of the limbus several changes
take place in the epithelium. The corneal epithelium more than doubles in thickness as it
approaches the sclera to become conjunctival
epithelium (Fig. 9–39 B). In darkly pigmented
individuals the basal cells contain melanin

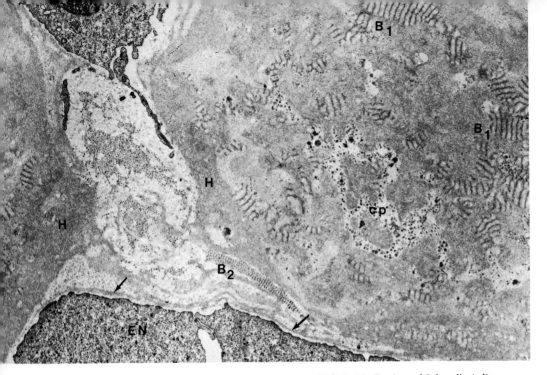

FIG. 9–37. Region of Schwalbe's line shows production of basement membrane in disarray. Note presence of thin basement membranes (**arrows**), homogeneous basement membrane (**H**), and banded basement membrane of both ~1000 A periodicity (**B₁**) and ~500 A periodicity (**B₂**). Debris of cell processes is still present within the mass (**cp**). **EN,** corneal endothelial cells. (× 16,500)

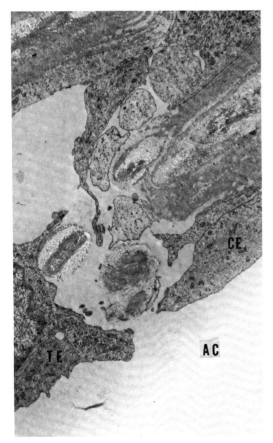

FIG. 9–38. Region of Schwalbe's line or ring where corneal endothelium (**CE**) alters to become endothelium of trabecular meshwork (**TE**). **AC,** anterior chamber. (× 5,400)

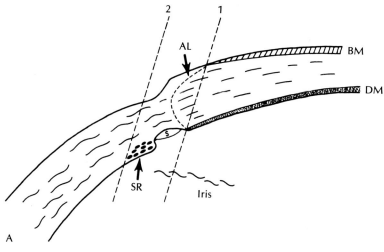

A

FIG. 9–39. Limbus. A. Histologically useful diagram of limbus. Line from end of Bowman's membrane (**BM**) to end of Descemet's membrane (**DM**) forms anterior border (**line 1**); parallel drawn through posterior edge of scleral roll (spur) forms posterior border (**line 2**). **AL,** arcuate line of *true* limbus; **S,** canal of Schlemm in inner scleral sulcus; **SR,** scleral roll. B. Transition of corneal epithelium on left to a thicker conjunctival epithelium on right takes place at end of Bowman's membrane (**arrow**). Note transition of regular, layered collagenous lamellas of cornea on the left to wavy, irregular collagenous lamellas of sclera on right. Vessels are present in tissues beneath the conjunctival epithelium. (H&E, × 115) (AFIP Neg. 62-2044)

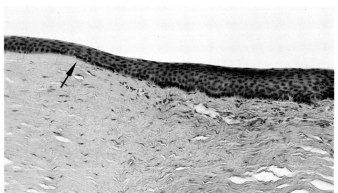

B

FIG. 9–40. Limbal epithelial basal cell in an infant. Clusters of small ovoid melanin granules are present within the apical cytoplasm. Note desmosomal attachments to adjacent cells (**arrows**). (× 16,000)

FIG. 9–41. Intraepithelial dendritic melanocyte lies freely between basal cells and lacks desmosomal attachments; **bm,** thin basement membrane of basal cells; **D,** desmosome of basal cells. (× 20,000)

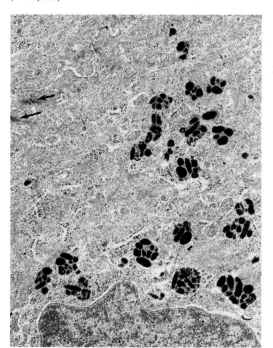

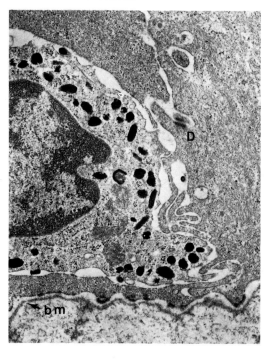

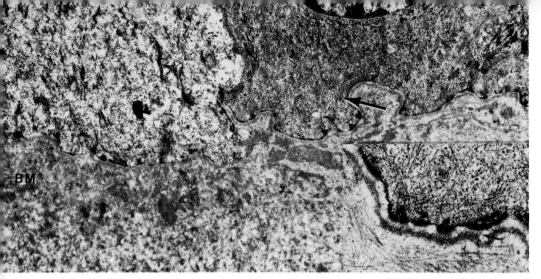

BM

FIG. 9–42. Limbus. Transition from corneal epithelium on the left to conjunctival epithelium on the right. A poorly formed multilaminar basement membrane (**M–BM**) lies beneath the corneal epithelial basal cell, while a typical thin basement membrane (**arrow**) lies beneath the conjunctival epithelial basal cell (× 5500). The inset shows conjunctival thin basement membrane and prominent hemidesmosomes. The hemidesmosomal cement substance is clearly seen at the **free arrow.** (× 30,000)

granules that are located characteristically in small clusters within the apical cytoplasm (Fig. 9–40). Dendritic melanocytes may also be present between the epithelial basal cells (Fig. 9–41).

Dendritic melanocytes here, as in epidermis, characteristically lie anterior to the epithelial basement membrane and lack desmosomal attachments. They, therefore, are free to wander between the somewhat loosened basal cells of the conjunctival epithelium. Langerhans' cells with their characteristic "tennis-racket" shaped granules have been described in this region (25).

There is abrupt transition of the basement membrane from the thickened multilaminar variety of the peripheral corneal epithelium to the typical thin basement membrane of the conjunctival epithelium (Fig. 9–42).

In the region of transition from cornea to conjunctiva, the epithelium is transformed rapidly into a more loosely arranged tissue, but the cells continue to be attached by desmosomes (Fig. 9–43). Degenerating cells about to desquamate are more commonly seen here than in the corneal epithelium.

Peripherally, where limbal epithelium becomes more noticeably conjunctival in nature, unicellular mucus-secreting glands or **goblet cells** (17, 24) appear (Fig. 9–44). They are more numerous nasally than in the other quadrants (17).

Beneath the epithelium lies a loose connective tissue (substantia propria) containing numerous nonfenestrated capillaries, lymphatics with their characteristic patchy or indistinct basement membranes, and a variety of cells, fibroblasts, and not infrequently, mast cells (8) with their highly characteristic granules (Fig. 9–45), which contain heparin and histamine.

Patches of variegated dense material also may be present in the substantia propria of normal eyes (Fig. 9–46). The material may represent either degenerating elastic tissue or foci of elastotic degeneration of collagen. Similar material has been described in the sclera as elastic fibers.

THE SCLERA

The white, collagenous sclera forms approximately five-sixths of the outer coat of the eye, with a radius of curvature of ~12 mm. As previously mentioned, the anteriormost one-fifth of this ocular layer is highly modified into the transparent cornea. Uniting the sclera to the cornea is a transition line or zone, the limbus, described above. Like the cornea, the sclera is composed mostly of extracellular materials.

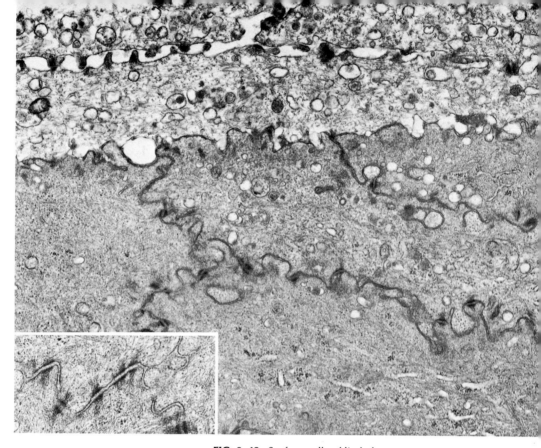

FIG. 9–43. Surface cells of limbal transitional epithelium. Desquamating surface cells are lucent and beginning to fragment. Note myriad desmosomes in underlying viable cells (better seen in inset). (× 18,000; inset × 30,000)

FIG. 9–44. Mucus-secreting goblet cell from bulbar conjunctiva. Mucus granules are being discharged onto the conjunctival surface. (× 6,000)

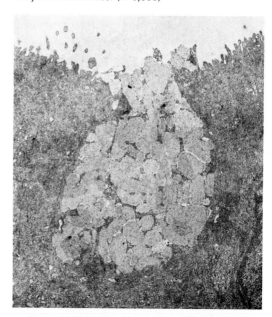

EMISSARIA

Vessels and nerves pass through canals or **emissaria** in varying degrees of obliquity en route to and from the interior of the eye. In addition to vessels and nerves, the emissaria contain uveal tissue that may be heavily pigmented in deeply pigmented individuals.

It is possible to have uveal nevi located partly or wholly within scleral canals. The emissaria may provide an avenue by which neoplasms, such as malignant melanomas of the uvea, and inflammations, such as sympathetic uveitis, may emerge from the globe.

Melanocyte-containing uveal tissue may extend out of the emissaria onto the scleral surface or episclera and in the living eye be clearly viewed anteriorly through the transparent conjunctiva. Episcleral uveal tissue, called **pigment spots** of the sclera (30), may be present 3–4 mm from the limbus. The spots are most commonly seen in eyes with darkly pigmented irises, usually in the superior episclera. Inferior,

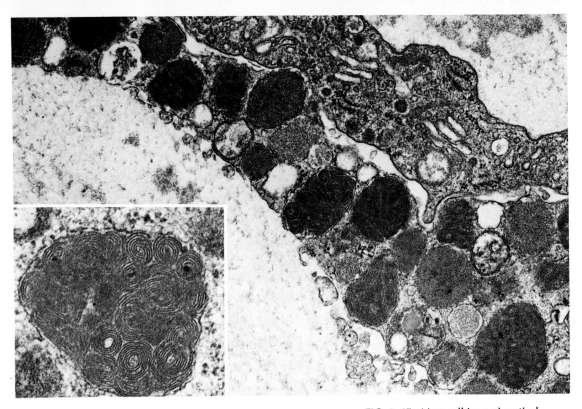

FIG. 9–45. Mast cell in conjunctival subepithelial tissues of limbus. Some granules contain a finely granular material while others contain the characteristic whorled or lamellar structures. The latter granule is seen at higher magnification in the inset. (× 24,500; inset × 55,000)

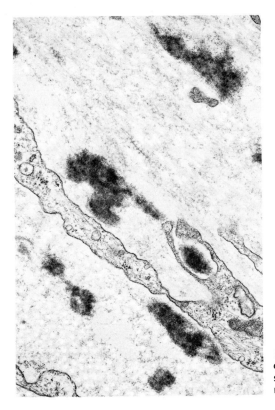

FIG. 9–46. Patches of dense material commonly present in conjunctival subepithelial tissues of young, otherwise normal eye. (× 16,200)

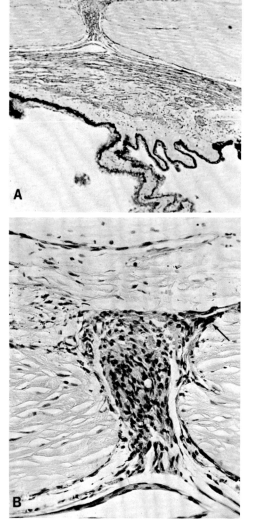

A

B

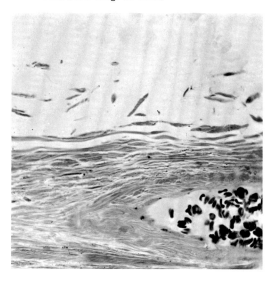

FIG. 9–47. A. Nerve loop of Axenfeld. (H&E, × 47) B. Higher magnification shows uveal tissue (**arrows**) in episclera. (H&E, × 125)

FIG. 9–48. Outer layers of scleral lamellas. A large blood vessel is passing through sclera. (Epon section, PD, × 305) (AFIP Neg. 63-6902)

FIG. 9–49. Scanning electron micrograph of full thickness of posterior fetal sclera to show its collagenous arrangement. (× 240)

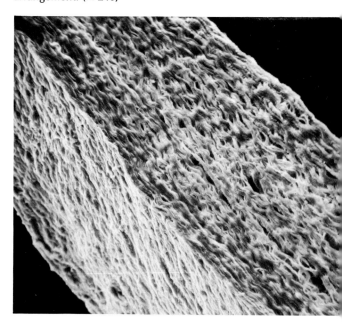

FIG. 9–50. Dense, interlacing collagenous lamellas of sclera. A large intrascleral nerve is present. (Epon section, PD, × 485) (AFIP Neg. 63-6900)

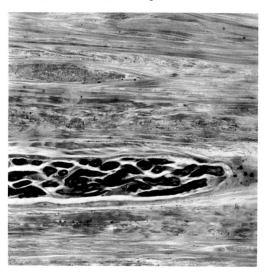

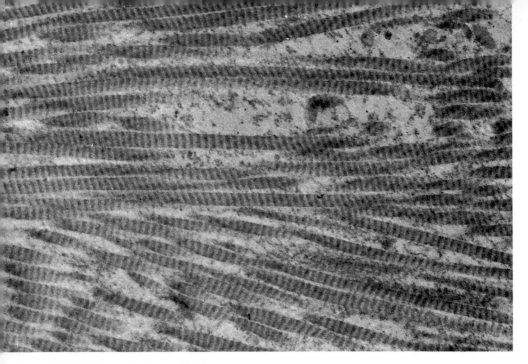

FIG. 9–51. Scleral collagen fibrils (longitudinal). ($\times$ 27,200)

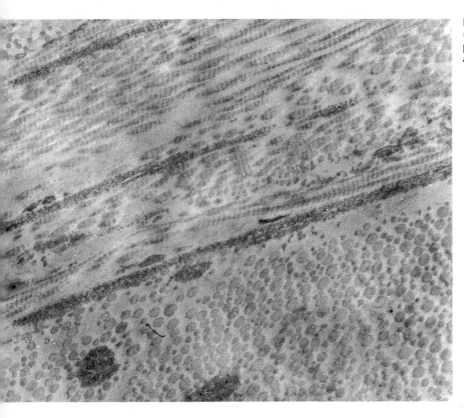

FIG. 9–52. Scleral collagen fibrils (oblique and cross-section). Dark patches are generally considered to be a form of elastic tissue. ($\times$ 24,000)

temporal, and nasal episcleral spots occur in decreasing frequency.

Largest among the apertures for the passage of nerves, arteries, and veins in the sclera is the one for the optic nerve. It lies just nasal to the posterior pole (Fig. 5–6) and is surrounded by a cluster of smaller apertures for passage of the adjacent short posterior ciliary arteries to the choroid. In the horizontal meridian are two additional oblique apertures for the passage of the two long posterior ciliary arteries and accompanying long ciliary nerves. The corresponding veins (vortex veins) that drain the posterior uveal tract traverse the sclera in the four posterior quadrants (Fig. 5–6).

Anteriorly, just behind the limbus but still well within the sclera, the anterior ciliary arteries perforate to reach the ciliary muscle. Approximately seven anterior ciliary arteries are derived from the blood supply to the four rectus muscles; the lateral rectus has the single vessel. The associated anterior ciliary veins are approximately 14 in number, at least two of which accompany each artery. Pigment spots are generally associated with perforating anterior ciliary vessels.

Branches or loops of the long ciliary nerves (nerve loop of Axenfeld, Fig. 9–47) often penetrate or even perforate the sclera just behind the limbus to form a small, often pigmented episcleral nodule.

These pigment spots and intrascleral nerve loops may be confused with nevi, cysts, or extensions of adjacent or underlying malignant melanomas. On clinical examination, the conjunctiva is freely movable over episcleral pigment spots, and the intrascleral nerve loops remain painful to touch even after the instillation of a topical anesthetic.

The collector channels from the canal of Schlemm perforate the sclera via a tortuous path through the region of the limbus. As mentioned in Chapter 11, some of these unite with anterior ciliary veins within the substance of the sclera (intrascleral plexus), whereas others reach the surface of the limbus (episclera) to appear clinically as aqueous veins.

EPISCLERA

The term episclera refers to the few loose, vascularized surface layers of scleral collagen beneath Tenon's capsule. Its vascularity differen-

tiates it from the avascular Tenon's capsule and its looser texture from scleral stroma.

STROMA

The stroma (Figs. 9–48 to 9–50) consists of obliquely arranged, interlacing bundles of collagen fibrils with a paucity of cells. By electron microscopy the fibrils possess the 640-A axial periodicity (Fig. 9–51) similar to corneal collagen but differ in their *nonuniformity* of fibril diameter (12) (Fig. 9–52). Patches of elastic tissue are scattered throughout the collagenous bundles (13). A combination of oblique arrangement, variability in collagen fibril diameter (32), and relative deficiency in water-binding substances probably helps account for scleral opacification.

It long has been known that white, opaque sclera, if dehydrated *in vitro*, becomes significantly translucent but not transparent.

A special circumferential arrangement of collagen fibrils is present at the posterior margin of the inner scleral sulcus (scleral roll); this is described in detail in Chapter 11.

The sclera is thickest at the posterior pole (~1.0 mm), thinner at the equator (~0.4–0.5 mm), and thinnest (~0.3 mm) just beneath the attachments for the rectus muscles (Fig. 9–53). With addition of the rectus muscle tendons, the thickness doubles to ~0.6 mm, and this

FIG. 9–53. Doubling of thickness of sclera at attachment of a rectus muscle. (H&E, × 35) (AFIP Neg. 70-1422)

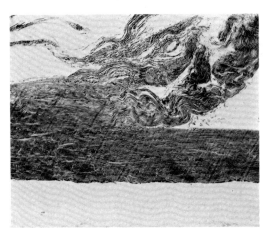

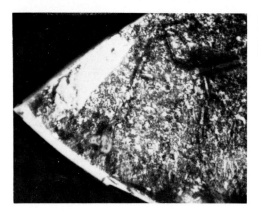

FIG. 9–54. Gross photograph of lamina fusca. Mechanical removal of choroid leaves thin pigmented layer attached to sclera.

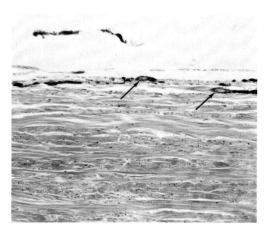

FIG. 9–55. Lamina fusca of sclera, formed by the few pigmented cells (**arrows**) that remain adherent to sclera after separation of choroid. (Epon section, PD, × 305) (AFIP Neg. 63-6901)

FIG. 9–56. Lamina fusca of sclera (**arrows**). Lamina is difficult to appreciate in sections where choroid has not separated from sclera. **SC,** interlacing bundles of scleral collagen. (H&E, × 265) (AFIP Neg. 68-9953)

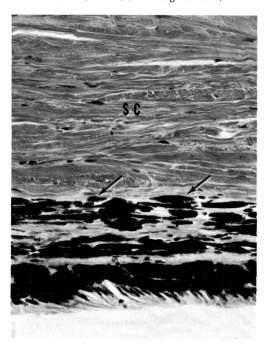

thickness continues to the limbus, where the sclera is again thinned, and thereby weakened, by the circumferential furrows (outer and inner scleral sulci).

The two "thin" regions of the sclera are of clinical importance. The surgeon engaged in muscle surgery must be constantly aware of the thinness of the sclera beneath the muscle attachment, to avoid penetrating the globe. Because of the two circumferential furrows present in the limbic area, that part of the globe is vulnerable to rupture in a contusion injury.

LAMINA FUSCA

If all the loose inner layers of an opened eye are stripped away from the sclera, the inner scleral surface remains pigmented (Fig. 9–54). In sections (Fig. 9–55), these few pigmented inner layers (**lamina fusca**) appear less conspicuous. They contain a number of scattered uveal melanocytes, which appear less flattened than those of the adjacent choroidal layers (Fig. 9–56). Their less conspicuous appearance, in sections, may give the false impression that this surface in the gross specimen should be less pigmented than it actually shows.

REFERENCES

1. Blümke S, Morgenroth K Jr: The stereo ultrastructure of the external and internal surface of the cornea. J Ultrastruct Res 18:502, 1967
2. Blümke S, Niedorf HR, Rode J, Kudszus G: Feinstrukturelle Veränderungen des Corneaepithels in der Gewebekultur. III. Die Desmosomen. Z Zellforsch 84:189, 1968
3. Bourne WM, Kaufman HE: Specular microscopy of human corneal endothelium in vivo. Am J Ophthalmol 81:319, 1976
4. Bourne WM, Kaufman HE: The endothelium of clear corneal transplants. Arch Ophthalmol 94:1730, 1976
5. Bruns RR: A symmetrical extracellular fibril. J Cell Biol 42:418, 1969
6. Feeney ML, Garron LK: Descemet's membrane in the human peripheral cornea: a study by light and electron microscopy. In Smelser GK (ed): The Structure of the Eye. New York, Academic Press, 1961, p 367
7. Gipson IK, Anderson RA: Actin filaments in normal and migrating corneal epithelial cells. Invest Ophthalmol 16:161, 1977
8. Iwamoto T, Smelser GK: Electron microscopic studies of the mast cells and blood and lymphatic capillaries of the human corneal limbus. Invest Ophthalmol 4:815, 1965
9. Jakus MA: Studies on the cornea. II. The fine structure of Descemet's membrane. J Biophys Biochem Cytol 2 [Suppl]:243, 1956
10. Jakus MA: The fine structure of the human cornea. In Smelser GK (ed): The Structure of the Eye. New York, Academic Press, 1961, p 343
11. Jakus MA: Further observations on the fine structure of the cornea. Invest Ophthalmol 1:202, 1962
12. Jakus MA: Ocular Fine Structure: Selected Electron Micrographs. Boston, Little, Brown, 1964
13. Kanai A, Kaufman HE: Electron microscopic studies of the elastic fiber in human sclera. Invest Ophthalmol 11:816, 1972
14. Kayes J, Holmberg A: The fine structure of Bowman's layer and the basement membrane of the corneal epithelium. Am J Ophthalmol 50:1013, 1960
15. Kayes J, Holmberg A: The fine structure of the cornea in Fuchs' endothelial dystrophy. Invest Ophthalmol 3:47, 1964
16. Kenyon KR, Maumenee AE: The histological and ultrastructural pathology of congenital hereditary corneal dystrophy: a case report. Invest Ophthalmol 7:475, 1968
17. Kessing SV: Mucous gland system of the conjunctiva —a quantitative normal anatomical study. Thesis, Copenhagen, 1968
18. Khodadoust AA, Silverstein AM, Kenyon KR, Dowling JE: Adhesion of regenerating corneal epithelium: the role of the basement membrane. Amer J Ophthalmol 65:339, 1968
19. Kikkawa Y, Hirayama K: Uneven swelling of the corneal stroma. Invest Ophthalmol 9:735, 1970
20. McTigue JW: The human cornea: a light and electron microscopic study of the normal cornea and its alterations in various dystrophies. Trans Am Ophthal Soc 65:591, 1967
21. McTigue JW, Fine BS: The basement membrane of the corneal epithelium. In Uyeda R (ed): Proceedings, Sixth International Congress for Electron Microscopy, Kyoto, Japan, 1966, vol 2. Tokyo, Maruzen, 1966, p 775
22. Ozanics V, Rayborn M, Sagun D: Some aspects of corneal and scleral differentiation in the primate. Exp Eye Res 22:305, 1976
23. Palade GE, Farquhar MG: A special fibril of the dermis. J Cell Biol 27:215, 1965
24. Ralph RA: Conjunctival goblet cell density in normal and dry eye syndromes. Invest Ophthalmol 14:299, 1975
25. Sugiura S, Matsuda H: Ultrastructure of Langerhans' cells in human corneal limbus. Trans Soc Ophthal Jap 72:2435, 1968
26. Walls GL: The vertebrate eye and its adaptive radiation. Cranbrook Institute Science Bulletin, No. 19, 1942
27. Weimer V: The transformation of corneal stromal cells to fibroblasts in corneal wound healing. Am J Ophthalmol 44:173, 1957
28. Witschell H, Fine BS, Grützner P, McTigue JW: Congenital hereditary stromal dystrophy of the cornea. A clinico-pathologic study. Arch Ophthalmol 96:1043, 1978
29. Wulle KG: Electron microscopy of the fetal development of the corneal endothelium and Descemet's Membrane of the human eye. Invest Ophthalmol 11:897, 1972
30. Yanoff M: Pigment spots of the sclera. Arch Ophthalmol 81:151, 1969
31. Yanoff M, Fine BS: Ocular Pathology: A Text and Atlas. Hagerstown, Harper & Row, 1975
32. Zinn KM: Changes in corneal ultrastructure resulting from early lens removal in the developing chick embryo. Invest Ophthalmol 9:165, 1970

chapter 10

THE UVEAL TRACT

THE IRIS   197

  UVEAL (MESODERMAL) PORTION   198

    ANTERIOR BORDER LAYER

    THE STROMA

  RETINAL (NEUROEPITHELIAL) PORTION   203

    SPHINCTER MUSCLE

    CLUMP CELLS

    DILATOR MUSCLE

    PIGMENT EPITHELIUM

THE CHOROID   215

  SUPRACHOROIDAL SPACE AND LAMINA
          FUSCA   215

  CHOROIDAL STROMA   216

    PIGMENTED AND NONPIGMENTED CELLS

    VESSELS

    BRUCH'S MEMBRANE

THE CILIARY BODY   226

  ZONES   226

  COMPONENTS   226

    RETINAL (NEUROEPITHELIAL) PORTION

      NONPIGMENTED EPITHELIUM AND INTERNAL
        BASEMENT MEMBRANE

      PIGMENT EPITHELIUM AND EXTERNAL
        BASEMENT MEMBRANE

    UVEAL (MESODERMAL) PORTION

The uveal tract is the pigmented vascular layer lying between corneoscleral and neuro-epithelial layers. It is conventiently divisible into three parts: the iris stroma anteriorly, the choroid posteriorly, and an intermediate part, the ciliary body.

The uveal tract is a tissue composed of a relatively even mixture of cells and extracellular materials.

Although the two-layered epithelium lining the inner surface of the ciliary body and posterior surface of the iris belongs embryologically to the neuroepithelia of the optic cup, the close association of the epithelia with the uveal tract in the iris and ciliary body makes it convenient to describe them together.

THE IRIS

The iris is a circular diaphragm separating the aqueous compartment into anterior and posterior chambers. Its central aperture, the pupil, is slightly nasal to center and controls the amount of light entering the eye. The iris diaphragm is thickest not far from the pupillary zone in the region of the *collarette* and thinnest at its periphery, the iris *root* (Fig. 10–1).

The thin periphery of the iris is subject to traumatic tearing or separation, **iridodialysis,** upon injury. Vascularity of the iris root may cause hemor-rhage into either the anterior or posterior chamber following ocular trauma. On the other hand, the pupillary margin rests on the lens anterior to the frontal plane of the iris root. This contact by the iris pigment epithelium may produce pigment cell adhesions to the lens capsule, as in inflammations or contusions. Absence of the supporting lens, as in subluxations, dislocations, or surgical removal due to cataract, allows the iris diaphragm to fall back to the plane of the iris root. The anterior chamber deepens and the iris looks flat and acquires a tremulousness (**iridodonesis**) with movement of the eye.

The color of the iris is determined for the most part by its content of pigmented cells in the stroma. Many irises appear blue at birth because the uveal tract is not maximally pigmented then. By 3–6 months of age, however, many blue irises have changed color because of increased stromal pigmentation. If the collagenous stroma of the iris lacks pigmented cells but its double layer of pigment epithelium is normally pigmented, the iris appears blue. In the albino, however, in whom the pigment is deficient not only in the stroma but also in the pigment epithelium, the red glow of the il-

FIG. 10–1. Meridional section of one leaf of iris diaphragm. **C,** edge of collarette; **CL,** clump cells anterior to sphincter muscle; **P,** pupillary border; **PC,** posterior chamber; **R,** iris root. (H&E, × 35) (AFIP Neg. 70-1424)

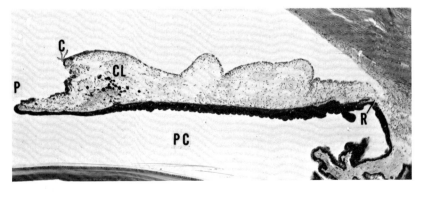

luminated fundus shows through, giving the iris a pink color.

Stromal pigmentation (*i.e.,* green or brown irises) obscures the finer morphologic detail of the iris that may be observed with the slit lamp.

UVEAL (MESODERMAL) PORTION

The iris stroma consists of two parts: the avascular *anterior border layer* and the *stroma proper* (Fig. 10–2), which is vascularized (18).

The presence of small blood vessels within the anterior border layer of the human iris suggests an abnormality, early neovascularization, which may progress onto the iris surface to be observed clinically as **rubeosis iridis,** a complication which occurs in a number of conditions, e.g., in long-standing diabetes mellitus. Unlike the human iris, small blood vessels are present normally in the anterior border layer of the rhesus monkey iris (Fig. 10–14).

Two cell types, *pigmented cells* and *nonpigmented cells* (31), are found in the iris stroma (Fig. 10–3 through 10–5). In the adult uvea, pigmentation appears to be almost all or none in any single cell (Fig. 10–4, 10–34A); in the pigmented cells every cell seems to have a maximum number of pigment granules.

The blue iris (Fig. 10–5) possesses amelanotic cells having a few small dense granules in their cytoplasm. The granules are not melanin and are typically found in blue irises, although their actual color *in vivo* is not yet defined. The cells containing the granules may represent potential melanocytes.

Anterior Border Layer

The anterior border layer (Fig. 10–6) consists of a dense packing of pigmented or nonpigmented cells (Fig. 10–7) similar in appearance to the cells present throughout the remainder of the stroma. Cell density in this surface layer varies from iris to iris. Within any particular iris there may be considerable variation from location to location. Absence of cells appears as **crypts** or "apertures" in the border layer (Fig. 10–5, 10–8). The crypts are usually more prominent in the thick pupillary zone and toward the iris root.

The iris surface, therefore, varies widely, from the smooth, heavily pigmented surface of a dark-brown iris to the irregular, crypt-marked surface of green or blue irises. In the latter

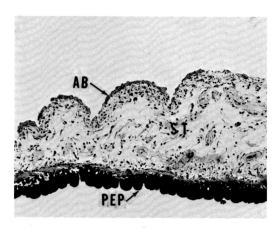

FIG. 10–2. Iris stroma and associated pigment epithelium (**PEP**). **AB,** anterior border layer; **ST,** stroma.(Epon section, PD, × 60) (AFIP Neg. 63-6907)

FIG. 10–3. Light micrograph of pigmented iris stromal cells. Large, circular nonpigmented portions of cells (**N**) represent nonstained nuclei. (Epon section, PD, × 1000) (AFIP Neg. 68-9945)

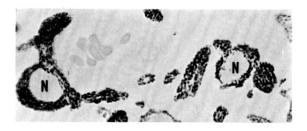

irises, groupings of surface cells together with more or less collagenous material bridge some of the spaces in the anterior border layer. These bridgelike tissue clusters are called **iris trabeculae.**

No continuous cell layer that can be defined as an endothelium lines the surface of the iris. The anterior border layer of the iris is a loose connective tissue whose surface has become visible, in part as a result of the very specialized cleft, the anterior aqueous chamber, that has been formed embryonically *entirely* within the predominantly mesodermal, *i.e.* middle ocular, layer (Fig. 10–9).

Peripherally, the anterior border layer ends abruptly at the iris root, except where spoke-like portions continue toward Schwalbe's line as iris processes (Fig. 11–34).

FIG. 10–4. Electron micrograph of typical pigmented iris stromal cell. A cilium (**CL**) is seen projecting from cell. (× 8500) Inset. Characteristic stromal melanin granules, sectioned in various planes at higher magnification. (× 23,400)

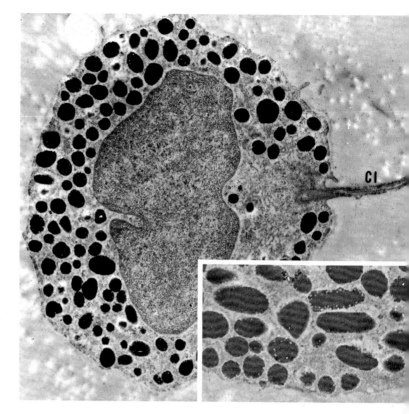

FIG. 10–5. Anterior border layer in blue iris. Note large space between two of surface cells. Dense granules are present (**arrows**) within nonpigmented stromal cells. Collagen fibrils (**C**) occupy much of intercellular space. **AC,** anterior chamber. (× 7000) Inset. Cilium projecting from nonpigmented stromal cell. (× 15,000)

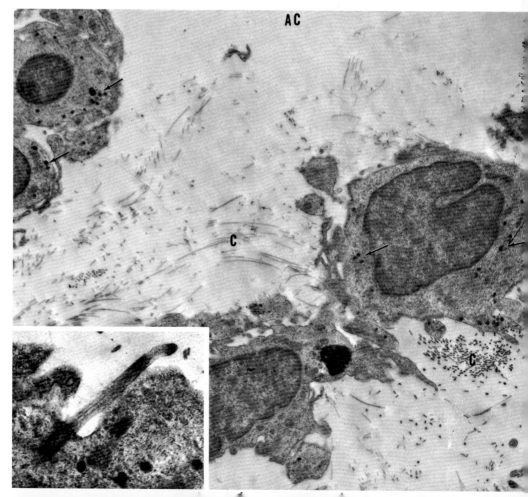

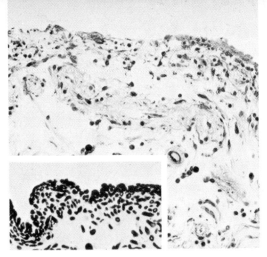

FIG. 10–6. Anterior border layer of iris. This layer may be lightly pigmented (main figure) or heavily pigmented (inset). (Main figure, Epon, PD, × 145) (AFIP Neg. 63-6906). (Inset, Epon, PD, × 180) (AFIP Neg. 65-6680)

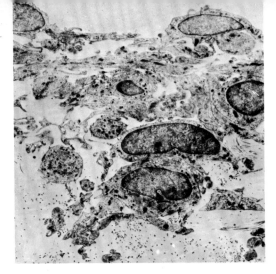

FIG. 10–7. Lower-power electron micrograph of nonpigmented anterior border layer of iris composed of a dense packing of stromal cells. (× 1500)

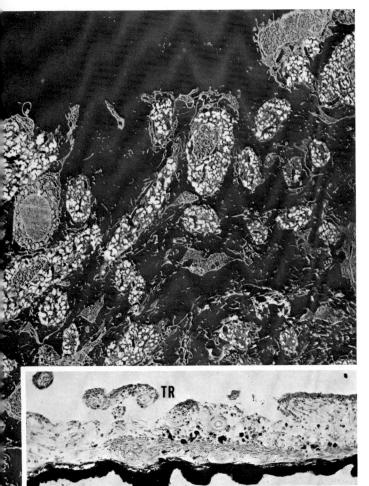

FIG. 10–8. Shadow-cast section of anterior border layer of iris, showing many surface apertures. Collagen fibrils are distributed in extracellular spaces. (U-shad, × 3000) Inset. Many larger crypts are seen within anterior border of pupillary zone as well as sections of surface trabeculae (**TR**). (H&E, × 85) (AFIP Neg. 70-1418). (Modified from Tousimis AJ, Fine BS: Arch Ophthalmol 62:974, 1959)

FIG. 10–9. A cleft, the anterior chamber (**arrow**), formed within mesodermal ("mesectodermal") tissue of a 4-month fetus (Masson, × 80) (AFIP Neg. 61-3078)

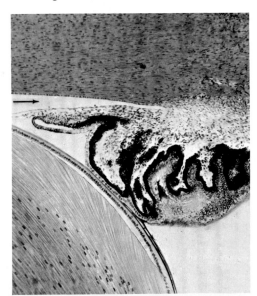

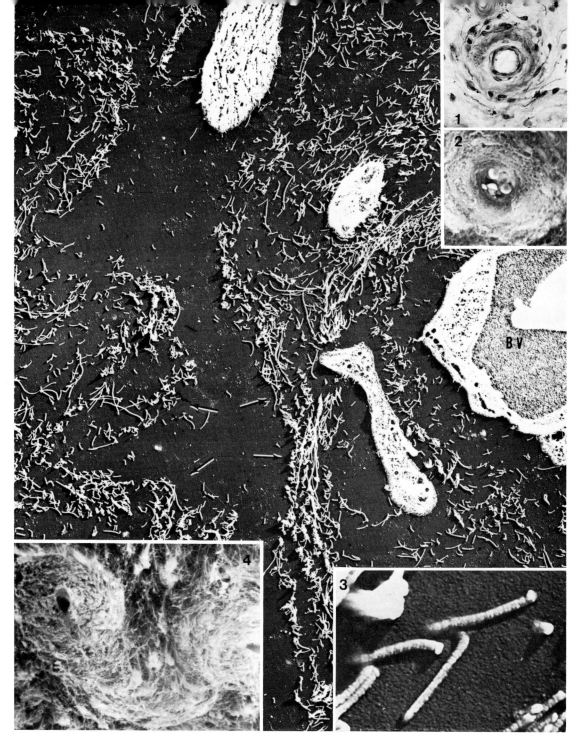

FIG. 10–10. Shadow-cast section of iris stroma. Collagen fibrils, acid mucopolysaccharides, and cells form columns or aggregates around blood vessels (**BV**) or nerves. **Arrows,** edges of two adjacent columns. Space between is occupied by mucinous drying patterns. (U-shad, × 5250) Inset 1. Light micrograph of "thick-walled" blood vessel. (H&E, × 220) (AFIP Neg. 70-1420) Inset 2. Scanning electron micrograph of similar vessel. (× 500) Inset 3. Typical banded collagen fibrils of iris stroma. (× 28,000) Inset 4. Scanning electron micrograph of sinuous collagenous columns. (× 600)

These normal processes are most noticeable when pigmented. The novice at gonioscopy sometimes confuses them with abnormal peripheral anterior synechias.

The Stroma

The loose stroma consists of pigmented and nonpigmented cells and extracellular materials, mainly bundles of collagen fibrils (inset 2, Fig. 10–10) in their matrix of hyaluronidase-sensitive mucopolysaccharides. The fibrils are generally arranged in cylindrical groupings, columns, or bundles around a number of nerves or a blood vessel (32) (Fig. 10–10). The collagenous columns have a characteristic arrangement, tending to radiate sinuously from the back of the iris toward the front and from the iris periphery toward the pupil (Col. Fig. 10–11). When iris blood vessels surrounded by the columns are observed in histologic sections, they are referred to as "thick-walled" blood vessels (Fig. 10–10, insets 1 and 2; Fig. 10–11 to 10–13).

The collagenous columns enclosing the cells, blood vessels, and nerves may be seen by slit lamp in blue irises as white stromal columns (Fig. 10–11). Occasionally a vessel deviates from its axial course and may be observed protruding from the white column. The nerves, lacking color, are not recognizable unless they are represented *in vivo* by the translucent central line that can be observed in many of the columns at higher magnification (*i.e.,* × 40). Because the space between adjacent columns is filled with transparent acid mucopolysaccharides, the entire thickness of the blue iris stroma as well as the pigmentation of the pigment epithelium can be examined directly. Defects in the pigment epithelial layer of light-colored irises can also be detected by transpupillary retroillumination.

These biomicroscopic observations may be clinically useful, as when determining if a retroiridal mass is simply pressing forward, as a cyst may do, is focally reducing the stromal thickness, as a more solid tumor may do, or is altering the stromal composition, as an infiltrating tumor may do.

Except for the great differences in cell and pigment density and surface trabeculae of the anterior border layer, the structure of the iris stroma appears identical in irises of all colors. Iris variation, therefore, is a property of stromal pigmentation and anterior border layer arrangement.

That the subsurface stromal arrangement of a blue iris is identical to that of a brown iris can be appreciated *in vivo* in a brown-eyed patient with *early* stromal atrophy. The white columnar arrangement of the collagen bundles can then be seen to be similar. Alterations in iris pigmentation (**heterochromia**) between the two irises of an individual (**heterochromia iridum**), or even within a single iris (**heterochromia iridis**) also may be acquired and so may indicate a pathologic change such as in Fuchs' heterochromic iridocyclitis or siderosis bulbi in the former or a segmental growth of nevus or melanoma of the iris in the latter.

Many stromal vessels are large (of the diameter of the choriocapillaris), endothelium-lined structures with the morphology typical of a nonfenestrated capillary. A basement membrane is present which blends with the surrounding matrix, except where it joins the basement membrane of an associated *pericyte* (Fig. 10–12). The endothelium possesses apical junctional complexes (terminal bars; see Ch. 6) as well as the pinocytotic vesicles, micro and macro (morphologic as well as functional), similar to those present in other nonfenestrated capillaries. To date a *minor* arterial circle analogous to the major arterial circle within the

---

FIG. 10–11. A. Radial, sinuous, collagenous columns are evident in the blue iris. An enclosed blood vessel can often be observed with the slit lamp. The zone of the sphincter muscle can be observed in the thinner pupillary zone beyond the collarette. B. Patches of pigmented anterior border layer focally screen underlying stromal columns. C. One sector of blue iris is heavily pigmented, effectively concealing the underlying stromal columns. D. The brown iris is the result of diffuse and dense pigmentation. Peripheral concentric rings are contraction furrows. E. Topography of iris may be irregular because of trabeculae formed within anterior border layer. F. Pigmentation of anterior border layer clearly outlines ring of collarette. G. Broad trabeculae of anterior border layer may course widely over the iris surface. H. Heterochromia iridis. Variation in topography combined with variation in pigmentation produces the assorted clinical appearances of the iris.

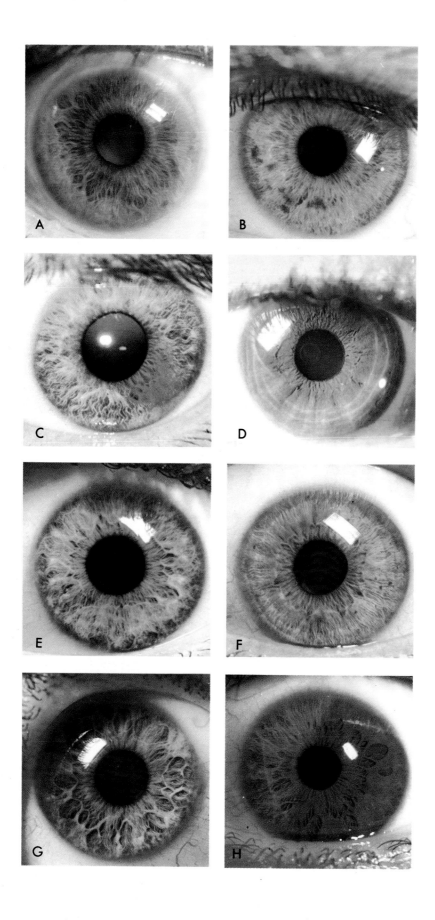

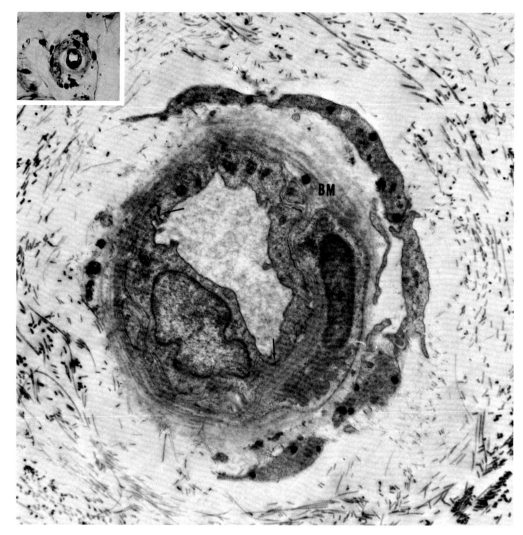

BM

FIG. 10–12. Iris blood vessel. Electron micrograph shows small stromal vessel. Apical junctional complexes (**arrows**) attach adjacent endothelial cells. A pericyte (**P**) is present. **BM,** basement membranes. (× 10,000) Inset. Arrangement of cells and collagen makes up "thick walls" of blood vessel seen in light micrograph. (H&E, × 220)

ciliary body has not been observed. It may be represented by the vascular arcades within the region of the collarette.

The radial, sinuous arrangement of the iris vasculature, and so indirectly the enveloping collagenous columns, are illustrated well in a fluorescein angiogram of a nonpigmented or lightly pigmented iris (Fig. 10–13B, C). The vascular arcades in the region of the collarette are also well demonstrated in a fluorescein angiogram (11).

RETINAL (NEUROEPITHELIAL) PORTION

Sphincter Muscle

Lying in the pupillary zone of the iris stroma is a ring of typical smooth muscle almost 1 mm

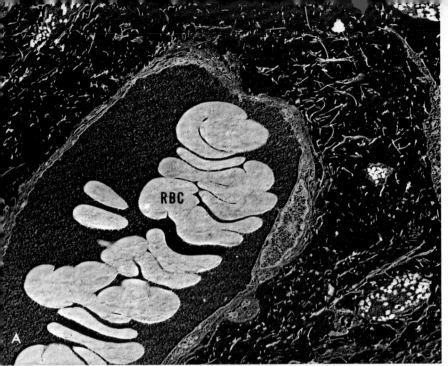

FIG. 10–13. Iris stroma. A. Shadow-cast section of large iris stromal vessel occupied by preserved plasma proteins in which red blood cells (RBC) are suspended. Collagen and stromal cells surround vessel. (U-shad, × 5000) (Tousimis AJ, Fine BS: Arch Ophthalmol 62:974, 1959) B. and C. Fluorescein angiograms of vessels in lightly pigmented iris stroma: B, early; C, late. (Courtesy Dr. J. W. Berkow)

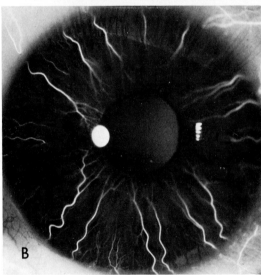

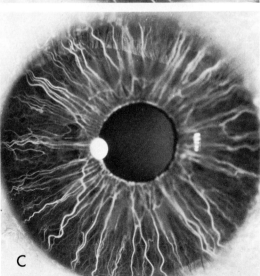

FIG. 10–14. Light micrograph of young rhesus monkey iris, cut along long axis of sphincter muscle (SM). Minimal connective tissue is present here between muscle and pigment epithelium. Pigmented septa (arrows) passing toward pigment epithelium are called Fuch's spurs. AB, anterior border layer. (Methacrylate section, toluidine blue, × 305) (AFIP Neg. 59-2588) (Tousimis AJ, Fine BS: Am J Ophthalmol 48:397, 1959)

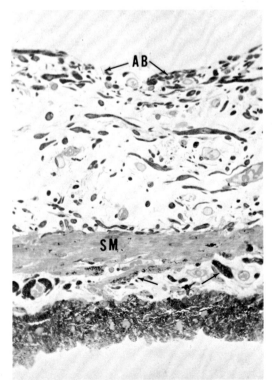

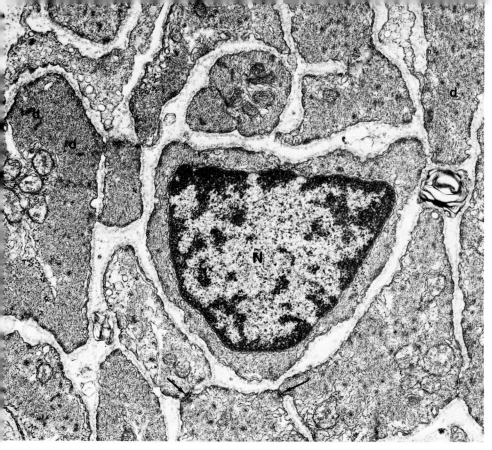

FIG. 10–15. Cross-section of bundle of sphincter muscle cells. Each cell is enveloped by a thin basement membrane and is filled with myofilaments and their associated densities (**d**). Plasmalemmal vesicles and associated densities also are present. Note short dense attachments (**arrows**) between adjacent smooth muscle cells, tying the cells close together. **N,** nucleus of muscle cell. (× 17,300)

wide, the **iris sphincter** (Fig. 10–1 and 10–11A). The smooth muscle cells are concentric with the pupil (Fig. 10–14), so that when the muscle contracts it causes the pupil to constrict. The muscle plate is separated from the pigment epithelium of the iris posteriorly by a layer of connective tissue which becomes increasingly dense with age.

It is probably this dense plate of retrosphincter connective tissue, occupying the area posterior to the muscle, that contributes most toward the ease with which the "periphery of the sphincter muscle" in the blue iris is observed biomicroscopically (Fig. 10–11A, B).

The muscle cells satisfy all the histologic criteria for smooth muscle (see discussion of ciliary muscle, later in this chapter) (Fig. 10–15). In the iris sphincter, however, they are unusual, for they are considered to be derived *wholly* from neuroectodermal cells that have migrated into the stroma from the neuroepithelium during embryonic life. Adding support to this belief is the presence within these smooth muscle cells of melanin granules that are characteristic in size and shape of neuroepithelial melanin (33). A series of pigmented projections from the plane of the dilator muscle remains in the adult (Fig. 10–16). These projections or "spurs" are known as Fuchs' or Michel's spurs in the vicinity of the sphincter muscle and as Grunert's spurs at the periphery of the iris (Fig. 10–17.

This muscle of neuroectodermal origin is innervated (17) by parasympathetic nerve fibers that originate in the Edinger-Westphal nucleus at the anterior aspect of the third nerve nucleus. The fibers are carried into the orbit by the branch of the third nerve that goes to the inferior oblique muscle. They branch off like small twigs to arrive at the ciliary ganglion, where a synapse occurs. Fibers from the ciliary ganglion enter the eye by way of the short ciliary nerves. There is some evidence that the sphincter muscle is supplied with inhibitory fibers by way of sympathetic nerves.

Clump Cells

Heavily pigmented, rounded cells are often present just anterior to the sphincter muscle (18, 31) (Fig. 10–18). Known as the **clump cells of Koganei,** they were once believed to have migrated into the stroma, as did the precursor cells of the sphincter muscle, but without having undergone further modification. More recent observations (35), however, supported by morphologic, embryologic, and experimental evidence, indicate that most of these cells are in reality macrophages, having engulfed melanin granules of both neuroepithelial and stromal varieties. A second type of cell grouping is less frequently present in these regions of stroma (Fig. 10–19). This latter type consists of a small grouping of cells completely surrounded by a basement membrane. The melanin granules are uniformly distributed within the cell cytoplasm and are all of the neuroepithelial type in size and shape. The macrophage-like cell has been designated the type 1 clump cell and the migrated neuroepithelial cell cluster the type 2 clump cell.

   Type 1 clump cells (Fig. 10–18) may be best observed *in vivo* in blue irises near the pupillary margin as tiny, spherical, deep-brown dots. They are best seen under 40 × magnification and can be easily distinguished from typical stromal melanocytes by their deeper brown color (identical with that of the cells of the pupillary pigment seam) and by their spherical shape (unlike the linear appearance of the stromal melanocytes). They are more common in older individuals and most noticeable when changes are also observable in the nearby pigment seam.

Dilator Muscle

The posterior boundary of the iris stroma, peripheral to the sphincter muscle, is demarcated by another sheet of smooth muscle, the **dilator muscle.** The fibers of the dilator muscle are derived from, and remain in continuity with, the cuboidal pigmented cell bodies that make up the anterior layer of iris pigment epithelium

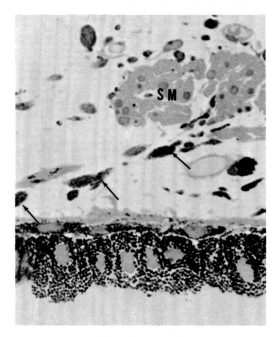

FIG. 10–16. Meridional section of young rhesus monkey iris showing peripheral edge of sphincter muscle (**SM**). A line of pigmented cells (**arrows**, Michel's spur) passes from this edge to pigment epithelium. (methacrylate section, toluidine blue, × 820) (AFIP Neg. 59-2552)

FIG. 10–17. Schematic drawing showing location of often pigmented "spurs" that project from region of dilator muscle of iris. (Wobmann PR, Fine BS: Am J Ophthalmol 73:90, 1972)

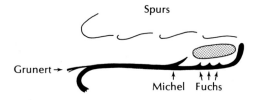

(Fig. 10–20). The dilator is therefore a *partial* specialization of cytoplasmic processes of the anterior layer of iris pigment epithelium into smooth muscle (neuroectodermal). The dilator processes are arranged in an overlapping manner somewhat like shingles on a roof. When the muscle elements contract, their radial direction causes pupillary dilation. Melanin granules typical of neuroepithelium may often be seen

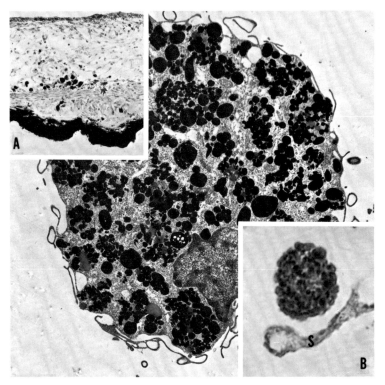

FIG. 10–18. Type 1 iris clump cells. Electron micrograph showing typical type 1 clump cell with its delicate villi and clusters of pigment granules which vary in size and shape. (× 4200) Inset A. Light micrograph of clump cells in region of sphincter muscle. (H&E, × 85) (AFIP Neg. 60-1421) Inset B. Light micrograph showing mulberry-like appearance of cell. A nearby branching stromal cell (**S**) is easily differentiated by its content of smaller granules of uniform size. (Epon section, PD, × 1040) (AFIP Neg. 70-8848) (Wobmann PR, Fine BS: Am J Ophthalmol 73:90, 1972)

FIG. 10–19. Type 2 iris clump cells. Less frequently observed in region of sphincter muscle, this type is recognized in light microscopy (insets A and B) by its multinucleated appearance and by uniformity of distribution of its melanin granules. By electron microscopy, type 2 clump cell is seen to consist of group of cells surrounded by continuous basement membrane (**BM**). **D,** desmosome. **Free arrow,** interdigitating apical villi. Melanin granules are all of neuroepithelial type. (× 5600) Inset A. **Upper arrow,** a type 1 clump cell anterior to sphincter muscle; **lower arrow,** a type 2 clump cell. (× 145) (AFIP Neg. 70-8836) Inset B. Multinucleate type 2 clump cell near iris root. (× 305) (AFIP Neg. 70-8850) (Wobmann PR, Fine BS: Am J Ophthalmol 73:90, 1972)

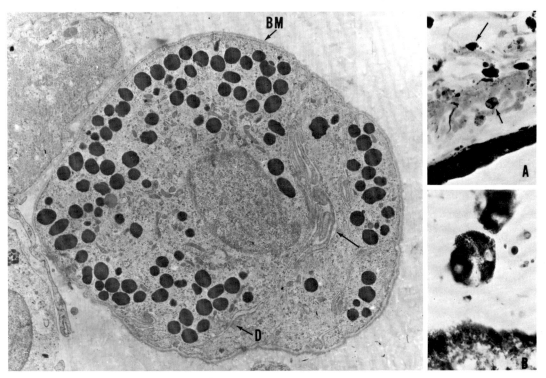

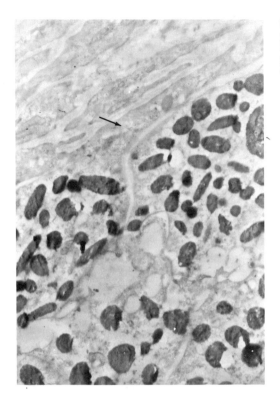

FIG. 10–20. Continuity of anterior pigment epithelium with dilator muscle of iris (**arrow**). (× 12,300) (Tousimis AJ, Fine BS: Am J Ophthalmol 48:397, 1959)

FIG. 10–21. Iris dilator muscle. Cell body with its nucleus (**N**), glycogen particles (**G**), and mitochondria (**M**) lies to the right. The melanin granules are typical neuroepithelial. Attenuated part of cell, on left contains most of the myofilaments and their associated densities. (× 13,000) Inset. A villous-filled focal enlargement ("canaliculus") between anterior (**above**) and posterior (**below**) pigment epithelial cell layers. (× 21,800)

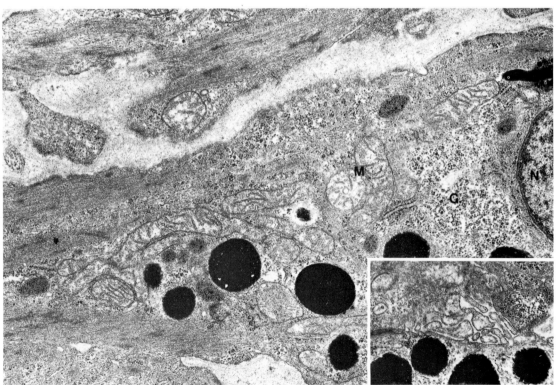

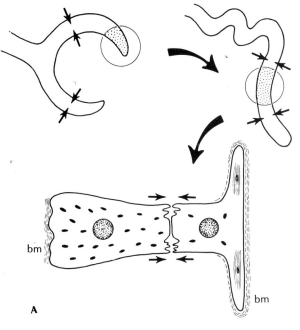

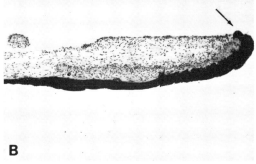

FIG. 10–22. Pigment epithelium. A. Schematic drawing, showing transformation of two epithelial layers at anterior margin of optic cup into two layers of ciliary and iris epithelium (**above**). The lower diagram shows the two epithelial layers of the iris as seen by TEM. Note apex-to-apex arrangement (**arrows**), basement membranes (**bm**) at opposite ends, and partial modification of anterior epithelial cells into smooth muscle (dilator). (AFIP Neg. 77-5860) B. Termination of iris pigment epithelium in pupil as pigment seam (**arrow**). (H&E, × 50) (AFIP Neg. 62-5287)

FIG. 10–23. Iris pigment epithelium. A. Meridional section showing clusters of cells on posterior surface (**arrows**). (Epon, PD, × 210) (AFIP Neg. 66-1290) B. Meridional section showing proliferations of posterior pigment epithelium. **D,** dilator muscle. (Epon, PD, × 165) (AFIP No. 66-1286) C. Meridional section showing evaginations through dilator muscle (**D**) and pigment epithelium possessing connective tissue cores, identified as vestigial iris processes that may occur near iris root. (Epon, PD, × 130) (AFIP Neg. 67-11207)

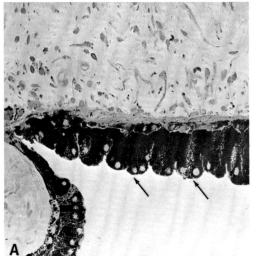

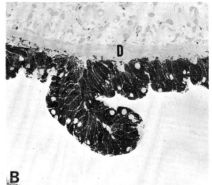

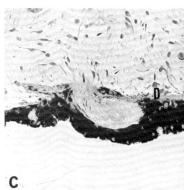

within the smooth muscle portions of the anterior pigment epithelial cells (Fig. 10–21).

As in other typical smooth muscle cells, the dilator cells have an investing membrane, cytoplasmic filaments, densities, and surface-connected vesicles.

Pigment Epithelium

The double layer of pigment epithelium that covers the posterior iris surface results from apposition of the two epithelial layers forming the anterior extremity of the embryonic cup (see Fig. 6–2, 6–3, and 10–22A).

The anterior border layer is separated from the pupil by a ridge of more heavily pigmented cells, which is the clinically visible portion of iris pigment epithelium, the **pigment seam** (1) (Fig. 10–22) or **ruff** (2). Under higher magnification this ridge can be observed as an apparent chain of little beads. With wide excursions of the pupil, the arrangement can be observed to indeed resemble a ruffle, which folds up like an accordion on pupillary constriction, opens to reveal more clearly the ruffle-like appearance on semidilation, and finally stretches to form an almost smooth ridge lining the pupillary margin on wide dilation. Why it has this appearance can be better appreciated on gross examination of the pigment epithelium lining the posterior surface of the iris.

In a meridional section of a dilated iris the posterior epithelial cells* appear to be arranged in small clusters (Fig. 10–23). Each cluster represents a cross-sectioned ridge lying between two *circumferential furrows* on the posterior iris surface (Fig. 10–24). The wedge-shaped configuration of the cells in each ridge often appears as an incomplete triangle because the cells are not only arranged radially across each ridge but are also staggered along its length (Fig. 10–25, 10–26).

The circumferential ridges do not form complete circles around the pupil but taper repeatedly to blend into adjacent furrows (Fig. 10–25, 10–27). This arrangement allows the posterior iris surface to be properly covered during contraction and dilation of the iris. The circumferential furrows are least prominent in the region behind the pupillary zone of the

---

* For convenience, in descriptions of the iris, the terms "anterior" and "posterior" replace the terms "inner" and "outer" that are used for most other ocular tissues.

FIG. 10–24. Posterior iris surface. A. Gross photograph of posterior surface and adjacent ciliary crests. Coarse longitudinal or radial furrows are clearly seen; finer circumferential furrows are seen with difficulty. B. Scanning electron micrograph of posterior iris surface from an infant, showing gross longitudinal furrows at pupillary margin (**below**) and along posterior iris surface. Circumferential ridges and furrows are also clearly seen. Anterior edges of infantile ciliary crests are seen above. (× 50) C. Adult iris. Circumferential ridges are lacking in the pupillary zone. (× 280) ▶

sphincter muscle and are most prominent at the iris root (Fig. 10–24).

The posterior layer of pigment epithelium is continuous with the *nonpigmented* epithelium of the ciliary body and ultimately with the neural retina.

The prominence of the circumferential ridges and furrows at the iris root may be related in some way to the high incidence of pigment cell proliferation in this region to form folds and processes (Fig. 10–23B) leading to the formation of pigment cysts or pigmented "balls" (3, 37), which may be observed clinically in the anterior chamber. On rare occasions such pigment epithelial cysts or clusters may even be confused with a malignant melanoma of the uveal tract (38).

Our own preliminary observations indicate that the circumferential ridges do not form until a few months after birth.

In the region of the sphincter muscle many short radial or longitudinal furrows replace the circumferential furrows (Fig. 10–24). They can be observed *in vivo,* terminating anteriorly, arranging the pigment epithelial cells of the pupillary border into the ruffle-like arrangement seen clinically.

This blind ending of the optic vesicle (pupillary pigment seam) projects slightly over the adjacent anterior border layer of the iris stroma, and the slight overhang is sometimes known clinically as the **physiologic ectropion** of the pigment epithelium. This appearance is in contrast to **pathologic ectropion,** often termed **ectropion uveae,** in which the pupillary border of the iris is sufficiently everted that much more pigment epithelium from the posterior surface becomes exposed to view. In histologic sections the pupillary margin of the sphincter

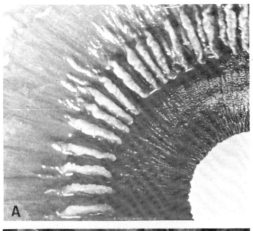

FIG. 10–25. Posterior iris surface. A. Posterior iris ridges and furrows as seen by SEM at higher magnification. Note tapering and blending of adjacent ridges. (× 500) B. In section from 4-month-old child, staggered arrangement of cells along each ridge is better seen. (× 750)

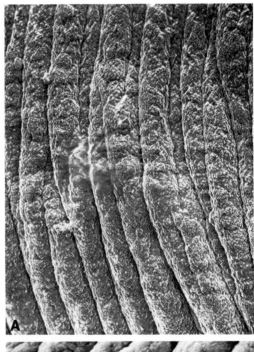

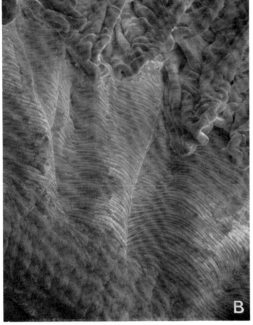

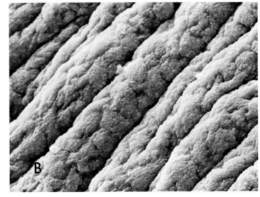

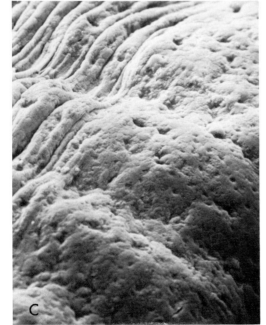

muscle generally is also everted in pathologic ectropion.

Peripheral to the sphincter muscle, the delicate pupillary radial furrows expand into the
structural furrows, which are less well demarcated and rapidly diverge. They traverse the
remainder of the iris to its root and become
continuous with the valleys between the ciliary
crests (Fig. 10–24).

The large melanin granules of the pigment
epithelium (spherical, ~0.8μ in diameter; ovoid
~0.5 by 1.3μ) permit adequate resolution by
oil-immersion light microscopy (Ch. 2) (Fig.
10–28). They contrast with the smaller (~0.2 by
0.6μ) uniformly ovoid granules of the pigmented cells of the iris stroma. The uniformity
and small size of the latter granules produce the

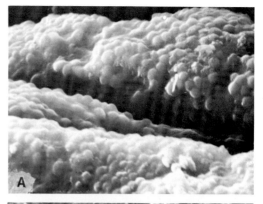

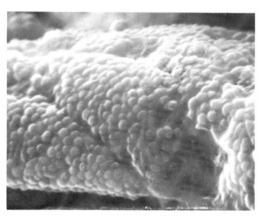

FIG. 10–26. Iris epithelial ridge, adult,
as seen by SEM at still higher
magnification. Note staggered
arrangement of cells (outlined by deep
grooves). Myriad small bumps are
produced by melanin granules. ($\times$ 2800)

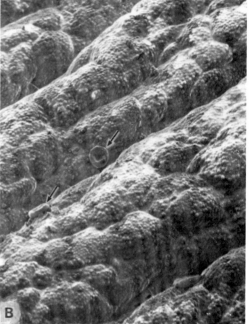

FIG. 10–27. Iris epithelial ridge. A.
Tapering out of one iris epithelial ridge
between two others (rhesus monkey
eye), as seen by SEM. ($\times$ 2800) B.
The staggered arrangement of cells
along each ridge can be better
appreciated in another view (rhesus
monkey eye). **Free arrows,** two
erythrocytes, one in surface view and
one in profile. These may serve as
internal measures of size. ($\times$ 900) C.
Cross sections of epithelial ridges
(human) to show incomplete pie-
shaped arrangement of sectioned cells.
(Epon, PD, $\times$ 440) (AFIP Neg. 71-7389)

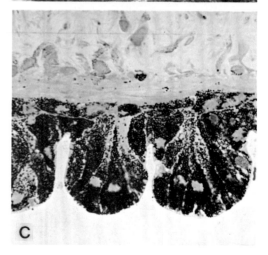

light-brown color characteristic of uveal pigmentation.

The melanin granules of iris stromal cells of the rhesus monkey are wholly unlike those of the human in that they are longer and straplike in shape (31, 35). Their arrangement can be appreciated easily not only in electron micrographs but also by light microscopy, where they can be seen as long pigment "needles." The pigment epithelial melanin granules, however, as well as those in the remainder of the uveal tract (*i.e.*, choroidal) resemble closely those of the human. Near the iris root (Fig. 10–29A) within the posterior layer of iris pigment epithelium as well as in adjacent "nonpigmented" ciliary epithelium

FIG. 10–28. Posterior edge of posterior layer of iris pigment epithelium. Electron micrograph shows free edge of cell with many villi (*i.e.*, basilar infoldings), some of which interdigitate with adjacent cells. Surface is covered by delicate, often multilaminar basement membrane (**BM**). (×14,500) Inset 1. Light micrograph of similar region of pigment epithelial cells. **PC,** posterior chamber. (Epon, × 1000) (AFIP Neg. 68-9949) Inset 2. Electron micrograph shows thin basement membrane (**arrow**) lining anterior pigment epithelium behind sphincter. (× 16,500)

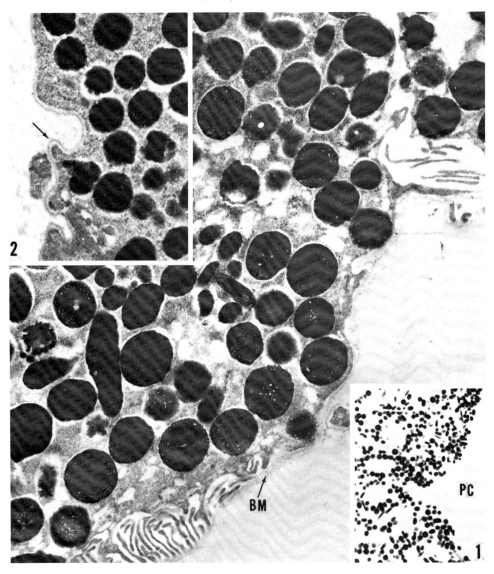

incompletely formed melanin granules are present frequently. These "transitional" granules (Fig. 10–29 B) which develop postnatally, appear to be forming from smaller particles that come together to produce a dense, more homogeneous granule. Such observations suggest that postnatal formation of melanin granules does not necessarily follow the sequence frequently observed in prenatal melanin formation (see Fig. 6–19).

The anterior layer of epithelium remains as a layer of pigmented cuboidal cells whose cytologic bases have expanded and specialized into the overlapping platelike smooth muscle "cells" that make up the dilator muscle, except in the region behind the sphincter muscle where dilator muscle is lacking. In this region a thin basement membrane is present (inset 2, Fig. 10–28). Where dilator muscle is present the basement membrane surrounds the basilar cytoplasmic expansions. The anterior layer is continuous with the layer of pigmented epithelium of the ciliary body and the retinal pigment epithelium.

The columnar cells of the posterior layer of pigment epithelium are arranged apex-to-apex with the cells of the anterior layer. Such an arrangement provides a delicate, often multilaminar, basement membrane on the posterior surface (33) and frequent clusters of apical villi on the anterior surface that project into small pockets or spaces between the two layers of epithelium (Fig. 10–21).

Remnants of the lumen of the optic vesicle persist throughout life. That the posterior layer and the anterior layer can be separated easily from each other is evidenced by the cysts that may form spontaneously in the pigment epithelium or be produced at the pupillary margin by the long-term use of strong miotic agents.

The posterior epithelial cells are attached to one another by very small and poorly formed desmosomes as well as by a terminal-bar-like arrangement. The cell attachments serve to hold the cells together in layers.

The thicker posterior layer of pigment epithelium is of relatively greater importance in maintaining the opacity of the iris, a property accentuated by folding into circumferential ridges.

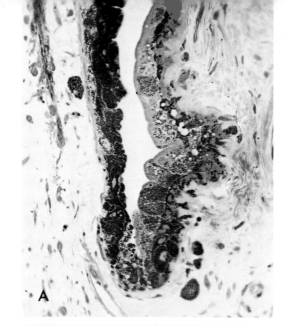

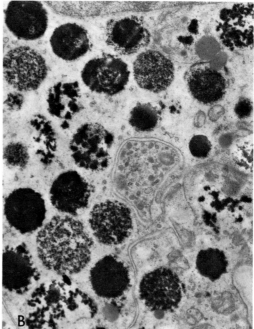

FIG. 10–29. Pigment epithelium. A. Transition from pigmented posterior iris epithelium on left to "nonpigmented" ciliary epithelium on right. Note gradual decrease of cell pigmentation along the ciliary crest declivity on the right. (Epon, PD, × 220) (AFIP Neg. 76-202) B. "Transitional" melanin granules frequently observed in posterior pigment epithelium of iris, near its root or in adjacent layer of "nonpigmented" ciliary epithelium. (× 15,500)

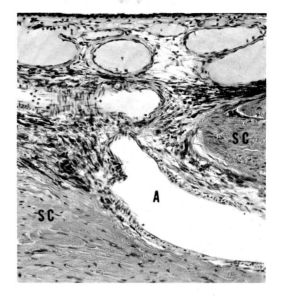

FIG. 10–30. Posterior choroid attached to sclera (**SC**) through which an artery (**A**) is passing.(H&E, × 115) (AFIP Neg. 62-5291)

THE CHOROID

The choroid is that part of the uveal tract extending from the edge of the nerve head to the ora serrata.

SUPRACHOROIDAL "SPACE" AND LAMINA FUSCA

The usually heavily pigmented posterior or choroidal portion of the uveal tract is loosely adherent to the overlying sclera. This plane of loose attachment is a zone of potential separation. When separated it is known as the suprachoroidal ("perichoroidal") space. This "space" is common to both the choroidal and ciliary portions of the uveal tract. Attachment of the longitudinal (meridional) ciliary muscle to the scleral roll limits the space (as in "choroidal detachments") anteriorly. The enlargement is limited posteriorly by attachment of the choroid to the sclera and by the outward passage of the vortex veins, by the perforating short posterior ciliary arteries (Fig. 10–30), and by border tissue at the scleral aperture for the optic nerve.

When the choroid is separated from the sclera (either *in vivo* or artifactitiously), delicate pigmented bands can be seen traversing the space from the choroidal stroma proper to the innermost few layers of the sclera (see Fig. 10–33). Delicate cytoplasmic extensions of nonpigmented cells parallel the pigmented cells (see Fig. 10–34) in the layers. A very small amount of detectable extracellular material accompanies the characteristic pigmented and nonpigmented uveal cells to make up a single choroidal lamella. Deeper within the choroidal stroma, additional quantities of collagen fibrils and other extracellular materials thicken the lamellas further. From behind forward, the multilaminar arrangement of loose, flattened, pigmented lamellas is diminished as the meridional ciliary muscle becomes thicker and elastic tissue becomes more noticeable.

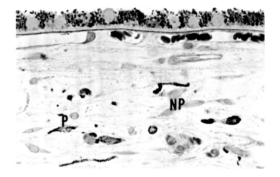

FIG. 10–31. Light micrograph of choroid. Pigmented (**P**) and nonpigmented (**NP**) cells are present in stroma. (Epon, PD, × 440) (AFIP Neg. 66-1298)

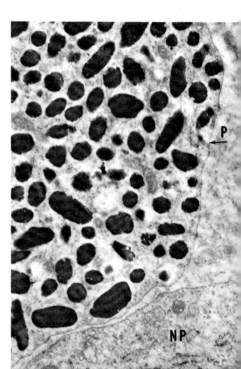

FIG. 10–32. Electron micrograph of choroidal cells from rhesus monkey. **P,** pigmented cells; **NP,** nonpigmented cell. (× 14,500)

The long posterior ciliary arteries and their corresponding long ciliary nerves lie within the suprachoroidal space in the horizontal plane, encased by collagenous tissue. Branches from the nerves to the adjacent choroid form small netlike arrangements where large ganglion cells may be observed.

Smooth muscle cells, at first single and then in small groupings, appear in the suprachoroid even as far posteriorly as the equator. These somewhat stellate cell groupings ("muscle stars") increase in number anteriorly until they form a detectable posterior border to the ciliary muscle.

CHOROIDAL STROMA

Pigmented and Nonpigmented Cells

As in the stroma of the iris, the resident cells are separable morphologically into pigmented and nonpigmented varieties (Fig. 10–31, 10–32). Because of the flattened or interconnecting lamellar arrangement, the pigmented cells, which are dendritic or branching on surface view, necessarily appear spindle-shaped in meridional section (Fig. 10–33, 10–34). The pigmented cells or melanocytes are easily observed and produce the deep-brown color of the choroid. Associated with these cells are varying amounts of collagen fibrils and watery mucinous intercellular materials whose composition has not yet been defined (Fig. 10–35).

On surface view the choroid is least pigmented where the larger vessels are located and most pigmented in the spaces between the vessels. The contrast between the pigmented zones and the vessels helps to produce the ophthalmoscopic choroidal pattern. In section, the outer layers are more heavily pigmented than the inner.

When the intervascular columns are moderately pigmented, the fundus appears ophthalmoscopically as a uniform red color. The uniformity is due to the layer of retinal pigment epithelium covering the vasculature.

Vessels

The venous drainage system is seen as four vortex systems, each located in a posterior quadrant. Each system converges to form a single vestibule, the **ampula,** which then exits through the sclera by a **vortex vein.**

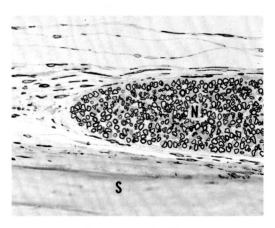

FIG. 10–33. Light micrograph of loose, pigmented suprachoroidal lamellas. Large nerve (**N**) lies in suprachoroidal space. **S,** sclera. (Epon, PD, × 225) (AFIP Neg. 66-1293)

The larger arteries are found most readily in the outer layers of the posterior choroidal stroma (Fig. 10–30). As elsewhere, the arteries and veins generally are differentiated by size, shape of lumen, and thickness of wall.

The capillary layer of the choroid, the **choriocapillaris** (Fig. 10–36), is very important. It nourishes the pigment epithelium and outer layers of the neural retina to approximately the level of the middle limiting membrane.

A lobular network (28) (Fig. 10–36), it lies in single plane and is formed by typical, fenestrated endothelial cells (Fig. 10–37). The fenestrations can be observed on both inner and outer walls.

At the posterior pole the choriocapillaris forms a distinct lobular pattern in which each lobule is supplied centrally by a precapillary arteriole and demarcated peripherally by a ring of postcapillary venules. The mosaic of functionally independent adjoining lobules can be observed best in the early phases of fluorescein angiography (16) (Fig. 10–36B).

A thin basement membrane surrounds the basal plasma membrane of the endothelial cells. Pericytes along the *outer* wall of the choriocapillaris are typically and completely invested by their own thin basement membranes. Similar cells are not normally observed along the *inner* surface of the choriocapillaris.

The cell body of the choriocapillaris endothelium protrudes as is the case in all vessels, into the lumen. The cell body is located mainly

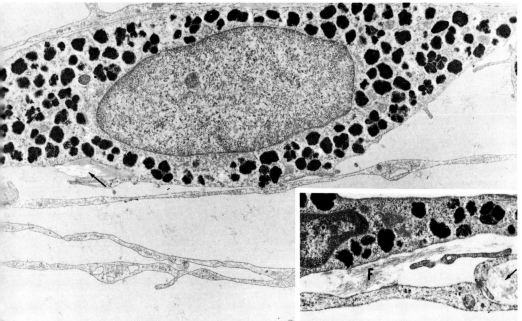

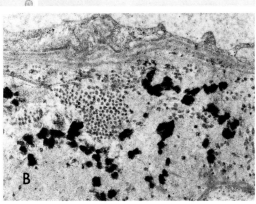

FIG. 10–34. Pigmented cells, stroma.
A. Electron micrograph of flattened
pigmented and nonpigmented cells,
that make up loose suprachoroidal
lamellas. Collagen is sparse in this
plane (**arrow**). (× 9600) Inset. Sample
of nasal choroid slightly deeper (*i.e.*,
internal) to that in main figure.
Filaments (**F**) (presumably collagen or
microfibrils of elastic tissue) are
present between the melanocyte above
and the nonpigmented cell process
below. At right (**free arrow**), a cluster
of negatively stained material (elastin)
is enveloped by filaments. (× 15,000)
B. From foveal region of 24-year-old
subject, sample of choroid near a
vessel (**above**) stained with TPPS for
elastic tissue (dark patches). (× 15,000)

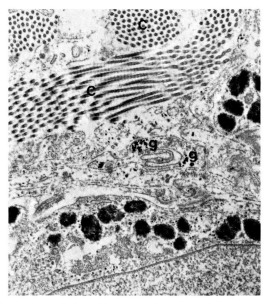

FIG. 10–35. Sample of choroid. Bundles
of collagen (**C**) are cut longitudinally
and in cross-section. Clusters of
glycogen particles (**g**) are present in the
nonpigmented cells, which also contain
filaments. Smaller isolated glycogen
particles are arranged diffusely in
cytoplasm of pigmented cells. (TSC,
× 15,000)

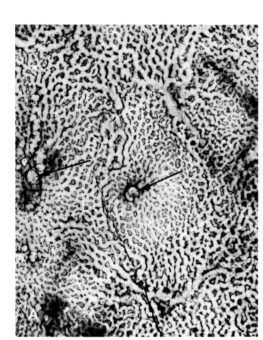

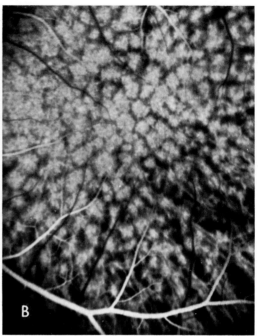

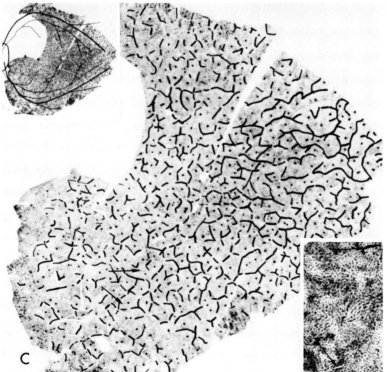

FIG. 10–36. Choriocapillaris. A. Flat preparation of choriocapillaris (posterior pole), to show lobular arrangement. Arrows indicate arteriolar openings. (PAS, × 50) (AFIP Neg. 63-5384) (Courtesy of Dr. M. O. M. Tso) B. Fluorescein angiogram of infant rhesus monkey in choroidal–early arteriolar phase at posterior pole. Note distinct lobular pattern of choriocapillaris. (Perry HD, Hatfield RV, Tso MOM: Am J Ophthalmol 84:197, 1977) C. Flat preparation of choroid from posterior pole (**upper inset**). Lobules of choriocapillaris are seen at higher power in **lower inset** (see also Fig. 10–36 A) and are marked out on photographic enlargement. Central dots in each lobule represent arteriolar openings to each lobule. (Torczynski E, Tso MOM: Am J Ophthalmol 81:428, 1976)

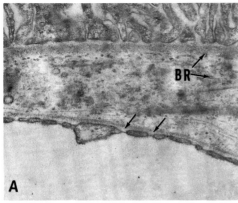
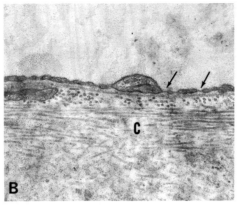
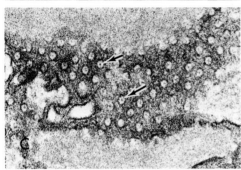

FIG. 10–37. Choriocapillaris, rhesus monkey. A. Fenestrated (**free arrows**) inner wall. **BR,** Bruch's membrane. (× 24,000) B. Fenestrated (**arrows**) outer wall. **C,** collagen fibrils of choroidal stroma. (× 24,000) C. Tangential section of choriocapillaris fenestrae to show their distribution. A small density (**arrows**) is present in the center of the fenestral diaphragm. (× 33,000)

along the outer wall, occasionally along the lateral walls, but only very rarely encroaches on the inner wall. Because of this, the number of endothelial fenestrae are greater per unit area along the inner wall when compared to the fenestrae per unit area along the outer wall. The junctions between adjacent endothelial cells of the choriocapillaris have a zonula adherens but a zonula occludens appears to be poorly formed or lacking.

"Leakiness" (e.g., fluorescein or horseradish peroxidase), a known characteristic of the choriocapillaris and other fenestrated capillaries (23, 24), may be due to the lack of a well-formed zonula occludens or to the permeability of *some* endothelial fenestrae or both. The precise function of endothelial fenestrae remains unclear.

A layer of acellular collagenous material occupies the plane between the endothelial and pigment epithelial basement membranes. The layer is in continuity with the remainder of the choroidal stroma through the spaces between adjacent segments of the choriocapillaris. The continuities or "columns" are necessarily thin or very delicate in the region of the posterior pole (Fig. 10–36A) where the segments of choriocapillaris are more numerous per unit

area than they are toward the equator and the retinal periphery.

With aging of tissues, the intervascular columns as well as the tissues anterior and posterior to the choriocapillaris endothelium (Fig. 10–38) become dense and thickened with masses of the many varieties of basement membrane. The early appearance of the masses of basement membrane adjacent to the endothelial cells and pericytes, as well as to its initial concentration in Bruch's membrane *external* to the elastic layer indicates that the masses of basement membrane are slowly produced by these cells, *i.e.,* endothelium-produced forms of basement membrane.

The midzone of Bruch's membrane may become exceedingly dense and even calcified, noted as an increase in basophilia by light microscopy (34) (see Fig. 6–11).

The various aging changes described here undoubtedly play a part in the pathogenesis of many forms of senile macular degeneration.

Bruch's Membrane

Bruch's membrane is most usefully considered as a continuous sheet composed of two layers: an inner cuticular layer or lamella (the **lamina vitrea** or basement membrane of the pigment epithelium) and an outer collagenous layer

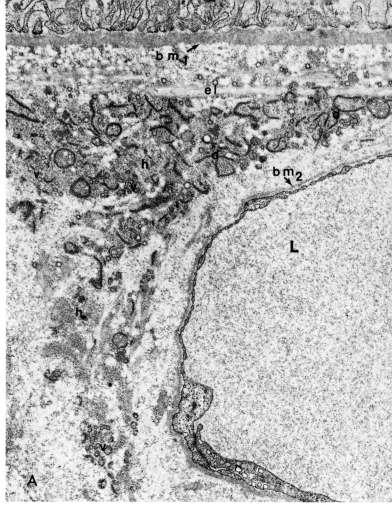

FIG. 10–38. Fovea of 24-year-old subject. A. Intervascular columns of choriocapillaris become dense with aging, as a result of massive accumulation of basement membrane materials (**h,** homogeneous; **v,** vacuolated; **d,** disordered banded). Note preferential accumulation external to midzonal elastic tissue (**el**). Basement membrane of pigment epithelium (**bm₁**) is thicker than basement membrane of choriocapillaris (**bm₂**). **L,** lumen of choriocapillaris. (× 17,000) B. Outer wall of choriocapillaris (**E**). Note masses of homogeneous (**h-bm**) to almost filamentous basement membrane associated with the thin basement membranes (**arrows**) of endothelium and pericytes (**P**). Double-membrane structures of disordered banded basement membrane are also present. **Ca,** calcium spherule. Note fenestrated endothelium of vessel deeper in choroid, a portion of a postcapillary collector venule (**fc,** lower right). **L,** lumen of choriocapillaris. (× 25,000) C. Choriocapillaris (**CH**) and postcapillary or collector venule (**PCV**). Note endothelial fenestrations (**free arrows**) along both walls of choriocapillaris as well as sporadically along both walls of postcapillary collector venules. **BR,** region of Bruch's membrane; **pe,** pigment epithelium. (18-year-old) (× 7200)

(lamina elastica) (6, 14, 15, 18, 27) (see section on Pigment Epithelium, Ch. 6).

The term **lamina elastica** is related to the affinity in the midzone for such stains as orcein or Weigert's elastic tissue stain. An aging process that occurs focally along the inner plane of this region is the development of basement membrane nodules, **drusen,** beneath the pigment epithelium. The nodules are eosinophilic and PAS-positive. By electron microscopy the nodules are found to be composed of aggregates of abnormally formed basement membrane materials (37) (Fig. 10–39). The abnormal quantities of basement membrane, differing somewhat in their appearance from "endothelial" produced basement membrane, also may be produced in sheets (Fig. 10–39C). Fluorescein is known to be taken up by drusen (12) as by a sponge, *i.e.*, staining. Because many of the aging changes along Bruch's membrane also consist of the accumulation of various forms of basement membrane, the rapid spread

and persistence of fluorescein along this plane in both the normal and abnormal eye is not surprising.

Just posterior to the ora serrata on the neural retina side in aging eyes, the choriocapillaris frequently extends through the interrupted lamina elastica to come to lie as a second layer of fenestrated large capillaries beneath the pigment epithelium (5, 19) (Fig. 10–40). The significance of this common senile form of subpigment epithelial neovascularization is not clear.

The neovascularization at the retinal periphery may result from a gradual decrease in already poor nutrition or oxygenation in the region. Recent work suggests that some nutrition of the extreme retinal periphery is maintained in the younger eye via pathways between the two layers of adjacent ciliary epithelium (pars plana), wherein also can be found

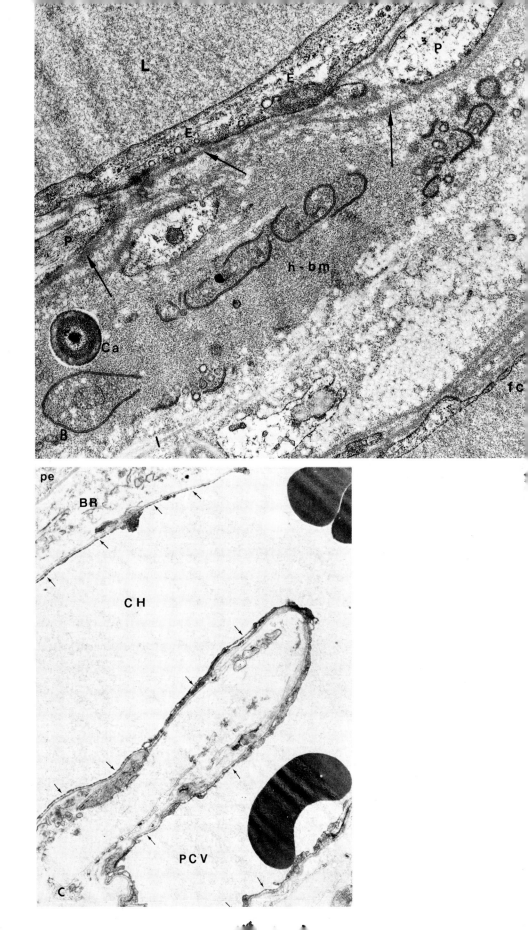

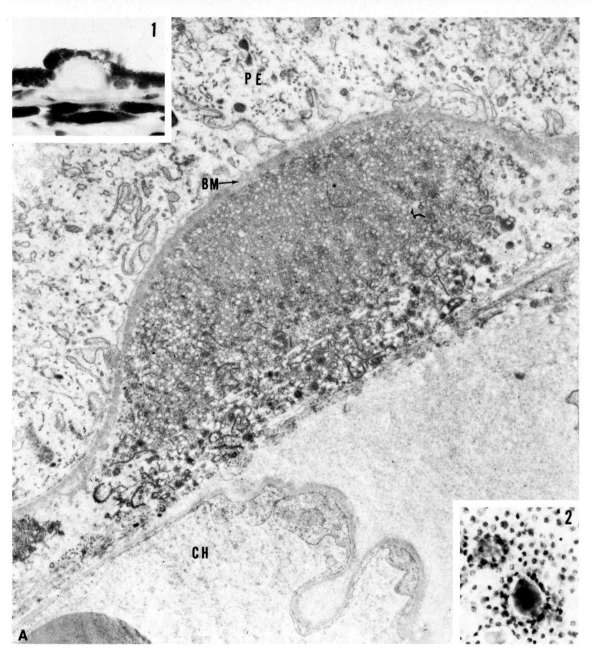

FIG. 10–39. Bruch's membrane. A. Drusen. Electron micrograph of very small simple druse formed beneath pigment epithelium (**PE**). Thin basement membrane characteristic of pigment epithelium (**BM**) follows basal contour of cells. Drusen accumulations appear similar to materials accumulating within intervascular columns containing homogeneous vacuolated basement membrane as well as areas of disordered banded basement membrane. **CH,** choriocapillaris. (× 11,000) Inset 1. Light micrograph section of a small druse. (H&E, × 575) (Neg. 70-3664) Inset 2. Light micrograph flat preparation of two small drusen. (H&E, × 245) (AFIP Neg. 60-1186) (Courtesy of Dr. M. O. M. Tso) B. Foveal region. Double mound of vacuolated basement membrane (**v**) is present beneath thin basement membrane of pigment epithelium. Patches of disordered banded basement membrane (**arrows**) as well as ordered banded basement membrane (~1000 A, **b-bm**) also are seen within the layers of Bruch's membrane. **CH,** choriocapillaris. (× 14,500) C. Foveal region. Sheet of vacuolated (**v**) basement membrane beneath pigment epithelium. Ordered banded basement membrane (~500 A, **b-bm**), as well as some disordered banded basement membrane, also is present. (× 14,400) *(continued)*

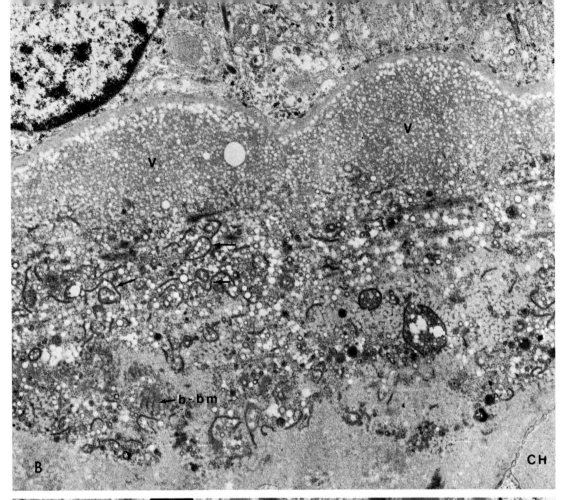

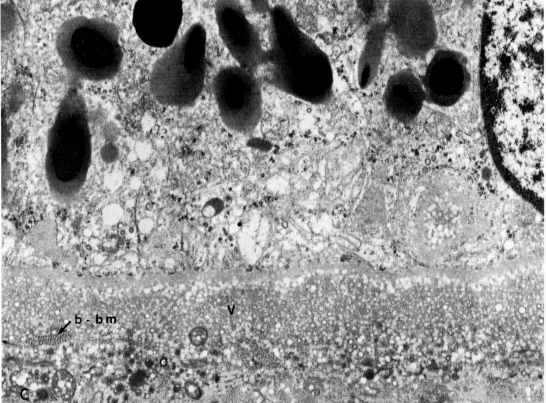

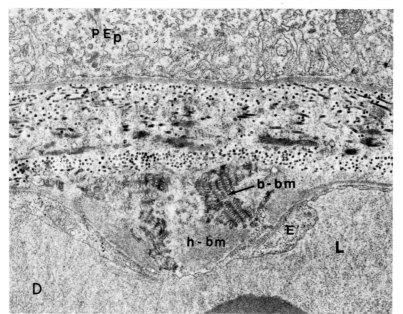

(continued) D. Foveal region, 24-year-old subject. Druse produced by endothelium (E) of choriocapillaris. Ordered banded basement membrane (~1000 A, b-bm) with an additional filamentous component has formed within a nodule of excess homogeneous basement membrane (h-bm). PE$_p$, retinal pigment epithelium. L, lumen of choriocapillaris. (TSC, × 16,000). E. Nodules (drusen) of abnormal basement membrane materials are present along external as well as internal walls of choriocapillaris (CH). The nodules consist of disordered banded basement membrane (arrows) and homogeneous (H) and vacuolated (v) basement membrane. PE$_p$, pigment epithelium. (× 10,800)

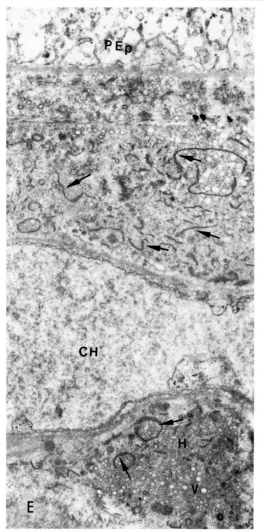

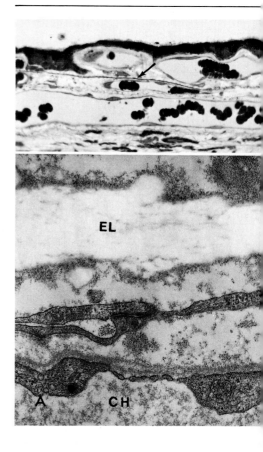

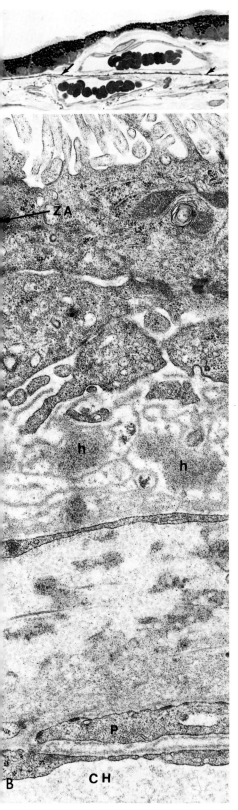

FIG. 10–40. Bruch's membrane. A. Upper figure shows two layers of vessels separated by elastic lamina (**arrow**) of Bruch's membrane. (Epon, PD, × 305) (AFIP Neg. 73-6966) The lower figure shows the typical fenestrated choriocapillaris (**CH**) lying in the usual plane external to the elastic lamina (**EL**). (× 20,000) B. Upper figure shows two layers of vessels separated by the elastic lamina (**arrows**). (Epon, PD, × 440) (AFIP Neg. 74-4413) The TEM shows layers internal to elastic lamina. Aberrant choriocapillaris (**CH**) has a fenestrated endothelium and an associated pericyte (**P**). The typically flattened pigment epithelium has produced a multilaminar basement membrane in which patches of homogeneous basement membrane (**h**) are also present. **ZA,** zonula adherens of pigment epithelium. (× 19,500)

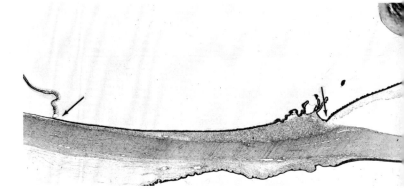

FIG. 10–41. Ciliary body, from infant. Structure extends from root of iris to ora serrata (**free arrows**). (H&E, × 15) (AFIP Neg. 62-5285) (Fine BS, Zimmerman LE: Invest Ophthalmol 2:105, 1963)

FIG. 10–42. Schematic representation of ciliary body. **A,** pars plicata (corona ciliaris); **B,** pars plana (orbiculus ciliaris). **Arrow at top** indicates anterior face of vitreous body.

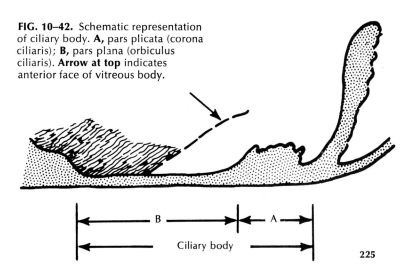

Ciliary body

focal villous-lined enlargements of the apical spaces ("interepithelial cisternae") (21). It also has been suggested that the apical spaces and pathways may represent an anatomic basis contributing to the common formation of peripheral cystoid degeneration of the retina as well as to some cyst formations in the posterior pars plana.

CILIARY BODY

The triangular ciliary body has its base at the iris root anteriorly and its apex at the ora serrata posteriorly (Fig. 10–41). It is formed by the two neuroepithelial layers internally and the intermediate portion of the uveal tract externally. It measures 6 mm* from its apex to its base, where it is thickened by large, smooth muscles.

The anterior surface (the "face") of the ciliary body forms part of the angle of the anterior chamber and continues anteriorly as the uveal trabecular meshwork and the root of the iris. Posteriorly, at the ora serrata, the ciliary body continues as the choroid.

ZONES

The ciliary body is clearly divisible into two parts (Fig. 10–42): an anterior ring, the **pars plicata** (corona ciliaris), and a wider posterior ring, the **pars plana** (orbiculus ciliaris).

The pars plicata consists of a ring of approximately 70 major crests ("processes," Fig. 10–24) meridionally arranged. Each crest measures ~2 mm long and is easily recognized by its usually whitish appearance along the free edge. In the valleys between the crests lie various smaller, uniformly pigmented folds that might be called **minor crests** (anteriorly, **plicae ciliares;** posteriorly, **warts**).

The pars plana is flat, extending from the posterior edges of the ciliary crests to the ora serrata (~4 mm). Thus, the ratio of width of pars plana to pars plicata in meridional section is 2:1.

The pars plana often is not uniformly pigmented. Frequently, a dark band (more prominent on the temporal side) can be observed posteriorly paralleling the toothlike configura-

---

* The total width of the ciliary body stated here for practical purposes as 6 mm is an average figure. In reality, the width is variable, being narrowest in the upper nasal quadrant (4.6–5.2 mm) and widest in the lower temporal quadrant (5.6–6.3 mm) (18).

tion of the ora serrata (see Fig. 6–101). Continuing the direction of the anterior toothlike projections from the retina at the ora serrata are *pigmented striae,* which course meridionally (radially) to blend with the pigmented minor ciliary crests lying in the valleys of the pars plicata. When proper light is reflected obliquely from the inner surface of the pars plana, a very fine meridional surface striation often can be appreciated (Fig. 10–59, inset 2). The striation is more delicate than the circumferential furrows present on the posterior iris surface.

COMPONENTS

For descriptive purposes the ciliary body may be subdivided in many ways. Separation into anterior (pars plicata) and posterior (pars plana) parts has already been described. Another method is to separate the ciliary body into at least six layers: 1) the suprachoroidal (potential) space, 2) the ciliary muscle, 3) the layer of vessels, 4) the external basement membrane, 5) the epithelium, and 6) the internal basement membrane. On the basis of embryonic development, the ciliary body may be separated into two layers: the inner retinal (neuroepithelial) and the outer uveal (mesodermal) portion. The latter is the classification used in the following discussion.

Retinal (Neuroepithelial) Portion

The two epithelial layers of the ciliary body derived from the embryonic optic vesicle retain their original orientation and are applied to one another, apex-to-apex (Fig. 10–43). The pigment epithelium of the retina is continuous with the pigment epithelium of the ciliary body without marked change, whereas the multi-layered retina ceases abruptly at the ora serrata (see Fig. 6–102, 6–103) to continue anteriorly the single-layered *nonpigmented* ciliary epithelium.

Here, the lumen of the optic vesicle becomes almost obliterated in contrast with persistence of the narrowed lumen posteriorly, between the sensory retina and its pigment epithelium, and anteriorly, between the two layers of iris pigment epithelium. The two epithelial cell layers become strongly attached to each other (Fig. 10–44) by a blending and modification of the two systems of terminal bars: the external limiting membrane of the neural retina and the

Ciliary epithelium

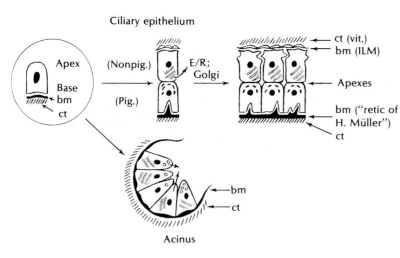

FIG. 10–43. Schematic drawing of arrangement of ciliary epithelium compared with that of an acinus of a more typical secretory tissue. **bm,** basement membrane; **ct,** connective tissue; **E/R** granular endoplasmic reticulum; **ILM,** internal limiting membrane; **vit**, vitreous filaments.

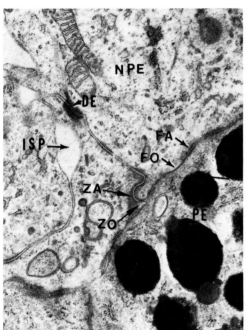

FIG. 10–44. Attachment between nonpigmented epithelium (**NPE**) and pigmented epithelium (**PE**). Attachment consists of three parts: fascia occludens (**FO**), fascia adherens (**FA**), and intercellular cement. Zonula adherens (**ZA**) of retinal external limiting membrane persists along apical plane of nonpigmented epithelium. An apical short zonula occludens (**ZO**) is added here to form a functional seal. **DE,** desmosome; **ISP,** enlarged intercellular space.(× 18,000)

FIG. 10–45. Tearing of apex of nonpigmented cell layer produced by mechanical separation. Enlarged intercellular spaces (**ISP**) and apical attachments remain behind. **PE,** pigment epithelium. (× 18,000)

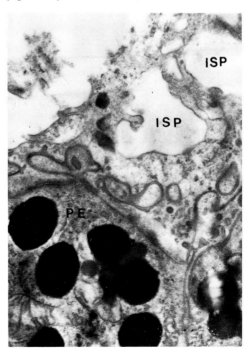

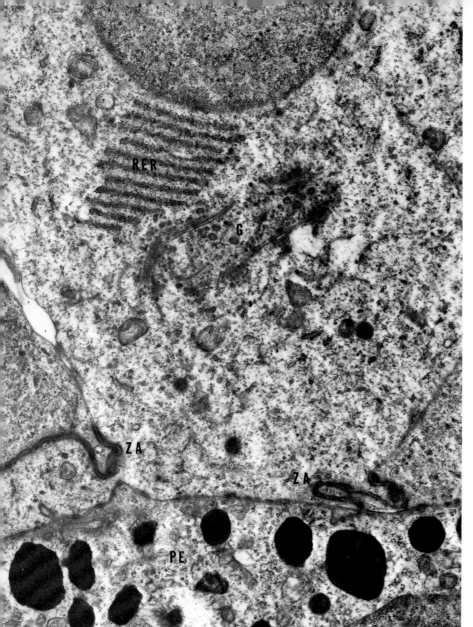

FIG. 10–46. Apical ends of nonpigmented epithelial cells linked by zonulae adherentes (**ZA**). The very short apical zonulae occludentes are not apparent here. Segments of granular endoplasmic reticulum (**RER**) and a Golgi complex (**G**) lie within apical cytoplasm. **PE,** pigment epithelium. (× 16,800)

fenestrated membrane of the pigment epithelium. Any attempt at mechanical separation of this attachment invariably tears the adjacent apical cell cytoplasm (Fig. 10–45).

Although the photoreceptor cells disappear at the ora serrata, the apical ends of the nonpigmented ciliary epithelial cells remain united to each other by a series of attachments resembling zonulae adherentes (Fig. 10–46), continuous with those of the external limiting membrane of the retina. A short zonula occludens is

added here (Fig. 10–44) to form a functional seal (Fig. 10–47) between apexes of the nonpigmented epithelial cells (20, 22, 26). Similarly, except for occasional foci, the apical villous processes of the retinal pigment epithelium disappear, and the terminal bar attachments, *both* occludens *and* adherens portions (Fig. 10–48), lie *between* the now-apposing surfaces of the two cell layers (*i.e.,* uniting pigmented epithelium to nonpigmented epithelium) (4).

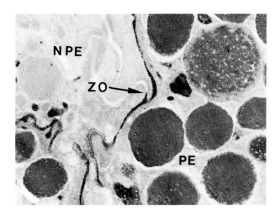

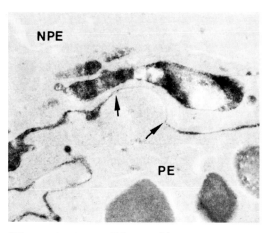

FIG. 10–48. Horseradish peroxidase passes freely between the two cell layers of the ciliary epithelium from rhesus monkey except for foci of fasciae occludentes (between **arrows**). **NPE,** nonpigmented epithelium. **PE,** pigment epithelium. (× 27,000)

FIG. 10–47. Intravascularly administered horseradish peroxidase passes between pigment epithelial cells (**PE**) in rhesus monkey tissue but is obstructed from passage between the nonpigmented epithelial cells (**NPE**) by the latter's apical zonulae occludentes (**ZO**). (× 18,000)

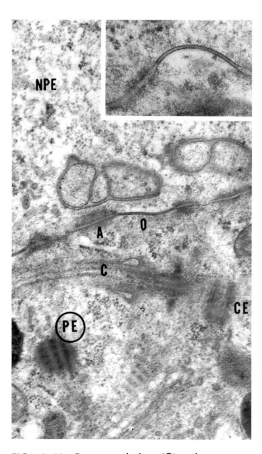

FIG. 10–49. Gap or occludens (**O**) and adherens (**A**) portions of fenestrated membrane of pigment epithelium now lying *between* two cell layers (**NPE** and **PE**). Note cilium (**C**), free centriole (**CE**), within apical cytoplasm of pigment cell. (× 30,000) Inset. Gap and/or occludens portion at higher magnification. (× 46,000)

Because the attachment zones between the two layers are observed segmentally in any single section (Fig. 10–44, 10–45, and 10–49), they presumably are incomplete girdles and therefore may also be termed **fasciae occludentes** (10) and **fasciae** or **puncta adherentes** (see Ch. 3). The zonulae adherentes of the neural retina (external limiting membrane) are carried over into the apical plane of the nonpigmented ciliary epithelium. A zonula occludens is added.

Lying between the two epithelia, in addition to the fascia occludens and fascia adherens, is a third component to the attachment plane, the **intercellular "cement" substance** (4) (Fig. 10–50). The cement substance lies extracellularly between the apical plasma membranes

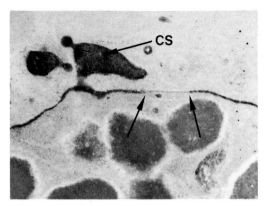

FIG. 10–50. Horseradish peroxidase passes between the two epithelial layers in tissue from rhesus monkey, filling "pockets" of intercellular spaces (**CS**). Foci of extreme intercellular attenuation (occludens or gap junctions) are present (between **arrows**). (× 27,000)

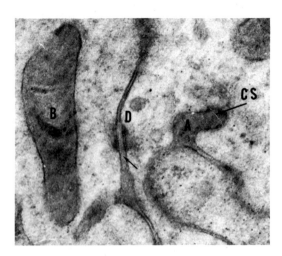

FIG. 10–51. Intercellular material (? cement) (**CS**) between apposing plasma membranes at **A.** The material (**free arrow**) is continuous with that of a nearby desmosome (**D**) or macula adherens. **B,** finger of intercellular material protruding from another plane. (× 59,000) (Fine BS, Zimmerman LE: Invest Ophthalmol 2:105, 1963)

and occasionally can be observed to be continuous with similar cement material of a nearby desmosome (Fig. 10–51). It is highly permeable to horseradish peroxidase.

The union of nonpigmented epithelium with pigmented epithelium is therefore tripartite: fascia (or macula or punctum) adherens, fascia (or macula) occludens, and an intercellular (?) cement. Desmosomes (**maculae adherentes**) attach adjacent cells to each other within a single epithelial layer (Fig. 10–51, 10–52).

Nonpigmented Epithelium and Internal Basement Membrane. At the ora serrata (Fig. 10–53) the delicate multilaminar basement membrane of the peripheral retina is carried over onto the nonpigmented epithelial cells as the **internal basement membrane** (internal limiting membrane). The basal surfaces of the cells are thrown into folds or processes, which intermingle with the multilaminar basement membrane. The intermingling is also continuous with the myriad collagenous filaments of the adjacent vitreous body (known as the base of the vitreous body).

Intercellular spaces of varying size between the nonpigmented cells (Fig. 10–54) reach to their apexes (4). The spaces (easily distinguishable from deep surface invaginations by lack of a basement membrane lining) are occupied by a lucent extracellular mucinous material that stains positively for acid mucopolysaccharides (Fig. 10–55).

In the region of the posterior pars plana, the apical cytoplasm of the nonpigmented epithelial cells possesses considerable quantities of organized granular endoplasmic reticulum (Fig. 10–56). Such quantities are lacking in all other

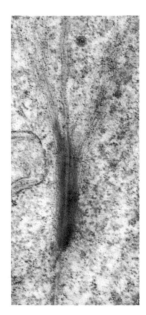

FIG. 10–52. Typical desmosome attaching adjacent nonpigmented epithelial cells to each other. (× 30,000)

FIG. 10–54. Posterior pars plana. Inset. Light micrograph of columnar nonpigmented cells of posterior pars plana. (Epon, PD, × 300) (AFIP Neg. 63-9615) Electron micrograph shows enlarged intercellular spaces filled with mucopolysaccharides (**MP**) between adjacent nonpigmented cells. Apical cell attachments to pigment epithelium are seen below. (× 14,000) (Fine BS, Zimmerman LE: Invest Ophthalmol 2:105, 1963)

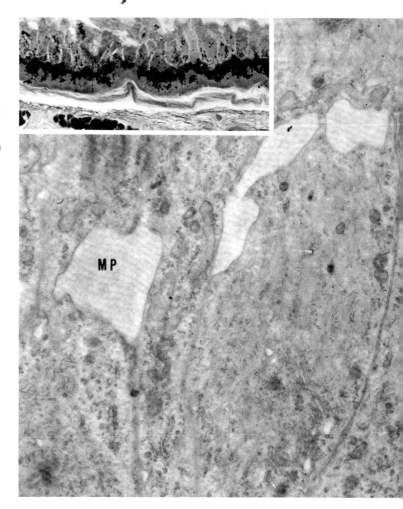

FIG. 10–53. Basement membrane of retina near ora serrata. Inset. Light micrograph showing density of vitreous base. (Wilder reticulum stain, × 70) (AFIP Neg. 70-1425) Electron micrograph shows multilaminar basement membrane (**arrows**). Many empty-appearing intercellular spaces (*i.e.*, not lined with basement membrane) are present in peripheral retinal tissue. (× 18,000)

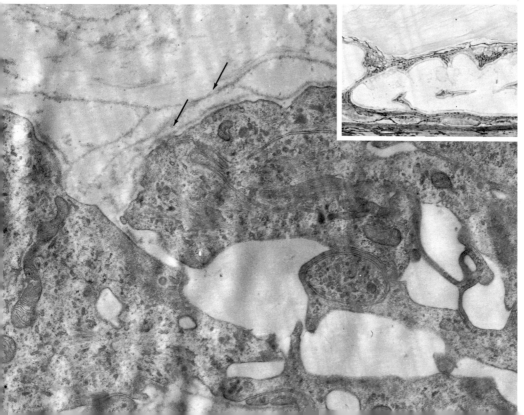

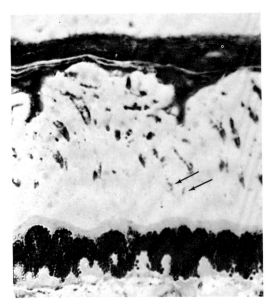

FIG. 10–55. Posterior pars plana of rhesus monkey eye stained for mucopolysaccharides. Blue-staining dots (**arrows**) are seen almost to apexes of nonpigmented cells. Blue-staining dots may be intra- or extracellular. (Methacrylate, Hale mucopolysaccharide stain, × 840) (Fine BS, Zimmerman LE: Invest Ophthalmol 2:105, 1963)

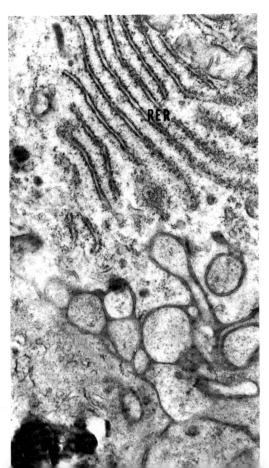

mature ocular tissues. In addition, the apical Golgi complex often may be observed to be enlarged with a lucent material, probably an acid mucopolysaccharide, that appears morphologically identical with the material present outside the cell in the enlarged intercellular spaces (Fig. 10–57).

The acid mucopolysaccharide component of the vitreous body is synthesized mainly by the nonpigmented epithelial cells of the pars plana. It is secreted into the adjacent lateral intercellular spaces (canaliculi) from whence it makes its way *basally* (Fig. 10–58) to enter the vitreous body at its base of attachment (4).

Flow of secreted materials toward the pigment epithelium is inhibited by the apical zonulae occludentes of the nonpigmented epithelium. Flow toward the vitreous base is not obstructed because only desmosomes join adjacent nonpigmented cells to each other. The vitreous body content of acid mucopolysaccharide is therefore maintained or replaced in the adult eye from the nonpigmented cells of the posterior pars plana, the rate of formation probably being very slow normally.

In the anterior pars plana (Fig. 10–59) the nonpigmented epithelium is cuboidal, whereas in the mid pars plana there is a transition zone of cuboidal to columnar epithelium. This transition region includes the attachment of the anterior face ("hyaloid") of the vitreous body. The multilaminar basement membrane of the cuboidal cells (Fig. 10–60) occupies the marked infoldings of their basilar surfaces. Issuing from many of the infoldings and attached to a thin basement membrane are the myriad collagenous filaments that, in aggregate, form the zonular fibers of the lens (Fig. 10–61).

It has long been known that the zonules are so strongly attached to the ciliary epithelium that a pull on them tears the epithelium. The firmness of this attachment is somewhat analogous to the attachment of hair to one's head; pulling out a single hair is relatively easy, whereas pulling out a handful is much more difficult. In addition, the basilar infold-

FIG. 10–56. Abundant granular endoplasmic reticulum (**RER**) in apical cytoplasm of posterior nonpigmented epithelium. (× 24,900) (Fine BS, Zimmerman LE: Invest Ophthalmol 2:105, 1963)

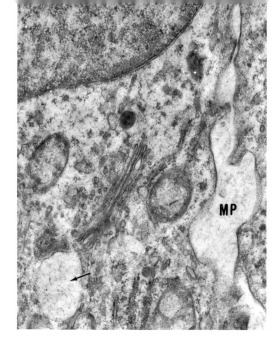

FIG. 10–57. Lucent material (**MP**) within intercellular space, morphologically similar to lucent material (**arrow**) within Golgi complex of adjacent nonpigmented epithelial cell. (× 32,000) (Fine BS, Zimmerman LE: Invest Ophthalmol 2:105, 1963)

FIG. 10–58. Intercellular canaliculus (**arrow**) carrying mucopolysaccharides synthesized within apical cytoplasm of nonpigmented epithelial cells into base of vitreous body (**V**). (× 12,480) (Fine BS, Zimmerman LE: Invest Ophthalmol 2:105, 1963)

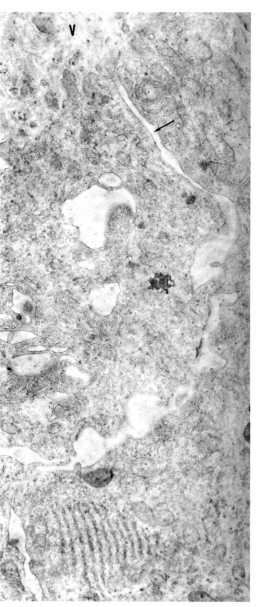

ings increase further the number of filament attachments per unit area of basilar surface, thus increasing the strength of adherence.

Zonular fibers in the anterior pars plana are considered vestigial, for few if any originate there. Fibers produced by similar cells found in the valleys of the pars plicata ("interciliary fibers," Fig. 10–62 through 10–65) are also considered vestigial.

That the major zonular fibers do not originate from the ciliary crests ("processes") but pass in the valleys between them (Fig. 10–66 through 10–70) is supported by clinical observations. When the equator of a subluxated lens is examined by slit lamp through a peripheral defect in the iris, the zonules can be observed to be taut, whereas the ciliary crests do not appear to be under any tension (1). Further clinical evidence in support of the anatomic observations is derived from iridocyclectomies where the zonules commonly remain untouched.

The nonpigmented epithelial cells of the pars plicata are cuboidal (25) (Fig. 10–63, 10–64). The nonpigmented cells lying on the apexes of the ciliary crests are covered by a minimum of

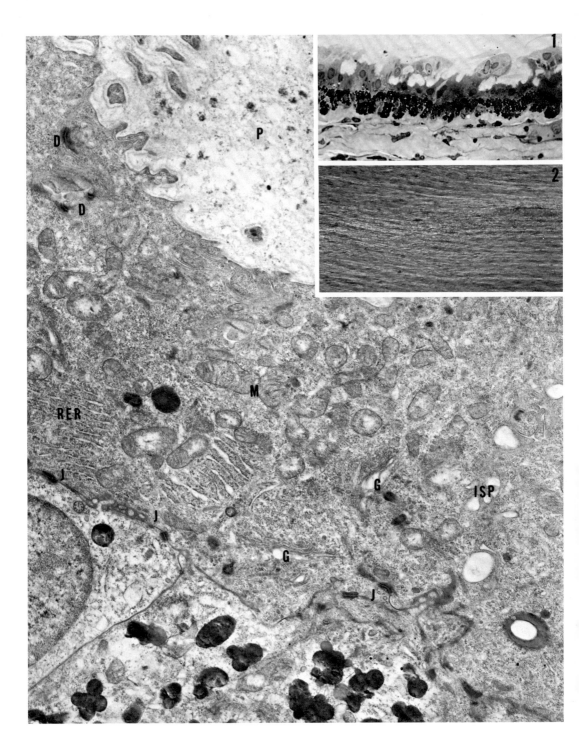

FIG. 10–59. Anterior pars plana. Electron micrograph shows large "pocket" (**P**) on basal surface of nonpigmented cells. Large spaces are occupied by expanded, multilaminar basement membrane, basement membrane materials, and vitreous filaments. Complex junctional regions (**J**) between nonpigmented and pigmented epithelia are seen, as well as desmosomes (**D**) between adjacent nonpigmented epithelial cells. Mitochondria (**M**) are abundant. Granular endoplasmic reticulum (**RER**) and a dilated Golgi complex (**G**) are present in apical cytoplasm of nonpigmented epithelium. Dilated intercellular spaces (**ISP**) are present. Pigment epithelial cells are joined to one another by small desmosomes. No enlarged intercellular spaces are present in pigment epithelial cell layer. (× 12,960) Inset 1. Light micrograph showing cuboidal appearance of epithelium. (Methacrylate, × 305) (AFIP Neg. 60-976) Inset 2. Scanning electron micrograph of "cleaned" inner surface showing delicate meridional surface striations apparently produced by "pocketing'" arrangement. (× 57) (Modified from Fine BS, Zimmerman LE: Invest Ophthalmol 2:105, 1963)

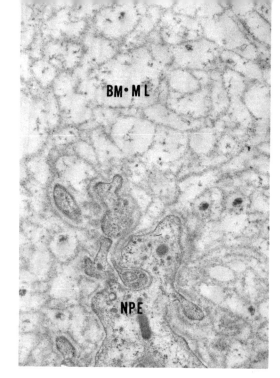

FIG. 10–60. Multilaminar basement membrane (**BM·ML**) characteristic of "internal limiting membrane" of nonpigmented ciliary epithelium (**NPE**). (× 19,800)

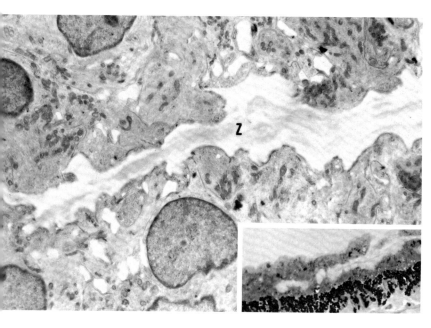

FIG. 10–61. Zonular fibers arising in basilar infoldings of nonpigmented epithelial cells. Electron micrograph shows thin basement membrane present along cell surface. Myriad filaments attached to basement membrane aggregate to form zonular fiber (**Z**). (× 5500) Inset. Light micrograph. (Methacrylate, × 305) (AFIP Neg. 60-972). (Fine BS, Zimmerman LE: Invest Ophthalmol 2:105, 1963)

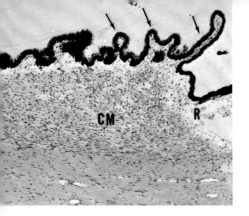

FIG. 10–62. Meridional section of pars plicata of infant, showing ciliary "processes" (**arrows**) on a ciliary crest. Large ciliary muscles (**CM**) thicken greatly this portion of uveal tract. Pars plicata extends from root of iris (**R**) to posterior extremity of ciliary crests (see Fig. 10–24). (H&E, × 55) (AFIP Neg. 65-234)

FIG. 10–63. Meridional section showing transition from anterior pars plana onto posterior edge of ciliary crest. "Motheaten" cuboidal cells characteristic of anterior pars plana (**arrows**) diminish in relative numbers, presenting anteriorly mostly in ciliary valleys (see Fig. 10–64). **CM,** ciliary muscle. (Epon, PD, × 165) (AFIP Neg. 66-1289)

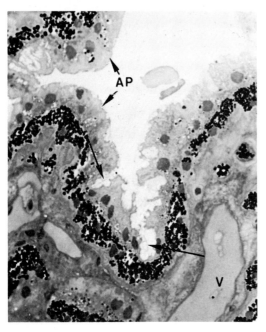

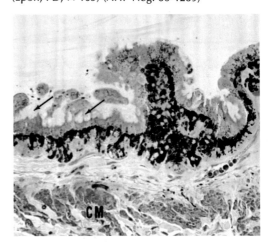

FIG. 10–64. Coronal section of pars plicata. "Motheaten" cells characteristic of anterior pars plana nonpigmented epithelial cells are present in ciliary valleys. Vestigial zonules (**free arrows**) are present. Nonpigmented epithelial cells at apex of crests (**AP**) possess smoother basal surface. **V,** blood vessel in connective tissue core. (Methacrylate, H&E, × 530) (AFIP Neg. 60-5331) (Fine BS, Zimmerman LE: Invest Ophthalmol 2:105, 1963)

FIG. 10–65. Ciliary processes. Their vascular collagenous core is covered by a double layer of epithelium, nonpigmented and pigmented. A small cyst (**C**) of nonpigmented epithelium is present at right, and two large granules of unknown composition (**arrows**) are present in nonpigmented epithelial layer at left. (Epon, PD, × 70) (AFIP Neg. 63-6909)

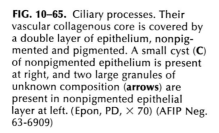

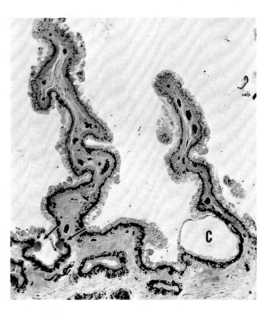

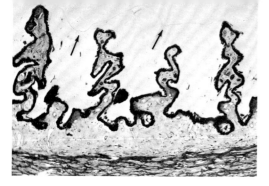

FIG. 10–66. Coronal section showing ciliary crests. Anterior border layer of vitreous body can be seen (**arrows**). (H&E, × 40) (AFIP Neg. 70-7287)

FIG. 10–67. Free surface of single ciliary crest as seen by SEM. Ciliary valley between crests is at right. (× 300)

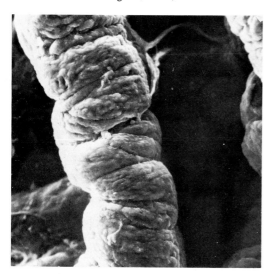

FIG. 10–69. Scanning electron micrograph of anterior zonules passing between ciliary crests. The lens has been pulled back to show zonules lifted from their valley beds. (× 23)

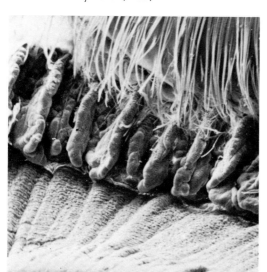

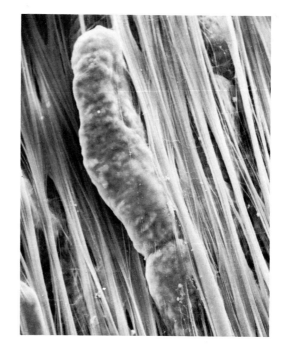

FIG. 10–68. Scanning electron micrograph of zonules passing alongside a small posterior ciliary process or wart. (× 200)

FIG. 10–70. Schematic representation of relation of orbiculoanterior zonular fibers to ciliary crests. Anterior border layer of vitreous body limiting posterior aqueous chamber posteriorly is indicated by **thick black line.**

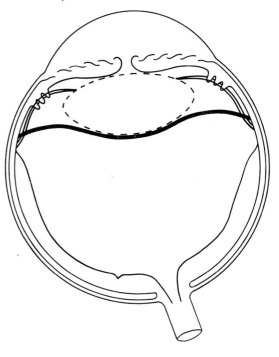

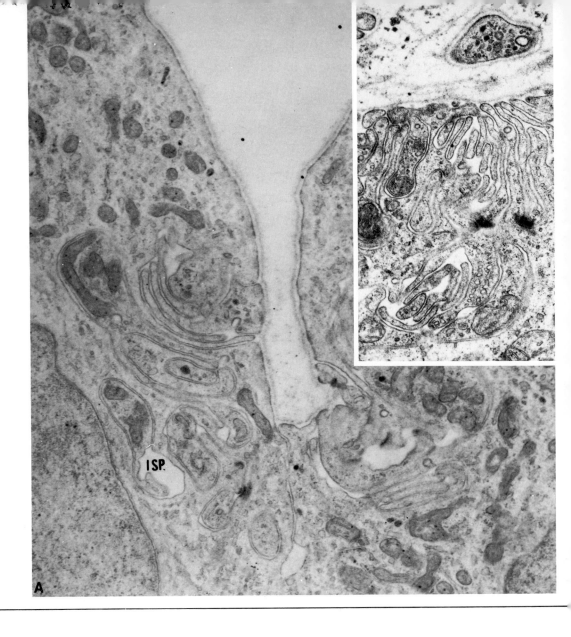

ISP.

A

basement membrane (Fig. 10–71). Although the basilar surfaces of these cells on the ciliary crests appear quite smooth by light microscopy, by electron microscopy, these surfaces show multiple deep infoldings, many of which are formed by interdigitation of myriad villous-like projections from adjacent epithelial cells (29, 30) (Fig. 10–71A). The white color of these apical regions (Fig. 10–24) is partly due to the high content of glycogen of the nonpigmented cells (Fig. 10–71B) as well as to the lesser pigmentation of the underlying pigment cell layer.

Focal enlargement of adjacent intercellular spaces between the nonpigmented cells is also present in the pars plicata, but since the content

of the spaces in this location is generally less well visualized than in the pars plana, the former is considered to be more watery.

On the anterior declivity of the ciliary crests (Fig. 10–72) the nonpigmented cells become more and more pigmented until they are completely altered into a layer of pigment epithelium *before* reaching the iris root.

Although the inner layer of ciliary epithelium is called nonpigmented, in the adult eye it may, in fact, contain a considerable amount of pigment, both lipofuscin and melanin granules (Fig. 10–72B), which bear a striking though not identical appearance to the neuromelanin granules of the substantia

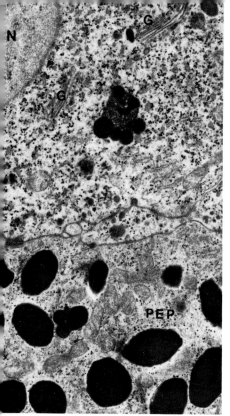

FIG. 10–71. Nonpigmented cells. A. Cuboidal nonpigmented epithelium present on free surface of ciliary crests. Basilar surfaces are lined by thin basement membrane. Infoldings are common along this basilar surface. Enlarged intercellular spaces (**ISP**), apparently empty, are present. (× 25,000) Inset. Another region in which basement membrane is multilaminar or "expanded." A few villi are embedded in this basement membrane. Tortuous basilar infoldings are due, in part, to interdigitation of basilar infoldings of adjacent cells. (× 16,500) Hogan M, Zimmerman LE: Ophthalmic Pathology: An Atlas and Textbook. Philadelphia, WB Saunders, 1962) B. Nonpigmented epithelium, 40-year-old subject. Myriad black dots show presence of glycogen in cells. The nonpigmented ciliary epithelial cell (**above**) contains a greater quantity of glycogen than the pigmented epithelium (**PEP**) below. **N**, nucleus of nonpigmented cell; **G**, portions of Golgi complex. (TSC only, × 14,000)

nigra (Fig. 10–72C). On occasion the granules may be so numerous in the apical cytoplasm that the nonpigmented cells of the pars plana appear markedly pigmented. Presumably, therefore, these cells retain some ability to synthesize melanin even in adult life.

Pigment Epithelium and External Basement Membrane. This layer of pigmented cells is continuous with the retinal pigment epithelium at the ora serrata, where the cell groups, as seen in section, form evaginations (Fig. 10–73) to give a thickened appearance to the layer. Grossly, this accounts for the heavily pigmented zone that parallels the ora serrata (see Fig. 6–101).

As in other epithelia, the melanin granules are located mostly apically and the basal plasma membranes are lined by a basement membrane (**external basement membrane,** cuticular lamella, or outer glass membrane of the pars ciliaris retinae; Fig. 10–74 through 10–77).

Anteriorly, in the region of the pars plicata, the pigment epithelial cells become more cuboidal than they are posteriorly. They are less pigmented on the apexes of the ciliary crests, where they rest upon the external basement membrane of the ciliary epithelium. This membrane becomes thicker in the anterior pars plana (Fig. 10–75, 10–76) and on the sides of the ciliary crests (Fig. 10–77A). It becomes so folded that on surface view of a suitable preparation of the pars plana, the appearance is that of a raised network or reticulum (reticulum of Heinrich-Müller [18] Fig. 10–76).

The thick basement membranes, like others, are all highly permeable to small molecules, such as horseradish peroxidase (Fig. 10–76B). The thick external basement membrane of the ciliary epithelium in reality is a continuation of the lamina vitrea of Bruch's membrane.

Uveal (Mesodermal) Portion

As elsewhere, the external basement membrane of the pigment epithelium is associated with collagen fibrils. In this region the fibrils are of considerable diameter (i.e., thick). A layer of vessels, continuous in a plane with those of the choriocapillaris, is separated from the pigment epithelium by a basement membrane and collagen fibrils (Fig. 10–74). Between these two aggregates may be found denser collagenous

FIG. 10–72. Ciliary crest. A. Anterior declivity of ciliary crest. Transition of nonpigmented epithelium to fully pigmented epithelium occurs here (**arrow**). (Epon section, PD, × 115) (AFIP Neg. 65-6684) B. Granules in apex of nonpigmented ciliary epithelium. Melanin-like particles (**arrows**) accumulate in the crevices between the homogeneous (?lipofuscin) bodies. By light microscopy the composite structures appear as melanin granules. (× 25,800) C. Substantia nigra of chimpanzee. Homogeneous dense material (neuromelanin) accumulates in close proximity to homogeneous, less dense granules (?lipofuscin). (× 20,400)

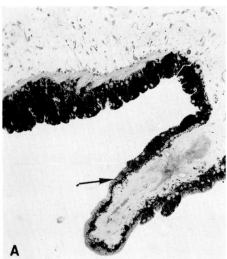

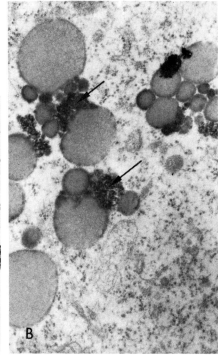

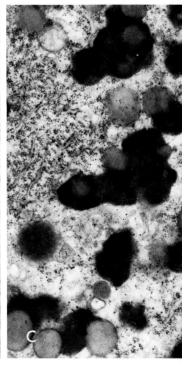

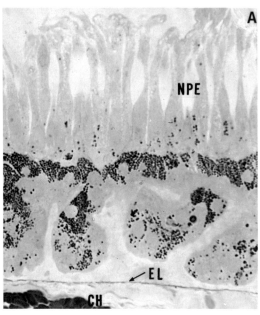

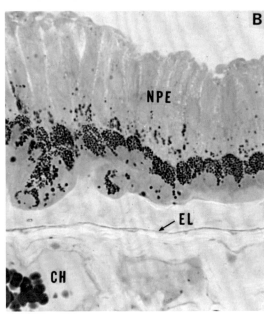

tissue or long patches of homogeneous elastic tissue, the **elastic lamina.** Anteriorly the vascular tissue is folded, forming the connective tissue cores of the ciliary crests ("processes"). The capillaries of the ciliary crests are large, and many possess *fenestrated* endothelia similar to those of the choriocapillaris (Fig. 10–77, 10–78).

In contrast with the situation in the pars plana (Fig. 10–73), the capillaries of the ciliary crests are not separated by a prominent elastic tissue layer from the very thick, more conspicuously multilaminar basement membrane (Fig. 10–64, 10–77) of the adjacent pigmented ciliary epithelium.

Excessive thickening of this normally thick multilaminar external basement membrane of the ciliary epithelium (37) is a characteristic histologic feature of the eye in many patients with long-standing diabetes mellitus (36).

FIG. 10–73. Pigment epithelium in eye of 40-year-old subject. Near ora serrata, pigment epithelium forms evaginations (**A**) which terminate rather abruptly (**B**) in line that roughly parallels ora serrata. In mid and anterior pars plana, pigment epithelium is a more uniform single layer (**C**). Note comparable transition in height of nonpigmented epithelium (**NPE**) from tall columnar to short columnar to more cuboidal cells. **CH,** choriocapillaris; **EL,** elastic lamina. Prominent elastic lamina of the pars plana appears "negatively stained" (**D**) when section is treated only with uranyl acetate and lead. With TSC treatment alone both elastic lamina and adjacent collagen fibrils become dense (**E**). With uranyl acetate, lead and Ag-TPPS (Ch. 1), the elastic tissue is densely stained with greater specificity (**F**). (**A**, Epon, PD, × 485) (AFIP Neg. 70-8858) (**B,** Epon, PD, × 485) (AFIP Neg. 70-8859) (**C,** Epon, PD, × 485) (AFIP Neg. 70-8857); (**D, E, F,** all × 21,000)

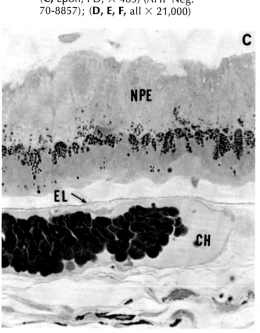

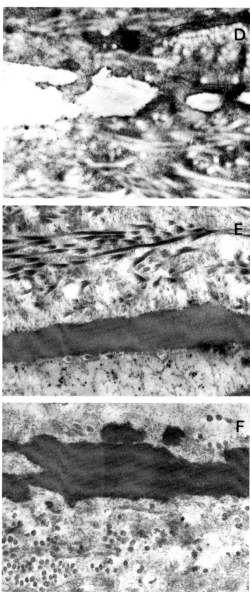

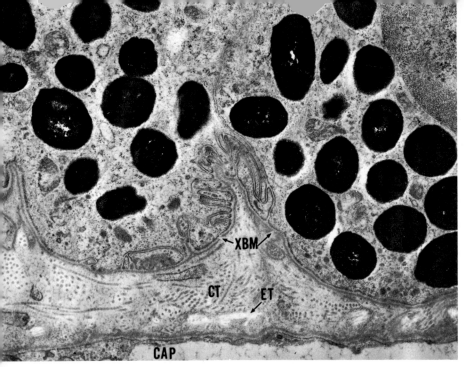

FIG. 10–74. Pigment epithelium of anterior pars plana from eye of 10-month-old infant. External basement membrane (**XBM**) is thin but markedly folded. Thin basement membrane is separated from similar thin basement membrane of adjacent fenestrated capillary layer (**CAP**) by collagenous connective tissue (**CT**), in which small patches of homogeneous-appearing elastic tissue (**ET**) are present. (× 16,500)

FIG. 10–75. Pigment epithelium from eye of 18-year-old subject. External basement membrane (**XBM**) is markedly thickened. A layer of elongated nonpigmented uveal cells (**arrows**) lines outer surface of this thick basement membrane. Collagenous connective tissue (**CT**) lies outside layer of nonpigmented uveal cells.(× 11,000) Inset. Close apposition (**arrow**) of thick basement membrane to cell plasmalemma. (× 15,000)

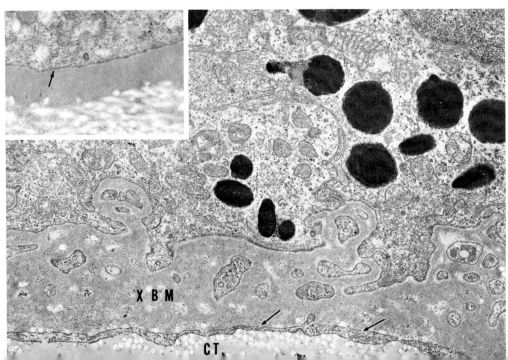

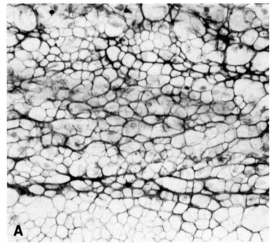

FIG. 10–76. External basement membrane. A. Flat preparation of ciliary body external basement membrane (anterior pars plana) showing its reticular topography (reticulum of Heinrich-Müller. (PAS, × 115) (Courtesy of Dr. G. de Venecia) B. Horseradish peroxidase in region of external basement membrane of ciliary epithelium (**double arrow**) and elastic lamina (**EL**). Note how peroxidase outlines the cell, the collagen fibrils (**CT**), and passes through the thick basement membrane into the intercellular space (**single arrow**) between pigment epithelial cells. (× 18,000)

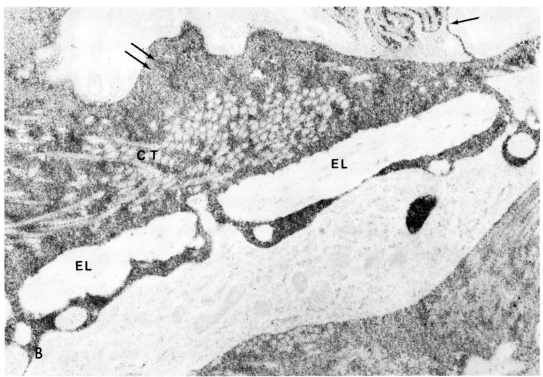

Continuous with the choroid proper and outside the plane of the ciliary crests lies the large mass of smooth muscle, the ciliary muscle (Fig. 10–79) that generally is subdivided into three parts: the meridional or longitudinal muscle externally; the circular, round, or radial muscle internally; and a variable oblique muscle in between.

The smooth muscle cells are typical of other smooth muscles (8) (Fig. 10–80), being enveloped by a continuous basement membrane (except for regions of apposition with another muscle cell or nerve ending) and having myriad surface plasma membrane infoldings (micropinocytotic vesicles or caveolae), surface densities, cytoplasmic filaments, and scattered densities among the cytoplasmic filaments.

When the criteria for a cell type are sufficiently numerous, as here for smooth muscle cells, they may

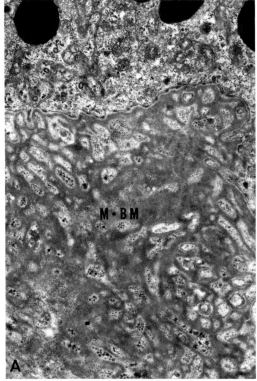

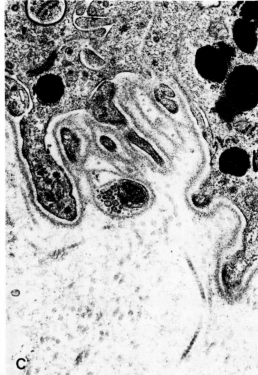

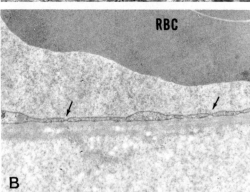

FIG. 10–77. External basement membrane. A. Prominent multilaminar basement membrane (**M·BM**) of pigmented ciliary epithelium of the pars plicata in 40-year-old man. ($\times$ 12,300) B. Fenestrated endothelium (**arrows**) of vessel in collagenous "core" of ciliary crest. **RBC,** red blood cell in lumen. ($\times$ 18,000) C. Multilaminar basement membrane of pigmented ciliary epithelium of pars plicata in a 4-month-old infant. ($\times$ 18,000)

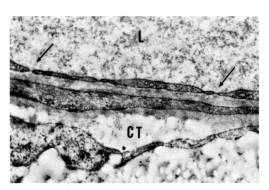

FIG. 10–78. Fenestrated (**arrow**) innermost capillary of pars plana. **CT,** connective tissue; **L,** lumen of vessel. ($\times$ 16,500)

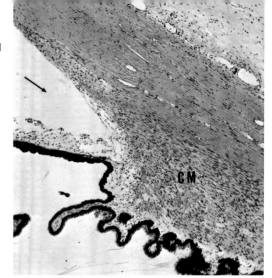

FIG. 10–79. Marked thickening of uveal tract in region of pars plicata is due to ciliary muscle (**CM**). **Arrow.** Drainage angle of anterior chamber. (H&E, × 55) (AFIP Neg. 65-233)

FIG. 10–80. Smooth muscle cells of ciliary muscle. **BM,** basement membrane; **P,** caveolae or micropino-cytotic vesicles; **FI,** intracellular filaments; **D,** densities among the filaments or (**D₁**) attached to cell plasma membranes; **M,** mitochondria. Circular profile containing myriad vesicles represents a nerve near its synaptic ending (**S**). Melanocyte (**ME**) is typical of uveal melanocytes. Inset. Smooth muscle cells in cross-section. Their basement membrane (**B**), filaments in cross-section (**F**), densities (**D**), vesicles (**P**), and nearby nerve endings (**S**) are clearly seen. (× 16,500)

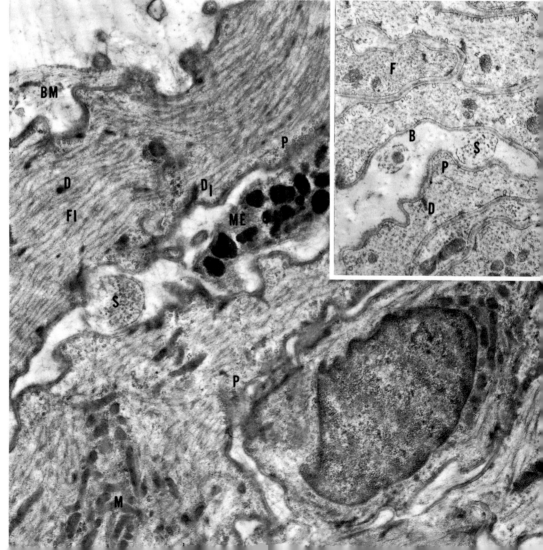
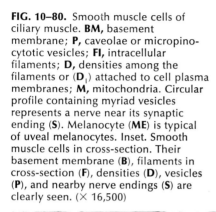

be useful in diagnosing a tumor (9) even if the material has been preserved inadequately (13).

The muscle cells are separated by delicate collagenous fibrils and spaces presumably occupied by watery intercellular mucinous materials. The muscles are liberally provided with arterial supplies from the long posterior ciliary and anterior ciliary arteries, whereas their drainage is mainly posteriorly, via the small vessels of the inner uveal layers, and externally (*i.e.*, laterally), via the anterior ciliary veins through the sclera. These latter veins also participate in drainage from the canal of Schlemm.

Lying within the loose uveal tissue anterior to the circular or oblique muscles and close to the root of the iris is a circumferential artery, the **major arterial circle.** This circle is formed from the terminal bifurcations of the two long posterior ciliary arteries, which also anastomose with branches from the anterior ciliary arteries. The iris and ciliary crests are supplied from this arterial circle.

Venous drainage from the uveal tract is somewhat unusual in that it does not accompany the arterial supply, but rather leaves the globe posteriorly as a separate and distinct system of four vortex veins, each located within one of the quadrants (see Fig. 5–6).

REFERENCES

1. Berliner ML: Biomicroscopy of the Eye. New York, Hoeber, 1949
2. Butler TH: An Illustrated Guide to the Slit-Lamp. London, Oxford University Press, 1927
3. Fine BS: Free-floating pigmented cyst in the anterior chamber. Am J Ophthalmol 67:493, 1969
4. Fine BS, Zimmerman LE: Light and electron microscopic observations on the ciliary epithelium in man and rhesus monkey, with particular reference to the base of the vitreous body. Invest Ophthalmol 2:105, 1963
5. Friedman E, Smith TR, Kuwabara T: Senile choroidal vascular patterns and drusen. Arch Ophthalmol 69:220, 1963
6. Garron LK: The ultrastructure of the retinal pigment epithelium, with observations on the choriocapillaris and Bruch's membrane. Trans Am Ophthalmol Soc 61:545, 1963
7. Hogan M, Zimmerman LE: Ophthalmic Pathology: An Atlas and Textbook. Philadelphia, WB Saunders, 1962
8. Ishikawa T: Fine structure of the human ciliary muscle. Invest Ophthal 1:587, 1962
9. Jakobiec FA, Font RL, Tso MOM, Zimmerman LE: Mesectodermal leiomyoma of the ciliary body. Cancer 39:2102, 1977
10. Kogan M, Pappas GO: Atypical gap junction in the ciliary epithelium of the albino rabbit eye. J Cell Biol 66:671, 1975
11. Matsui M, Parel J-M, Weder H, Justice J: Some improved methods of anterior segment fluorescein angiography. I. Basic system. Am J Ophthalmol 74:1075, 1972
12. McMahon RT, Tso MOM, McLean IW: Histologic localization of sodium fluorescein in choroidal malignant melanomas. Am J Ophthalmol 83:836, 1977
13. Meyer SL, Fine BS, Font RL, Zimmerman LE: Leiomyoma of the ciliary body: electron microscopic verification. Am J Ophthalmol 66:1061, 1968
14. Nakaizuma Y: The ultrastructure of Bruch's membrane. I. Human, monkey, rabbit, guinea pig, and rat eyes. Arch Ophthalmol 72:380, 1964
15. Nakaizuma Y, Hogan MJ, Feeney L: The ultrastructure of Bruch's membrane. III. The macular area of the human eye. Arch Ophthalmol 72:395, 1964
16. Perry HD, Hatfield RV, Tso MOM: Fluorescein pattern of the choriocapillaris in the neonatal rhesus monkey Am J Ophthalmol 84:197, 1977
17. Richardson KC: The fine structure of the albino rabbit iris, with special reference to the identification of adrenergic and cholinergic nerves and nerve endings in its intrinsic muscles. Am J Anat 114:174, 1964
18. Salzmann M: The Anatomy and Histology of the Human Eyeball in the Normal State. Brown EVL (trans). Chicago, University of Chicago Press, 1912
19. Sarks SH: New vessel formation beneath the retinal pigment epithelium in senile eyes. Br J Ophthalmol 57:951, 1973
20. Shabo AL, Maxwell DS: The blood aqueous barrier to tracer protein. A light and electron microscopic study of the primate ciliary process. Microvasc Res 4:142, 1972
21. Shabo AL, Maxwell DS: Structural organization of the pars plana-ora serrata transition in the human and monkey eye with emphasis on protein barriers. Lab Invest 29:511, 1973
22. Shabo AL, Maxwell DS: Electron microscopic localization of occluding junctions in the primate ciliary process and pars plana. Invest Ophthalmol 12:863, 1973
23. Simionescu M, Simionescu N, Palade G: Segmental differentiations of cell junctions in the vascular endothelium. The microvasculature. J Cell Biol 67:863, 1975
24. Simionescu N, Simionescu M, Palade G: Permeability of intestinal capillaries. Pathway followed by dextrans and glycogen. J Cell Biol 53:365, 1972
25. Smelser GK: Electron microscopy of a typical epithelial cell and of the normal human ciliary process. Trans Am Acad Ophthalmol Otolaryngol 70:738, 1966
26. Smith RS, Rudt LA: Ocular vascular and epithelial barriers to microperoxidase. Invest Ophthalmol 14:556, 1975
27. Takei Y, Ozanics V: Origin and development of Bruch's membrane in monkey fetuses: an electron

microscopic study. Invest Ophthalmol 14:903, 1975

28. Torczynski E, Tso MOM: The architecture of the choriocapillaris at the posterior pole. Am J Ophthalmol 81:428, 1976

29. Tormey J McD: Relationship between the structure of the ciliary epithelium and the secretion of aqueous humor. In Rohen JW (ed): The Structure of the Eye. Stuttgart, Schattauer, 1965, p 237

30. Tormey J McD: The ciliary epithelium: an attempt to correlate structure and function. Trans Am Acad Ophthalmol Otolaryngol 70:755, 1966

31. Tousimis AJ, Fine BS: Ultrastructure of the iris: an electron microscopic study. Am J Ophthalmol 48:397, 1959

32. Tousimis AJ, Fine BS: Ultrastructure of the iris: the intercellular stromal components. Arch Ophthalmol 62:974, 1077, 1959

33. Tousimis AJ, Fine BS: Electron microscopy of the pigment epithelium of the iris. In Smelser GK (ed): The Structure of the Eye. New York, Academic Press, 1961, p 441

34. Verhoeff FH, Sisson RJ: Basophilic staining of Bruch's membrane. Arch Ophthalmol 55:125, 1926

35. Wobmann PR, Fine BS: The clump cells of Koganei: a light and electron microscopic study. Am J Ophthalmol 73:90, 1972

36. Yamashita T, Becker B: The basement membrane in the human diabetic eye. Diabetes 10:167, 1961

37. Yanoff M, Fine BS: Ocular Pathology: A Text and Atlas. Hagerstown, Harper & Row, 1975

38. Yanoff M, Zimmerman LE: Pseudomelanoma of anterior chamber caused by implantation of iris pigment epithelium. Arch Ophthalmol 74:30, 1965

chapter 11

THE ANTERIOR CHAMBER ANGLE

THE AQUEOUS COMPARTMENT   251
  ANTERIOR CHAMBER
  POSTERIOR CHAMBER
THE AQUEOUS   251
THE LIMBUS   251
THE DRAINAGE ANGLE   252
THE TRABECULAR MESHWORK   261

THE AQUEOUS COMPARTMENT

The opened eye (Fig. 11–1) clearly separates into two unequal *compartments:* The smaller or **aqueous compartment** lies anteriorly, in front of the vitreous face, and the larger or **vitreous compartment** lies posteriorly, behind the lens (Fig. 11–2).

The anterior (aqueous) compartment is further subdivided by the iris diaphragm into two *chambers:* the anterior and the posterior (Fig. 11–3). The anterior chamber is bounded by the anterior surface of the iris and the pupil posteriorly, by the corneal endothelium anteriorly, and by the arciform boundary of the drainage angle laterally.

At the periphery of the anterior chamber the corneoscleral and uveal coats of the eye unite (Col. Fig. 11–4) to form the iridocorneoscleral angle of the anterior chamber, or drainage angle. The angle consists of a circumferential furrow or groove in the mesodermal (ectomesenchymal, see Ch. 5) tissue at the periphery of the anterior chamber. In meridional section, therefore, this iridocorneoscleral *angle*, sometimes called the **angular sinus,** appears as a concavity lying on the "face" of the ciliary body whose blunt end faces the anterior chamber. Histologically, this concavity or arc extends from the end of Descemet's membrane (Schwalbe's anterior border ring or line) to the iris root, where the anterior border layer of the iris also terminates abruptly.

THE AQUEOUS

The aqueous appears to be actively secreted mostly by the nonpigmented ciliary epithelium that lines the posterior chamber. It flows continuously from the posterior to the anterior aqueous chamber via the pupil, and within the anterior chamber it flows in at least two directions (Fig. 11–5): first, from the pupillary entrance toward the drainage angle in the chamber periphery; and second, from where it rises as it becomes warmed by the iris posteriorly to

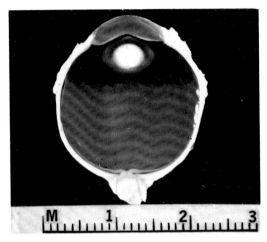

FIG. 11–1. An opened, fixed globe. Temporal part of globe has been removed by cut running through optic nerve and just temporal to pupil.

where it falls anteriorly as it is cooled by the cornea.

These currents of flow can be best appreciated clinically when small amounts of material such as the products of inflammation, are present in the aqueous. Excessive accumulation of such materials may even halt the currents of flow. In such a case resumption of motion by these materials in the anterior chamber may be the first sign of improvement.

THE LIMBUS

In the region of the limbus (see Ch. 9) where clear cornea alters into opaque sclera, a deep inner circumferential groove, the **inner scleral sulcus** or **furrow,** and a shallow outer one, the **outer scleral sulcus** or **furrow** (Fig. 11–6) can be seen on gross examination of a dissected preparation (20). On meridional section, the transition line from cornea to sclera extends from the end of Bowman's membrane to the end of Descemet's membrane and appears as an arcuate line with its convexity directed laterally and posteriorly.

This "convexity" of peripheral transparent corneal tissue within the "concavity" of the adjacent opaque sclera can also be well appreciated clinically by slit-lamp examination (gonioscopy). The radius of curvature of this union is shorter superiorly and inferiorly than laterally.

THE DRAINAGE ANGLE

The posterior boundary of the inner scleral sulcus is a collagenous ridge, composed mainly of circumferentially oriented bundles of collagen fibrils, the **scleral roll** (5, 20) (Fig. 11–7, 11–8) or Schwalbe's posterior border ring. After continuing for a short distance posteriorly, the ridge tapers and finally blends with the more predominant, obliquely arranged collagenous lamellas of the sclera.

Deep within this sulcus (Fig. 11–4, 11–9) and applied closely to the collagenous tissue of the corneosclera lies the large vessel known as the **canal of Schlemm.** This circumferentially arranged vessel (or complex of vessels, for it branches frequently,* Fig. 11–26A) is formed by a continuous layer of nonfenestrated endothelial cells (Fig. 11–10 through 11–13) with a rather patchy or diffuse basement membrane (Fig. 11–14, 11–21). The structure of the canal of Schlemm closely resembles the structure of a lymphatic (see section Conjunctiva, Ch. 13). It is called an aqueous vessel because *in vivo* it contains aqueous fluid alone.

The canal of Schlemm is lined by endothelial cells whose bodies protrude into the lumen (Fig. 11–17A) and whose basal cytoplasm is attenuated into large area-covering sheets. The endothelial cells abut one against the other in a number of forms, which vary from simple end-to-end apposition to more complex arrangements resembling interlocking mortise-and-tenon joints (Fig. 11–14). The cell-to-cell appositions form an attachment zone resembling a zonula adherens (Fig. 11–15) which can be easily separated by a reflux of red blood cells and plasma proteins (17, 19). Near the attachments, the cytoplasm often is thrown into large villi or folds The folds project either into the lumen of the canal or into the adjacent

---

* The projections of tissue intervening between segments of the canal are called **septa.** Each septum contains a dense collagenous core resembling closely those of the adjacent corneoscleral tissue.

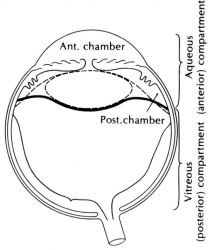

FIG. 11–2. Aqueous and vitreous compartments. Compartments are separated by anterior face of vitreous body (**heavy black line**), which also demarcates posterior boundary of posterior (aqueous) chamber.

FIG. 11–3. Chambers of aqueous compartment. Aqueous compartment is subdivided into two chambers by iris diaphragm. Anterior chamber in front of diaphragm is indicated by stippling; the posterior chamber behind iris diaphragm is indicated in solid black.

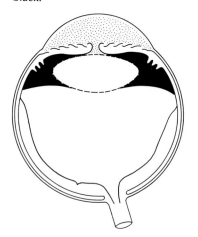

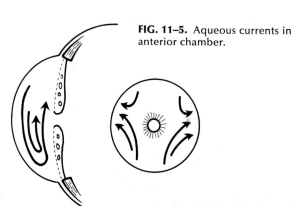

FIG. 11–5. Aqueous currents in anterior chamber.

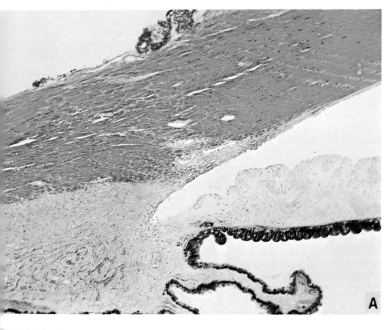

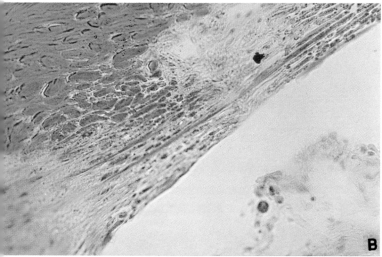

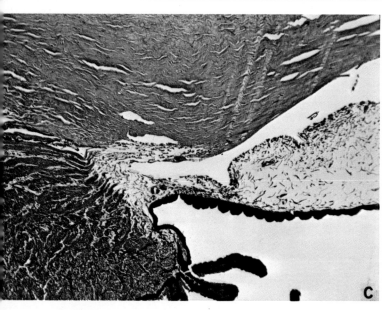

FIG. 11–4. The drainage angle. A. Iridocorneoscleral angle is formed by union of corneoscleral and uveal coats at periphery of anterior chamber. Trabecular meshwork fills inner scleral sulcus (Fig. 11–6), posterior boundary of which is scleral roll.(Masson, × 60) (AFIP Acc. 84029) B. High magnification of region of adult scleral spur, showing its bipartite composition of circumferentially arranged bundles of collagen from scleral roll and more meridionally arranged bundles of collagen from adjacent trabecular (uveal) meshwork. (Masson, × 300) C. Rhesus monkey drainage angle. Most of trabecular meshwork extends from deep corneal periphery to become continous with uveal tract. A small outer portion (corneoscleral) blends with scleral roll. Compare drainage angle of infant (Fig. 11–26A). (Masson × 80) (AFIP Neg. 60-4865) (Fine BS: Invest Ophthalmol 3:609, 1964)

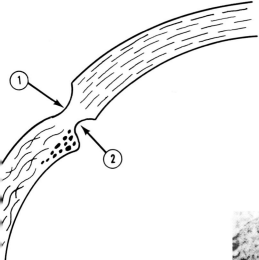

FIG. 11–6. Schematic representation of meridional section of corneoscleral coat. Circumferential shallow outer sulcus (**1**) and deeper inner sulcus (**2**) are present in region of union of cornea with sclera. Posterior boundary of inner sulcus is thickened by scleral roll (posterior border ring of Schwalbe).

FIG. 11–7. Light micrograph of region of scleral roll, showing cross-sectioned bundles of circumferentially arranged collagen (**arrows**) characteristic of this region. Contrast these collagen bundles with those of adjacent sclera (**S**) and with nearby ciliary muscles (**CM**). **CS,** canal of Schlemm. (Meridional section, H&E, × 265) (AFIP Neg. 68-9954)

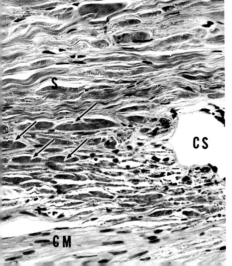

FIG. 11–8. Scleral roll. A. Electron micrograph shows collagen fibrils, though varying in diameter, all circumferentially arranged within each collagen bundle. A number of cells are present, as well as patches of elastic tissue. (Meridional section, × 16,000) B. Patch of elastic tissue forming in scleral roll of 4-month-old infant. Most of the elastic tissue here consists of microfibrils. Elastica (**free arrows**) is not prominent. **C,** collagen fibrils. (× 35,400)

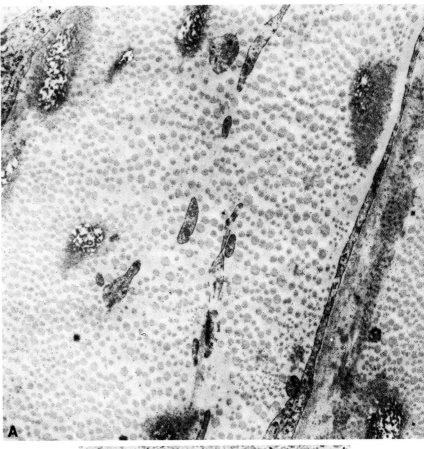

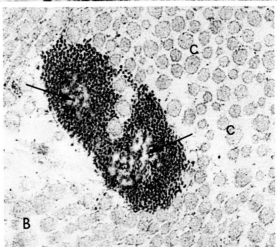

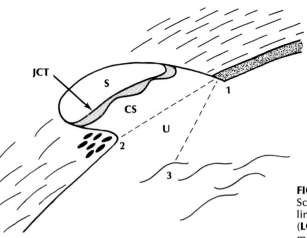

FIG. 11–9. Schematic drawing of drainage angle. **1,** end of Descemet's membrane; **2,** tip of scleral roll; **3,** end of anterior border layer of iris; **CS,** corneoscleral meshwork; **JCT,** juxtacanalicular connective tissue layer; **S,** canal of Schlemm; **U,** uveal meshwork. (Fine BS: Trans Am Acad Ophthalmol Otolaryngol 70:777, 1966)

FIG. 11–10. Drainage angle of adult. Scleral roll (**SR**) is outlined by dotted line. Adjacent longitudinal ciliary muscle (**LCM₁**) is partially "hyalinized," more markedly in anterior and outer parts of longitudinal ciliary muscle (**LCM**). **TR** indicates imaginary line extending from scleral roll to Schwalbe's line. Meshwork is separable into inner or uveal (**U**) portion and outer or corneoscleral (**C**) portion. A special region, the juxtacanalicular connective tissue (**JCT**), variable in thickness, lies adjacent to endothelium-lined (**EN**) canal of Schlemm (**CS**). **AC,** anterior chamber; **CL,** canaliculus of canal of Schlemm; **SC,** sclera. (1.5-μ meridional section, hematoxylin-phloxine, × 420) (AFIP Neg. 63-4155) (Fine BS: Invest Ophthalmol 3:609, 1964)

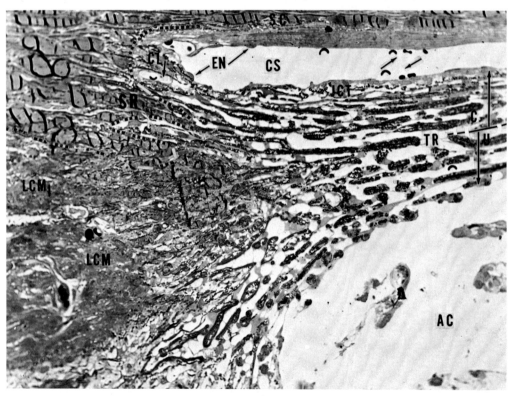

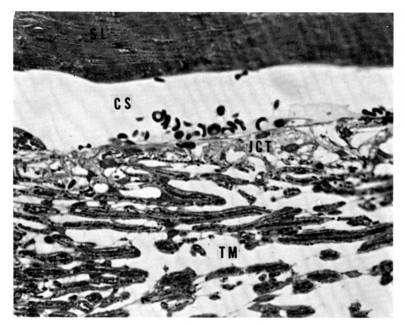

FIG. 11–11. Region of canal of Schlemm (CS). Density of adjacent scleral lamellas (SL) is apparent. Trabecular meshwork (TM) blends with irregular juxtacanalicular connective tissue (JCT). Red blood cells are present in lumen of canal of Schlemm. (1.5-μ section, hematoxylin-phloxine, × 530) (AFIP Neg. 63-4154) (Fine BS: Trans Am Acad Ophthalmol Otolaryngol 70:777, 1966)

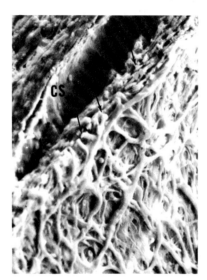

FIG. 11–12. Scanning electron micrograph of cut-open canal of Schlemm (CS) and anterior chamber surface of adjacent uveal meshwork of young adult. A few red blood cells lie on smooth outer endothelial lining of canal, and cut edges of full thickness meshwork can be seen at arrows. (× 310)

FIG. 11–13. Electron micrograph showing canal of Schlemm (CS), adjacent juxtacanalicular connective tissue (JCT), and corneoscleral meshwork with intertrabecular spaces (IT). (× 4000)

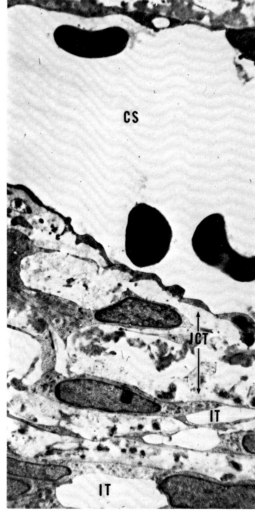

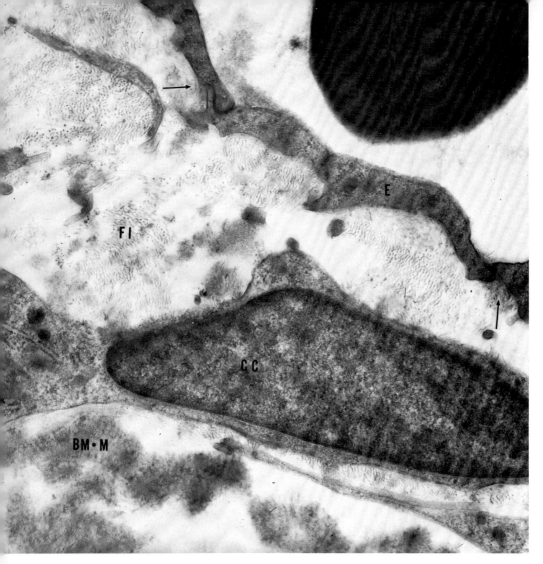

FIG. 11–14. Electron micrograph of endothelium (**E**) lining inner wall of canal of Schlemm. Endothelial basement membrane is diffuse and patchy (**arrows**). Endothelial cell-to-cell abutments are present. Juxtacanalicular connective tissue contains cells surrounded by extracellular materials varying from delicate filaments (**FI**) of collagen or elastic tissue to patches of banded basement-membrane-like material (**BM•M**). **CC,** connective tissue cell. (× 21,500) (Fine BS: Invest Ophthalmol 3:609, 1964)

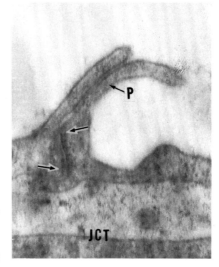

FIG. 11–15. Zonula adherens type of attachment (**free arrows**) between endothelial cells of inner wall of canal of Schlemm, from rhesus monkey. **JCT,** juxtacanalicular connective tissue; **P,** villous projections or flaps into lumen. (× 41,600) (Fine BS: Trans Am Acad Ophthalmol Otolaryngol 70:777, 1966)

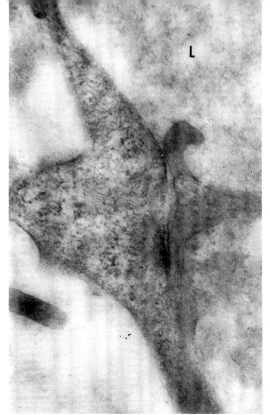

FIG. 11–16. Endothelial cell villi or folds projecting into lumen of canal of Schlemm (**L**) or into adjacent juxtacanalicular connective tissue. (× 40,500) (Fine BS: Invest Ophthalmol 3:609, 1964)

FIG. 11–17. Inner wall of canal of Schlemm in adult. A. Protrusion of cell bodies into the canal lumen can be seen by SEM (**free arrows**). (× 1300) B. Endothelium of inner wall of canal of Schlemm (**CS**) contains large numbers of micropinocytotic vesicles (seen enlarged in inset, × 36,000). Note adherens type of junctions between adjacent endothelial cells (**arrows**). **JCT,** juxtacanalicular connective tissue. (× 17,500)

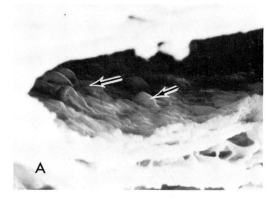

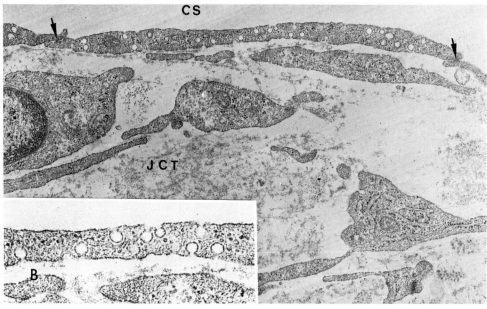

juxtacanalicular connective tissue (5) (Fig. 11–16) and often assume bizarre configurations. There is some evidence that they may even participate in a form of *macropinocytotic* transport mechanism across the endothelial cell barrier (5, 24–26).

It is likely that some of the large "cytoplasmic vacuoles" (11–14, 24) that are often reported to be present within the endothelial cells are formations produced by the large endothelial villi, folds, or "flaps" during fixation (6, 21).

All the endothelial cells lining the canal of Schlemm (Fig. 11–17A) possess small invaginations of the plasmalemma (Fig. 11–17B). Because of their appearance and their pinocytotic-like activity they have been termed **micropinocytotic** vesicles (4–6). They are present at both the apical and basal surfaces of the endothelial cells. Free forms of these vesicles also are present and functional within the cell cytoplasm.

Pinocytotic vesicles often may be *induced* in a cell by contact of its plasmalemma with a foreign substance such as a tracer material. Vesicles observed in normal tissues, otherwise untouched except by fixation procedures, generally are considered to be present *in vivo* and presumably carrying out some normal function. Demonstration of uptake of a small amount of tracer material by these preexistent, surface-connected vesicles on one side of the cytoplasmic barrier and its presence in "free" vesicles within the cytoplasm as well as in lumen-connected vesicles suggests transport of the tracer material together with its supporting milieu (18) (Fig. 11–18). Larger quantities of tracer material may be transported by the *macropinocytotic* mechanism presumably similar to the proposed mechanism of "endothelial vacuolation" (26). In the normal eye, the milieu alone (*i.e.*, the aqueous) would be transported.

Not infrequently, red blood cells are present in the lumen of the canal of Schlemm in histologic material, because blood can reflux easily into this vessel. The red blood cells often separate endothelial cells and thus gain access to the underlying loose connective tissue and even to the anterior chamber. Such histologic observations indicate that the endothelial cell-to-cell attachments are not excessively strong and that they can be separated with comparative ease. Such observations are compatible with the cytologic observations of a zonula adherens type of attachment as well as with more recent experimental observations.

The transport of aqueous across the endothelium (both inner and outer [5]) of Schlemm's canal is undoubtedly similar to transport mechanisms found

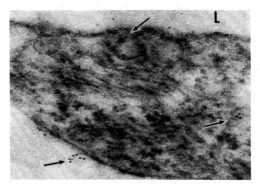

FIG. 11–18. Ferritin particles being transported across endothelial cell by micropinocytotic vesicles (**arrows**), rhesus monkey. **L,** lumen of canal of Schlemm. (× 86,500)(Fine BS: Invest Ophthalmol 3:609, 1964)

FIG. 11–19. Proliferation of cells into a portion of the lumen of the canal of Schlemm (**arrows**) is seen commonly in aging eyes. This section is from a 48-year-old subject. (PD, × 210) (AFIP Neg. 76-9322) Inset. The cell proliferation, endothelial and/or juxtacanalicular, into the lumen of the canal, as seen at higher power. (PD, × 350) (AFIP Neg. 76-9323)

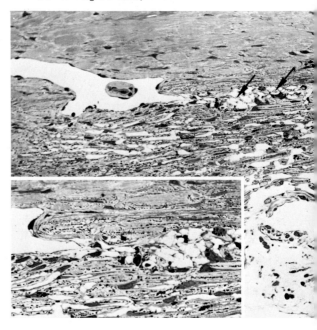

elsewhere in vessels of similar structure. The precise mechanisms of transendothelial passage have not been widely agreed upon except that there appear to be both a large (physiologic) "pore" system and a small (physiologic) "pore" system (see Ch. 6, The Vascular System). In addition to the canal of Schlemm, the "pore" systems would apply to the vasculature at the root of the iris and within the ciliary muscle (especially the longitudinal muscle), *i.e.,* all structures lying *within* the drainage angle.

Two prominent aging changes occur in this region: 1) development of a scleral spur from the scleral roll (Fig. 11–4), and 2) proliferation of cells from the inner endothelial lining and/or from the juxtacanalicular connective tissue into the canal of Schlemm (Fig. 11–19). Obstruction of aqueous outflow occurs with age as well as a concomitant decrease in aqueous secretion. Imbalance of the two will result in an elevation of intraocular pressure.

The outer wall of the canal rests on a basement membrane that is separated from the dense collagenous lamellas of the cornea and the sclera by a few loose cells (Fig. 11–20). The "looser" arrangement is more prominent posteriorly than anteriorly.

FIG. 11–20. Canal of Schlemm. A. Endothelium (**E**) lining outer wall. Patches of basement membrane are present as well as a few loose connective tissue cells (**CC**). **L,** lumen of canal. (× 11,000) B. Outer wall of canal of Schlemm in an infant eye. Endothelial cells (**E**) of canal of Schlemm lie on a thin basement membrane. Microfibrils and elastica of patches of elastic tissue are present (**EL**), as are bundles of collagen fibrils (**COL**). (× 18,000)

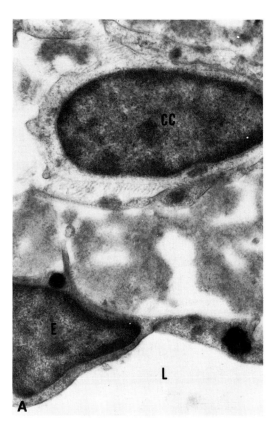

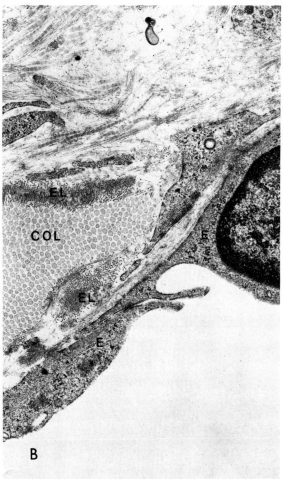

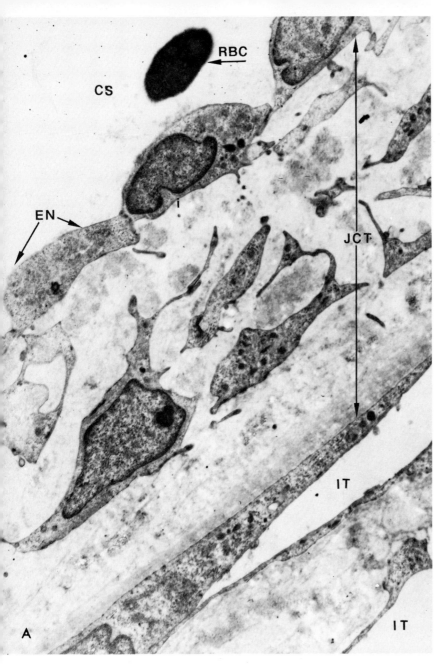

FIG. 11–21. Juxtacanalicular connective tissue. A. Region of juxtacanalicular connective tissue (**JCT**) in an adult. Tissue separates endothelial cell lining (**EN**) of canal of Schlemm (**CS**) from intertrabecular spaces (**IT**) in this plane of section. Intertrabecular spaces represent distalmost extensions of anterior chamber space. **RBC**, red blood cell in lumen of canal of Schlemm. (× 12,000) (Fine BS: Trans Am Acad Ophthalmol Otolaryngol 70:777, 1966) B. Region of juxtacanalicular tissue in 4-month-old infant. The extracellular materials are less prominent and appear more watery than in older individuals. **EN**, endothelium of canal of Schlemm; **IT**, distalmost intertrabecular space. (× 7400) C. Another portion of juxtacanalicular connective tissue region in 4-month-old infant. The endothelial basement membrane is thin and patchy. Masses of elastic tissue microfibrils and elastica are present near the collagen (**C**) fibrils. Endothelial junction is that of a zonula adherens (**arrow**). **CS**, lumen of canal of Schlemm. (× 17,400)

The inner wall rests on a thinner or patchy basement membrane that is associated with a zone of delicate connective tissue, the **juxtacanalicular connective tissue** (4, 5) (Fig. 11–13, 11–14, and 11–21). This is a special zone of the corneoscleral trabecular meshwork and consists of cells surrounded by a variety of fibrous and mucinous extracellular materials. The juxtacanalicular connective tissue is irregular in thickness from front to back in any single meridional section; it is more delicate in the younger eye (Fig. 11–21B) and more prominent in the adult eye (Fig. 11–21A).

The cells embedded within this tissue are mesodermal (ectomesenchyme, see Ch. 5) and presumably retain the capacities of fibroblasts. Excessive increase in density of this connective tissue layer in the aging eye may produce disease.

Large endothelium-lined channels (collector channels; Fig. 11–22 and 11–23) connect the canal of Schlemm either anteriorly or, more

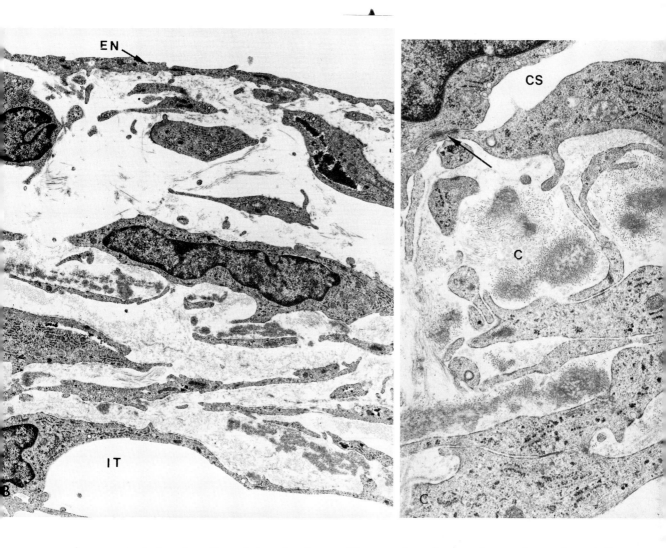

commonly, posteriorly to the intrascleral venous plexus (Fig. 11–24), which drains both the canal of Schlemm and the longitudinal ciliary muscle. If the collector channels reach the surface of the sclera unconnected, they can be observed *in vivo* as the clear aqueous veins described by Ascher (1) (Fig. 11–25).

THE TRABECULAR MESHWORK

In meridional section of a young eye a loose collagenous meshwork can be seen to fill the inner scleral sulcus and extend as an open fan to the root of the iris (Fig. 11–26). The "handle" of this fan is located just anterior to the end of Descemet's membrane, where a few layers of meshwork enter into and blend with the deep peripheral corneal stroma (Fig. 11–27).

The meshwork may be easily and usefully separated into two parts by an imaginary line extending from the scleral roll to the end of Descemet's membrane (Fig. 11–9, 11–10).

The meshwork lying external to the line and extending from cornea to sclera is known as the **corneoscleral meshwork;** the meshwork lying internal to the line and in continuity with the uveal tract posteriorly is known as the **uveal meshwork.**

A single trabecula of uveal meshwork (Fig. 11–28) consists essentially of a collagenous core surrounded by a single layer of cells ("endothelium," in reality a mesothelium). A basement membrane separates the endothelial cells from the underlying collagenous core, and not infrequently, patches of this basement membrane present a periodic structure that measures 1000 A (5, 9, 10), banded basement membrane (see Ch. 4) inset 1, Fig. 11–28A).

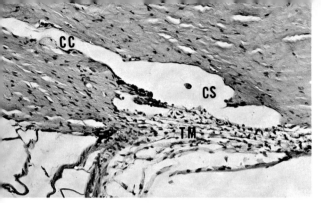

FIG. 11-22. Large collector channel (**CC**) continuous with canal of Schlemm (**CS**), rhesus monkey. **TM,** trabecular meshwork. (Alcian blue, × 115) (AFIP Neg. 60-4872) (Fine BS: Trans Am Acad Ophthalmol Otolaryngol 70:777, 1966)

FIG. 11–23. Canal of Schlemm. A. Large collector channel (**CC**) draining posterior extremity of canal of Schlemm (**CS**). **C,** adjacent corneoscleral meshwork. Cornea is to left. (Epon, PD, × 530) (AFIP Neg. 60-4569) B. Scanning electron micrograph of drainage angle showing surface of uveal trabecular meshwork (**U**), canal of Schlemm (**CS**), and collector channel (**free arrow**). (× 260)

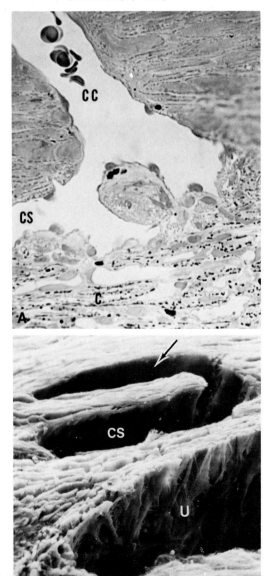

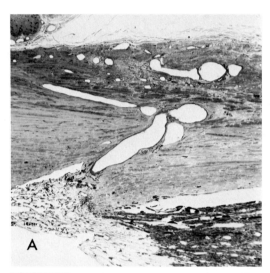

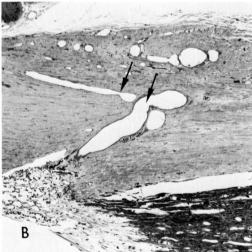

FIG. 11–24. A. Intrascleral vascular plexus in rhesus monkey. (PD × 70) (AFIP Neg. 76-9319) B. Intrascleral vascular plexus in rhesus monkey. Deeper section shows connection (**arrows**) of a few of the very tortuous vessels in this region. (PD × 70) (AFIP Neg. 76-9320)

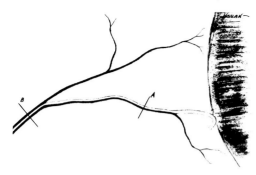

FIG. 11–25. Aqueous veins of Ascher observed biomicroscopically as clear layer uniting with and running parallel to blood-filled layer (or vein), as at **A,** and more noticeably further downstream as central clear or faintly pink band within larger vein formed by union of two adjacent vessels, as at **B.** (Ascher KW: Am J Ophthalmol 25:31, 1942)

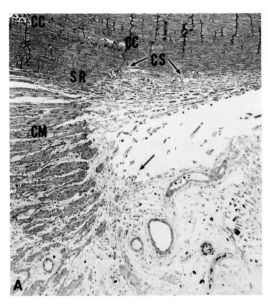

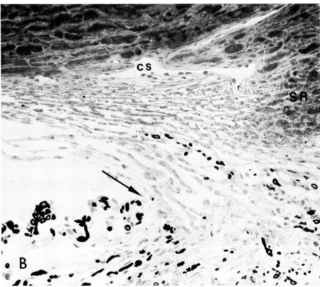

FIG. 11–26. A. "Open fan" arrangement of trabecular meshwork in infant. **CC,** collector channels; **CM,** ciliary muscle; **CS,** branches of canal of Schlemm; **SR,** scleral roll; **free arrow,** root of iris. (Epon meridional section, PD, × 90) (AFIP Neg. 63-4363) (Fine BS: Invest Ophthalmol 3:609, 1964) B. Higher magnification of trabecular meshwork in 4-month-old infant. Canal of Schlemm (**CS**), scleral roll (**SR**), and end of anterior border layer of iris (**arrow**) are seen clearly. Note slight continuity of pigmented uveal tissue from ciliary muscle into uveal meshwork. (TB, × 165) (AFIP Neg. 76-206)

FIG 11–27. Trabecular meshwork (**arrows**) lying anterior to periphery of Descemet's membrane (**DM**). Meshwork ultimately blends centrally with corneal stroma (**C**). (Epon, PD, × 395) (AFIP Neg. 65-12339)

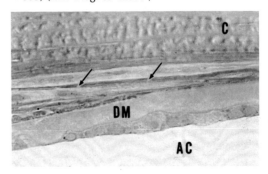

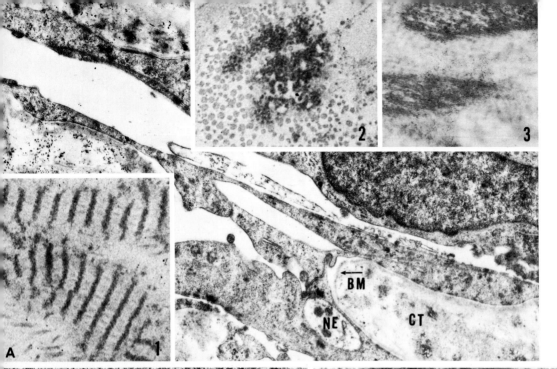

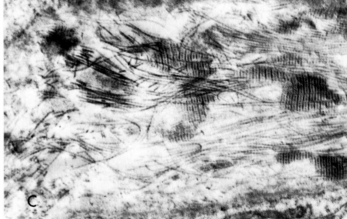

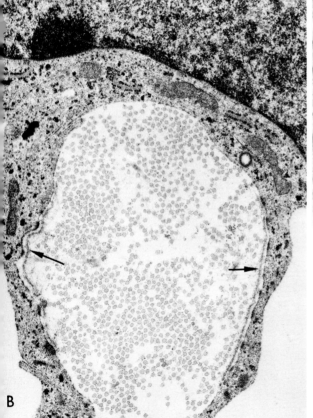

BM

NE

CT

A

1

2

3

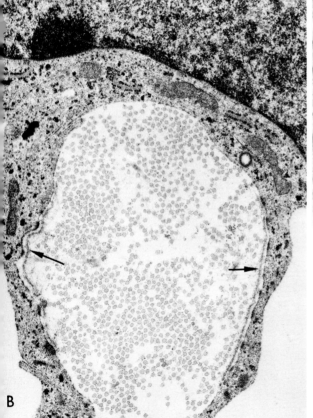

B

C

FIG. 11–28. A. Uveal trabecular meshwork, showing "endothelial" cells with basement membranes (**BM**) and associated connective tissue (**CT**). Apical surfaces line intertrabecular spaces, which are prolongations of anterior chamber space. **NE,** neurite enveloped by trabecular endothelial cell. (× 13,500) Inset 1. Banded basement membrane. (× 39,500) Inset 2. Density of elastic material within collagen cores is shown in cross-section. (× 39,000) Inset 3. Oblique section of elastic material (× 23,400) (Modified from Fine BS: Invest Ophthalmol 3:609, 1964) B. Uveal trabecula of infant. Collagenous core is composed of collagen fibrils of relatively uniform diameter and loose arrangement. The thin basement membrane (**arrows**) of endothelium is incomplete. (× 17,700) C. Spiraling collagen fibrils within a trabecula from rhesus monkey produce another form of 1000-A periodic structure. (× 18,000) (Fine BS: Trans Am Acad Ophthalmol Otolaryngol 70:777, 1966)

The core of a trabecula is formed of packed collagen fibrils frequently twisted in spiraling fashion (6). Thin sections of such spiraling fibrils often produce another form of 1000-A periodicity measured from fibril to fibril (Fig. 11–28C). This latter variety of banding is more prominent in the tissue of the monkey eye.

Lying within the tightly packed collagenous cores of the trabeculae are many aggregates of filamentous and homogeneous elastic tissue whose density increases with age (insets 2 and 3, Fig. 11–28A). The aggregates also take the stains for elastic tissue (15, 27). As in other connective tissues, additional ground substance materials are probably present, but their identification and quantitation remain obscure.

The endothelial cells covering the connective tissue core have apical surfaces, line intertrabecular spaces, and are therefore bathed by aqueous.

The trabeculae of the meshwork are roughly arranged into circumferential sheets lying superimposed one upon the other (7). They can be fairly easily separated from one another mechanically, especially in the uveal meshwork. The spaces between adjacent sheets are **intertrabecular** spaces. Large oval apertures traverse each trabecular sheet and are also called intertrabecular spaces but should be more properly called **transtrabecular** spaces (Fig. 11–29, 11–30). The latter or transtrabecular apertures are not superimposed and decrease in size in the direction of the corneoscleral meshwork.

The corneoscleral sheets differ only slightly from the uveal in having somewhat flatter trabeculae as observed in cross section and in lacking the staining characteristics for elastic fibers. The transtrabecular apertures here are more circular and smaller than those of the uveal meshwork.

Spaces *between* individual sheets are well seen on proper meridional section (Fig. 11–4, 11–10, 11–21), and here are termed the *inter-*

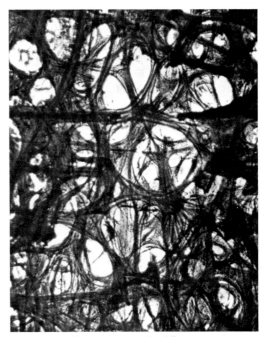

FIG. 11–29. Light micrograph of flat preparation of trabecular meshwork from rhesus monkey, viewed from anterior chamber side. Transtrabecular apertures are not superimposed and decrease in size away from anterior chamber. (Silver carbonate, × 275) (AFIP Neg. 60-6100)

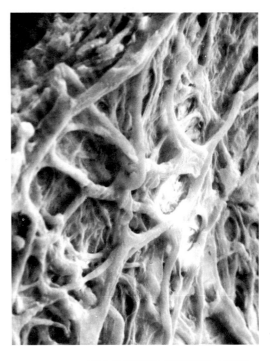

FIG. 11–30. Scanning electron micrograph of uveal meshwork from anterior chamber side in young adult human. Heavy beams of trabecular meshwork are clearly seen, as are large transtrabecular spaces. Cut edges of layers of trabecular mehhwork are seen in upper left. Spaces between adjacent sheets (*i.e.*, intertrabecular) are visible. (× 780)

trabecular spaces. In the uveal meshwork, the intertrabecular spaces are observed frequently to pass the scleral roll to be continuous with the tissue spaces lying between the smooth muscle cells of the ciliary muscles (especially those of the meridional ciliary muscle). If serially sectioned in a frontal or coronal plane, the spaces can be seen as large-apertured, relatively straight, short tubes (Fig. 11–31). Such a grouping of tubes with apertured walls might be termed a system of compound **aqueous tubes** (5, 8). In the corneoscleral meshwork, which blends posteriorly with the region of the scleral roll, the intertrabecular spaces (tubes) abut upon the canalicular extensions of the canal of Schlemm (Fig. 11–32). Such extensions are frequent in this region.

The blind inpouchings of the canal of Schlemm (canals of Sondermann) here termed canaliculi, are endothelium-lined and do not appear to be in continuity with the intertrabecular spaces. On the basis of light microscopy, however, they were once thought to be in such continuity, but acceptable electron microscopic evidence in support of this belief has not yet been obtained. Their function presumably is to drain off aqueous passing laterally along the corneoscleral trabecular meshwork (*i.e.,* along the intertrabecular spaces).

Not infrequently, various trabecular sheets have some interconnection from one level to another, an arrangement that occurs sporadically around the circumference of the globe. Such regions of interconnection appear most prominent within the corneoscleral meshwork, and therefore the transition of corneoscleral trabecular connective tissue "cores" into the looser juxtacanalicular connective tissue may be observed.

All transtrabecular and intertrabecular spaces may thus be considered extensions of the anterior chamber space and can be recognized in any single micrograph by locating the apex (*i.e.*, non-basement-membrane or non-connective-tissue-related surface) of the endothelial cell. "Endothelium" of the canal of Schlemm appears capable of producing collagen (Fig. 11–33).

Where the transtrabecular extensions of the anterior chamber space terminate in any single plane of section, therefore, is defined as the place where the lining cells abruptly depolarize and become completely surrounded by extracellular materials (*i.e.*, the juxtacanalicular connective tissue). The quality and quantity of the nonfibrous extracellular materials present normally in this juxtacanalicular connective tissue layer are not clear. In the normal primate eye, the region is highly permeable to such tracer materials as ferritin.

The collagenous "cores" of the uveal meshwork blend wtih the looser collagen of the intercellular spaces posteriorly between the smooth muscle cells of the ciliary body. They are also continued somewhat axially as the collagenous bundles or columns within the iris stroma.

It should be understood that anatomic subdivisions of the drainage angle region are somewhat arbitrary and are used to simplify and improve our understanding of the arrangements in this region. All the tissues and layers involved are *mesodermal* (or ectomesenchymal, including the so-called endothelia). The anterior chamber represents essentially an exaggerated cleft within this tissue lying between corneal stroma in front and iris stroma behind. The two tissue layers reunite at the periphery of the anterior chamber to form the loose tissues of the "drainage angle." Outflow from the anterior chamber is without doubt mainly via the drainage angle (5, 16). There is no doubt that aqueous passes into the canal of Schlemm, much of it exiting via the collector channels. There is evidence (5) that the canal also functions as a source for nourishment of the adjacent deep peripheral corneal and scleral stroma, which lie at some distance from the aqueous of the anterior chamber as well as from the limbal vasculature. The precise or relative *quantities* that pass 1) toward, into, or exit from the canal of Schlemm, 2) along the uveal meshwork, and 3) into the root of the iris are incompletely known.

Functionally, the drainage angle is quantitatively the most significant region for aqueous outflow in the normal primate eye. This is well supported by the clinical fact that removal of the entire iris diaphragm (as has occurred as a surgical accident on occasion) does not immediately or significantly produce an elevation in the intraocular pressure. *Quantitation* of flow into the three anatomic regions of the drainage angle (iris root, uvea, and canal of Schlemm) has not yet been determined.*

* Attempts have been made (2, 3) to quantitate aqueous outflow with the anatomic structures present in the drainage angle. "Conventional outflow," a term proposed for the *assumed* quantity of outflow via the canal of Schlemm exclusively, is determined by placing a radioactive tracer into the anterior chamber and subsequently measuring the dilution in the systemic bloodstream. This, of course, determines not only tracers leaving the anterior chamber via the canal of Schlemm but rather *all* anterior chamber tracers that manage to
(*continued*) ▶

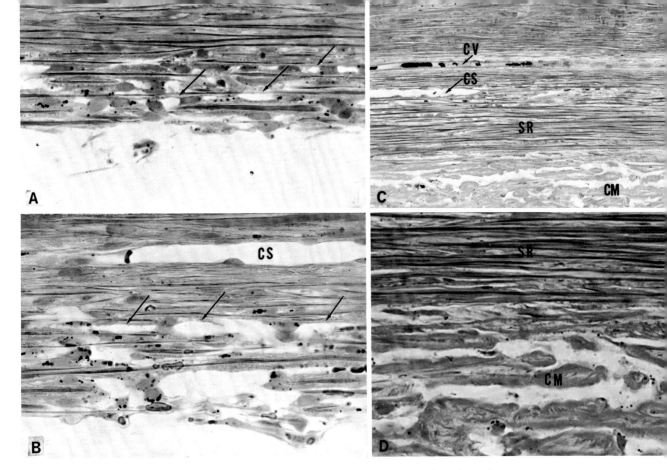

Obstruction of flow at one or more of the sites (*i.e.*, entryway, within, or near the final drainage mechanisms) along these three anatomic pathways when *quantitatively* sufficient, and accompanied by a normal inflow, will produce an imbalance, raising the intraocular pressure such that the nerve tissues at the optic disc may be damaged (*i.e.*, glaucoma [28]).

The anterior border layer of the iris stroma (with or without pigmentation) may occasionally fail to end abruptly at the iris root and continue as short bands or processes along the surface of the uveal meshwork (Fig. 11–34), reaching even to attach to the end of Descemet's membrane (line of Schwalbe). Such ana-

(continued)

reach the systemic blood. "Uveoscleral" outflow, a term proposed for the amount that passes into the uveal tissues and thence out of the eye through scleral tissues, is separate from any vascular drainage (5, 22, 23) that may occur, such as in the root of the iris or via the anterior ciliary veins, which drain the region of the longitudinal ciliary muscle.

FIG. 11–31. Coronal sections of trabecular meshwork. A. Anterior meshwork. Arrows point to spaces between trabecular sheets (intertrabecular spaces). (Epon, PD, × 530) (AFIP Neg. 64-563) B. Spaces (**arrows**) between adjacent trabecular sheets posterior to those in A. Spaces are large and circular to oval in cross-section. Anterior extremity of canal of Schlemm (**CS**) has appeared in this section. (Epon, PD, × 530) (AFIP Neg. 64-562) C. Low magnification of posterior region of trabecular meshwork showing posterior extremity of canal of Schlemm (**CS**), circumferentially oriented collagen bundles of scleral roll (**SR**), and cross-sectioned layers of longitudinal ciliary muscle (**CM**); **CV,** collector vessel. (Epon, PD, × 195) (AFIP Neg. 64-558) D. Higher magnification showing region of scleral roll (**SR**) and its relation to adjacent longitudinal ciliary muscle (**CM**). (Epon, PD, × 530) (AFIP Neg. 64-559) (Fine BS: Invest Ophthalmol 3:609, 1964)

FIG. 11–32. Canaliculi from canal of Schlemm (**CS**) projecting into corneoscleral meshwork anterior to scleral roll (**SR**) in infant. (Epon, PD, × 100) (AFIP Neg. 68-5146) Inset. Canal and its canalicular extension (**arrow**) at higher magnification. (× 265)

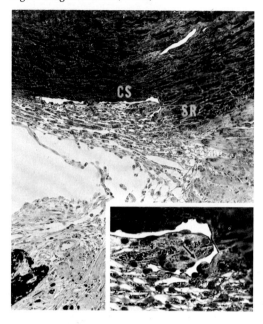

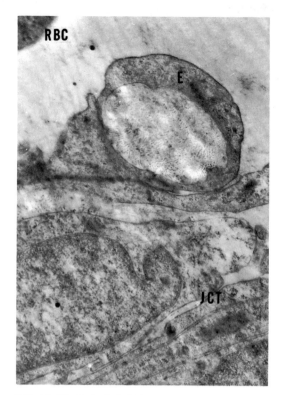

FIG. 11–33. Endothelial "loop" (**E**) along inner wall of canal of Schlemm enveloping a cluster of filaments. A basement membrane is only questionably present. **JCT,** juxta-canalicular connective tissue; **RBC,** red blood cell in lumen of canal of Schlemm. (× 17,400)

FIG. 11–34. Iris process (**arrow**) is a sporadic continuation of anterior border layer beyond iris root. Processes are most easily appreciated when pigmented, as here. (H&E, × 110) (AFIP Neg. 70-1415)

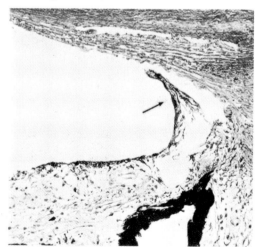

tomic variations intermittently distributed around the circumference of the drainage angle are known as **iris processes** and are best seen when pigmented and when observed clinically by gonioscopy (Fig. 11–35).

In histologic sections, the end of Descemet's membrane may vary from a delicate tapering out beyond visibility by light microscopy to an enlarged nodule (Fig. 11–36) that may be clinically visible as a thickened circumferential cord, Schwalbe's anterior border ring or line (Fig. 11–37). The thickened line generally is composed of a mixture of basement membranes and collagen fibrils or filaments with the contribution of each component being variable (Fig. 11–38) (see Ch. 9, Peripheral Cornea).

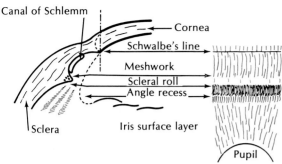

Canal of Schlemm
Cornea
Schwalbe's line
Meshwork
Scleral roll
Angle recess
Sclera
Iris surface layer
Pupil

FIG. 11–35. Schematic drawing to illustrate histologic landmarks in drainage angle (**left**) and comparable zones that may be seen from anterior chamber side by gonioscopy (**right**).

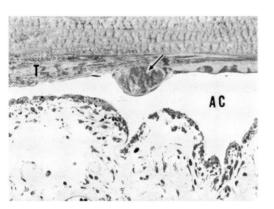

FIG. 11–36. Termination of Descemet's membrane may occur as thickened band (Schwalbe's anterior border ring), which appears as a large nodule (**arrow**). **AC,** anterior chamber; **T,** trabecular meshwork. Anterior border layer of iris and adjacent stroma lie in lower half of figure. (Epon meridional section, PD, × 130) (AFIP Neg. 67-11208)

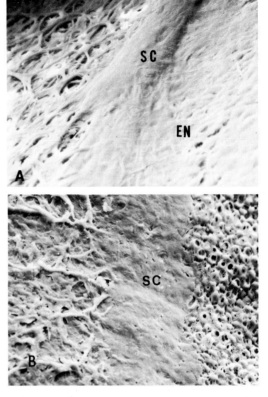

FIG. 11–37. A. Scanning electron ▲ micrograph of region of thickened Schwalbe's "anterior border ring'" (**SC**) in young adult. Uveal meshwork on left disappears anterior to ridge (see Fig. 11–27 and 11–36), while corneal endothelium (**EN**) continues over free surface of roll. (× 320) B. Flat Schwalbe's anterior border ring (**SC**) in infant's eye. Corneal endothelial cells on right are artifactitiously vacuolated and ruptured. (SEM, × 300)

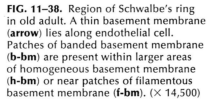

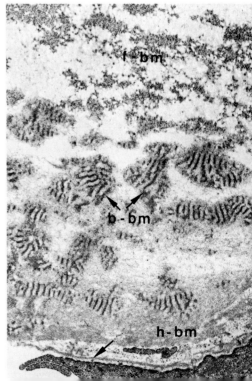

FIG. 11–38. Region of Schwalbe's ring in old adult. A thin basement membrane (**arrow**) lies along endothelial cell. Patches of banded basement membrane (**b-bm**) are present within larger areas of homogeneous basement membrane (**h-bm**) or near patches of filamentous basement membrane (**f-bm**). (× 14,500)

REFERENCES

1. Ascher KW: Aqueous veins: preliminary notes. Am J Ophthalmol 25:31, 1942
2. Bill A: Conventional and uveo-scleral drainage of aqueous humour in the cynomologus monkey (*Macaca irus*) at normal and high intraocular pressures. Exp Eye Res 5:45, 1966
3. Bill A: Blood circulation and fluid dynamics in the eye. Phys Rev 55:383, 1975
4. Feeney L, Wissig S: Outflow studies using an electron-dense tracer. Trans Am Acad Ophthalmol Otolaryngol 70:791, 1966
5. Fine BS: Observations on the drainage angle in man and rhesus monkey: a concept of the pathogenesis of chronic simple glaucoma: a light and electron microscopic study. Invest Ophthalmol 3:609, 1964
6. Fine BS: Structure of the trabecular meshwork and the canal of Schlemm. Trans Am Acad Ophthalmol Otolaryngol 70:777, 1966
7. Flocks M: The anatomy of the trabecular meshwork as seen in tangential sections. Arch Ophthalmol 56:708, 1956
8. Frey-Wyssling A: Submicroscopic Morphology of Protoplasm. Amsterdam, Elsevier, 1953
9. Garron LK, Feeney ML: Electron microscopic studies of the human eye. II. Study of the trabeculae by light and electron microscopy. Arch Ophthalmol 62:966, 1067, 1959
10. Garron LK, Feeney ML, Hogan MJ, McEwen WK: Electron microscopic studies of the human eye. I. Preliminary investigations of the trabeculae. Am J Ophthalmol 46:27, 1958
11. Grierson I, Lee WR: Light microscopic quantitation of the endothelial vacuoles in Schlemm's canal. Am J Ophthalmol 84:234, 1977
12. Holmberg A: The fine structure of the inner wall of Schlemm's canal. Arch Ophthal 62:956, 1959
13. Holmberg A: Schlemm's canal and the trabecular meshwork: an electron microscopic study of the normal structure in man and monkey (*Cercopithecus ethiops*). Doc Ophthalmol 19:339, 1965
14. Inomata H, Bill A, Smelser GK: Aqueous humor pathways through the trabecular meshwork and into Schlemm's canal in the cynomolgus monkey (*Macaca irus*). Am J Ophthalmol 73:760, 1972
15. Iwamoto T: Light and electron microscopy of the presumed elastic components of the trabeculae and scleral spur of the human eye. Invest Ophthalmol 3:144, 1964
16. Kaufman PL, Bill A, Barany EH: Formation and drainage of aqueous humor following total iris removal and ciliary muscle disinsertion in the cynomologus monkey. Invest Ophthalmol 16:226, 1977
17. Okisaka S: Effects of paracentesis on the blood-aqueous barrier: a light and electron microscopic study on cynomologus monkey. Invest Ophthalmol 15:824, 1976
18. Palade GE, Bruns RR: Structural modulations of plasmalemmal vesicles. J Cell Biol 37:633, 1968
19. Raviola G: Effects of paracentesis on the blood-aqueous barrier: an electron microscopic study on macaca mulatta using horseradish peroxidase as a tracer. Invest Ophthalmol 13:828, 1974
20. Salzmann M: The Anatomy and Histology of the Human Eyeball in the Normal State. Brown EVL (trans). Chicago, University of Chicago Press, 1912
21. Shabo AL: Reese TS, Gaasterland D: Postmortem formation of giant endothelial vacuoles in Schlemm's canal of monkey. Am J Ophthalmol 76:896, 1973
22. Sherman SH, Green K, Laties A: The fate of anterior chamber fluorescein in the monkey eye. Presented at the Annual Meeting of the Association for Research in Vision and Ophthalmology, Sarasota, FL, 1976 (in preparation)
23. Green K, Sherman SH, Laties AM et al.: The fate of anterior chamber tracers in the living rhesus monkey eye with evidence for uveo-vortex outflow. In Cant JS (ed): Intraocular Fluid Dynamics. Oxford, Oxford University Press (in press)
24. Tripathi RC: Ultrastructure of Schlemm's canal in relation to aqueous outflow. Exp Eye Res 7:335, 1968
25. Tripathi RC: Ultrastructure of the trabecular wall of Schlemm's canal. Trans Ophthalmol Soc 89:449, 1969
26. Tripathi RC: Mechanism of the aqueous outflow across the trabecular wall of Schlemm's canal. Exp Eye Res 11:116, 1971
27. Yamashita T, Rosen DA: The elastic tissue of primate trabecular meshwork: a histologic and electron microscopic study. Invest Ophthalmol 3:85, 1964
28. Yanoff M, Fine BS: Ocular Pathology: A Text and Atlas. Hagerstown, Harper & Row, 1975

chapter 12

THE OPTIC NERVE

INTRAOCULAR (BULBAR) PORTION   274
   RETINAL LAYER   274
   CHOROIDAL LAYER   278
   SCLERAL LAYER   278
ORBITAL (RETROBULBAR) PORTION   281
   SHEATHS AND THEIR SPACES   281
   INTRANEURAL COMPONENTS   282
VASCULAR SUPPLY   283

The term **optic nerve** is in reality somewhat of a misnomer, for it is unlike a peripheral nerve, in that it is actually a nerve fiber tract of the central nervous system, a tract formed by axons of the retinal ganglion cells. Although once considered to differ greatly from peripheral nerves, which have a close relation to a layer of Schwann cells (the neurilemmal sheath), the structural differences between peripheral and central nerves appear to be relative. A peripheral nerve is enveloped by a continuous layer of Schwann cells (the neurilemmal sheath) thick enough to be observed by light microscopy. Spiral wrapping of the axon by the doubled plasmalemma of Schwann cells produces the myelin sheath, which therefore is produced in segments by the individual cells (Fig. 12–1A). The doubled plasmalemma, which connects the layers of myelin with the rest of the Schwann cell cytoplasm, is termed the mesaxon (outer and inner) (see also Fig. 6–63).

In the optic nerve, as in the white matter of the brain (23), the ganglion cell axons also are enveloped by a sheath of doubled plasma-lemma, to form the myelin. The outer layer of enveloping cytoplasm is derived in this location from oligodendrocytes (Fig. 12–1B). The cytoplasmic sheath is exceedingly thin and cannot be appreciated by light microscopic examination. In addition this *quantitative* difference in neurilemmal thickness between a peripheral nerve and the optic nerve, there is further difference, in that the Schwann cell is enveloped by a thin basement membrane, a structure that is lacking in the oligodendrocyte.

Since the optic nerve is a tract of the central nervous system, it is subject to many of the same diseases that affect other such tracts and reacts similarly to disease processes.

FIG. 12–1. Formation of myelin sheath. A. In peripheral nerve spiral, envelopment of a neurite by Schwann cell cytoplasm produces myelin sheath. Schwann cell has a thin basement membrane. B. In central nervous system, myelin sheath is formed by oligodendrocyte spirally enveloping a neurite. Oligodendrocyte lacks basement membrane. (Courtesy of Dr. Peter W. Lampert)

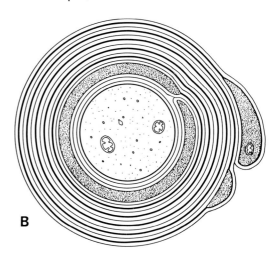

A

B

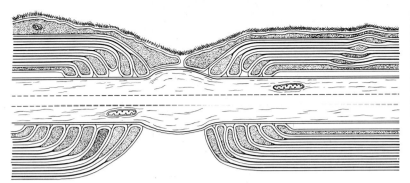

FIG. 12–2. Node of Ranvier from peripheral nerve (**above**) and node of Ranvier in central nervous system (**below**). Ends of adjacent myelin segments fall short of touching one another, and a basement membrane is lacking in node of central nervous system. (Courtesy of Dr. Peter W. Lampert)

Foci of attenuated myelin, the nodes of Ranvier (6, 23), are present in *both* central and peripheral nerves and represent the endings of adjacent segments of myelin.

Adjacent segments of myelin abut in peripheral nerves but fall short of each other in the central nervous system, leaving short segments of axon exposed (Fig. 12–2).

INTRAOCULAR (BULBAR) PORTION

The intraocular portion of the optic nerve can be conveniently divided into three parts or layers: the inner retinal, the middle choroidal, and the outer scleral, each continuing the plane of an ocular coat across the opening of the scleral canal (Fig. 12–3).

The retinal and choroidal layers are frequently lumped together and called the **prelaminar** part of the nerve head while the scleral lamina is then called **laminar** (3, 10, 11, 17).

RETINAL LAYER

The aggregated nerve fibers (ganglion cell axons) of the retinal nerve fiber layer exit from the eye through a circular to slightly oval aperture measuring ~1.5 mm in diameter. Clinically and grossly, it is represented by the *optic disc*. (An older term, optic papilla, is presumably histologic in origin and relates to the slight elevations present in this region in the mature eye, especially to the prominence of the nerve fibers on the nasal side.)

A smaller, disc-shaped depression, the **physiologic cup,** whose edge parallels that of the optic disc, lies slightly temporal to the center of the optic disc. The depression (Fig. 12–3) or excavation is lined by a glial plaque, the **central supporting tissue meniscus** (27) (of

Kuhnt)* (inset 1, Fig. 12–4), which may remain developmentally exaggerated as a **Bergmeister's papilla** or may appear relatively empty. In the latter situation, the ophthalmologist can see deeply into the cup and may recognize the sievelike perforations (inset 1, Fig. 12–3) of the scleral lamina cribrosa, the apertures through which the nonmyelinated nerve fiber bundles pass out of the globe. The glial cells of the central supporting tissue meniscus, mostly fibrous astrocytes (Fig. 12–4), are covered on their anterior surface by a thin basement membrane. They are attached to one another by desmosome-like structures, puncta adherentes (Fig. 12–13 and also possess typical gap junction separations (26).

Where the periphery of the physiologic cup joins with the remainder of the optic disc, the thin basement membrane of the fibrous astrocytes lining the inner surface of the central supporting tissue meniscus changes over into the thicker basement membrane of the neural retina (inset 2, Fig. 12–4). This ring of transition apparently outlines a ring of strong attachment of the (secondary) vitreous body to the nerve head and also the area (Martegiani) exposed to the lumen of the **canal of Cloquet** (primary vitreous).

The ring of heavily vascularized retinal layer between the physiologic cup and the outermost

---

* The thickened glial plaque is continuous with a wider thinner glial plaque (the inner limiting membrane of Elschnig) lining the surface of the nerve head. It also has been referred to as the *glial* limiting membrane of the optic nerve head and is analogous to the external glial limiting membrane (32) of the cerebral cortex. It should not be confused with the internal limiting membrane of the nerve head (*i.e.,* the thin basement membrane covering the optic nerve head and continuous with the thicker basement membrane or internal limiting membrane of the adjacent retina).

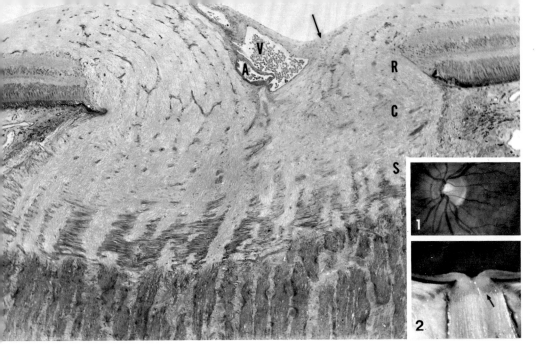

FIG. 12–3. Components of intraocular portion of optic nerve: retinal layer (**R**), choroidal layer (**C**), scleral layer (**S**). Plaque of glial tissue (**arrow**) lies in floor of physiologic cup adjacent to central retinal vessels. Artery (**A**) lies nasal to vein (**V**). Note continuity of some of supporting tissue meniscus (Kuhnt) with that around adjacent vein. Latter tissue, called intercalary tissue (Elschnig), separates collagenous vascular adventitia from adjacent nerve fibers. (Epon, PD, × 56) (AFIP Neg. 69-10521) Inset 1. Clinical appearance of nerve head or optic disc. Inset 2. Nerve head on gross section. Abrupt termination of myelinated part of optic nerve at scleral lamina cribrosa is clearly seen (**arrow**).

FIG. 12–4. Central supporting tissue meniscus (Kuhnt) in floor of optic cup. Electron micrograph of astrocytes (**AS**) whose thin basement membranes line floor. (Glutaraldehyde fixation. × 15,000) Inset 1. Light micrograph showing astrocytes (**AS**) that make up tissue. (Epon, PD, × 220) (AFIP Neg. 69-10520) Inset 2. Transition (**arrow**) from thin basement membrane of cup to thicker basement membrane (**BM**) near periphery of optic disc. (× 18,000)

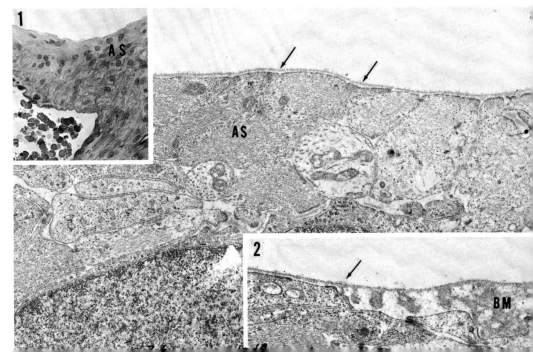

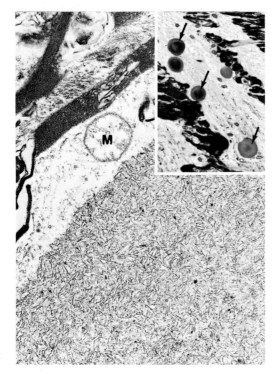

FIG. 12–5. Electron micrograph shows short needlelike filaments, of which a corpus amylaceum is composed, accumulating within an astrocyte. Note presence of adjacent myelinated nerve fibers. **M,** astrocyte mitochondrion. (× 18,000) Inset. Numerous corpora amylacea (**arrows**) within nerve substance of optic nerve. Some have denser staining centers or cores. (PD, × 180) (AFIP Neg. 75-8326)

FIG. 12–6. Thin basement membrane (**arrow**) of astrocytes (**AS**) lining optic cup overgrown by layer of free cells. Filamentous (**F**) cytoplasm of these free cells indicates that they are fibrous astrocytes. (Glutaraldehyde fixation, × 18,000)

edge of the optic disc (Fig. 12–3, inset 1) appears pink on clinical examination and is known as the **rim** of the optic disc.

The innermost retinal layers are occupied by the basal ends of the large atypical specialized fibrous astrocytes known as the Müller cells. About the footplates of these cells are interspersed a number of more typical astrocytes which apparently produce only short segments of thin basement membrane, in contrast to the thick basement membrane produced by the Müller cells. Another apparent difference between these two varieties of fibrous astrocytes is the relative ease with which the typical small astrocytes can undergo proliferation, while the Müller cells undergo swelling, condensation, or elongation with somewhat less tendency to proliferate. Glial proliferations, therefore, are observed more frequently in the nerve fiber layer of the retina and in the region of the nerve head, where the small astrocytes are most abundant, than elsewhere in the retina. A common aging change is the formation of myriad *corpora amylacea* ("brain dust") (Fig. 12–5) from degenerating astrocytes, quite similar to those that occur in the inner layers of the retina (see Ch. 6) and in the white matter of the brain. Corpora amylacea differ from the concentrically laminated concretions called *corpora arenacea* produced by the arachnoidal meningothelial cells in the meninges surrounding both the optic nerve and the brain. Detachments of the vitreous from the internal limiting membrane of the retina usually terminate at the strong ringlike attachment at the optic disc. A new surface or posterior hyaloid comes into continuity with the nerve head. Glial proliferations or neovascularizations can readily gain access to the vitreous compartment by proliferating from the nerve head (Fig. 12–6) along the adjacent retinal surface or along this posterior hyaloid. Such new growths can produce a variety of secondary complications.

When the optic nerve head is viewed in meridional section, the nerve fiber bundles can be seen to be much thicker on the nasal side

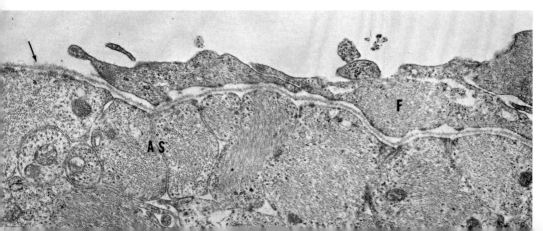

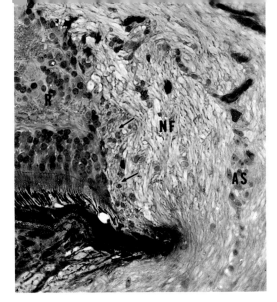

FIG. 12–7. Intermediary tissue (Kuhnt) (arrows) separating retina (R) from adjacent nerve fiber bundles (NF). Columns of nuclei represent astrocytes (AS), which separate nerve fiber bundles in the retinal layer. Note swelling of nerve fibers and slight displacement of both retina and intermediary tissue laterally. (Epon, PD, × 220) (AFIP Neg. 69-10517)

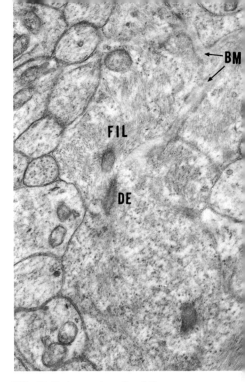

FIG. 12–9. In osmium-fixed tissue, intracellular filaments (FIL) of astrocyte are clearly seen. BM, astrocytic basement membranes; DE, obliquely sectioned punctum adherens. Adjacent axons appear to contain mostly filaments. (Dalton's fixation, × 24,000)

FIG. 12–8. Astrocytes (AS) separating bundles of nonmyelinated nerve fibers (NF) or axons in region of choroidal layer. Astrocyte is characterized by its cytoplasmic content of filaments. Axons do not possess microtubules in this preparation. (Dalton's chrome-osmium fixation, × 18,000)

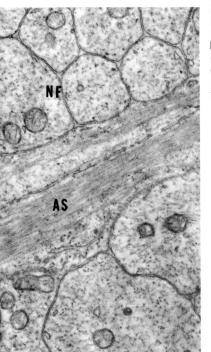

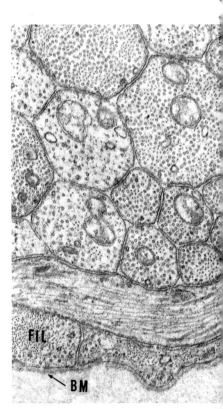

FIG. 12–10. In rhesus monkey tissue initially fixed in glutaraldehyde by perfusion, astrocytes contain mostly filaments (FIL), while adjacent axons contain mostly tubules. BM, thin basement membrane of astrocytes. (Glutaraldehyde perfusion, × 30,000)

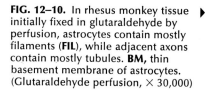

than on the temporal. The situation is often exaggerated by the slight obliqueness of the nerve head toward the temporal side. At the periphery of the nerve head, the greatly thickened nerve fiber layers of the retina are separated into large bundles by columns of fibrous astrocytes (Fig. 12–3). The posterior retinal layers are separated from the adjacent nerve fiber bundles by a thin delicate sheet of glial tissue, the **intermediary tissue** (27) (of Kuhnt, Fig. 12–7). In this plane of the nerve head, the bundles of nerve fibers (axons) are nonmyelinated and closely approximated to one another.

Histologically the earliest sign of pathologic edema (*i.e.*, papilledema) of the nerve head is a swelling of the nerve fibers in this region near the intermediary tissue. The swelling not only alters the linear appearance of the axons, but also displaces adjacent retinal tissue laterally from its usual correspondence with its pigment epithelium (Fig. 12–7).

The axonal bundles are separated by columns of fibrous astrocytes (2, 6, 15) (Fig. 12–8) recognized by their high content of cytoplasmic filaments (15, 21, 24).

Although the intracytoplasmic appearance of astrocytes varies little with the method used for initial fixation, being mostly filamentous under all conditions, the axonal cytoplasm varies widely in appearance. Initial fixation of axons in osmium tetroxide produces a high percentage of intracytoplasmic filaments (Fig. 12–9), while initial fixation in glutaraldehyde produces a high percentage of intracytoplasmic tubules (Fig. 12–10). This fixation-related change reaches its maximum in well-fixed retinas where all the filaments and tubules of the ganglion cell axons appear to be interconvertible (8).

Centrally, within the physiologic cup, the retinal artery and vein enter the eye along the nasal side, with the artery lying nasal to the vein. Both vessels lie closely apposed to the surface of the adjacent thick layer of nasal nerve fibers but separated from them by their collagenous adventitia and by fibrous astrocytes. Occasionally, a thin glial sheet extends from the central meniscus deeper along the vessel bundle and is sometimes called the **intercalary** tissue (of Elschnig). The vessels then divide into their major upper and lower, nasal and temporal branches that lie within and nourish the inner retinal layers.

CHOROIDAL LAYER

Approximately in line with the choroidal coat, the nonmedullated nerve fiber bundles are even more clearly recognizable as bundles or columns. It is in this region that the lamina cribrosa begins.

Lamina cribrosa (Fig. 12–11), a term generally applied to the striated portions of the bulbar optic nerve, is separable into two parts: the choroidal lamina (lamina choroidalis), present in the choroidal layer, is composed mostly of astrocytes, and the scleral lamina (lamina scleralis), present in the scleral layer (see next section), is composed of astrocytes, collagenous connective tissue, and small blood vessels (1, 27).

In meridional section the entire lamina cribrosa shows a slight bowing outward. The concavity may be related to a normal intraocular pressure, but chronic increases in intraocular pressure, as in the chronic glaucomas, usually exaggerate it. Separation of the axonal bundles is here maintained by heavy lines of fibrous astrocytes whose filament-laden processes pass at right angles to the axons and so parallel to the direction of the choroidal plane (Fig. 12–11). The astrocytes are identified in conventional microscopic sections by long columns of nuclei, the nuclear columns (Fig. 12–7, 12–11). Collagenous connective tissue is absent or sparse in the choroidal region except in the area around the central vessels (vessel adventitia). Peripherally, a thick looser tissue, the border tissue (inset, Fig. 12–11) separates the neural elements from the choroid. The border tissue is separable into two additional parts, a larger mainly collagenous portion adjacent to the choroid, the **border tissue of Elschnig,** and a narrower mainly glial-like zone more closely related to the tissues of the optic nerve, the **border tissue of Jacoby.** The latter may be continuous with the intermediary tissue of Kuhnt lining the nearby retinal layer. The border tissue may also contain a number of pigmented cells.

SCLERAL LAYER

In continuity with the scleral coat, the bundles of nonmyelinated nerve fibers are separated by clearly recognizable heavier columns formed by glial cells and collagenous tissue (inset, Fig. 12–11) the lamina scleralis. The glial cells, mostly fibrous astrocytes, separate the nerve fibers from the collagenous septa (Fig. 12–12).

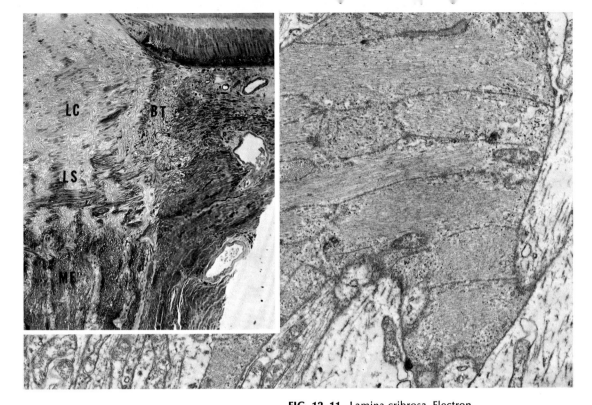

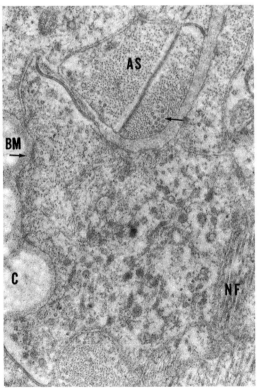

FIG. 12–11. Lamina cribrosa. Electron
micrograph shows dense packing of
fibrous astrocytes that make up lamina
choroidalis. Axons contain microtubules
in this preparation. (Glutaraldehyde-
osmium fixation, × 18,000) Inset. Light
micrograph showing division of lamina
cribrosa into lamina choroidalis (**LC**),
composed mostly of astrocytes, and
lamina scleralis (**LS**), composed of
astrocytes, collagen, and small blood
vessels. Border tissue (**BT**) separates
choroid proper from lamina choroidalis.
MF, myelinated nerve fibers
(retrobulbar). (Epon, PD, × 80)
(AFIP Neg. 69-10518)

FIG. 12–12. Rhesus monkey tissue,
showing astrocytes (**AS**) separating
nonmyelinated nerve fibers (**NF**),
recognized here by their microtubular
content, from adjacent collagen (**C**) in
region of lamina scleralis. **BM,** thin
basement membrane of cells whose
cytoplasmic content is mostly
filamentous. A few microtubules (**free
arrow**) are present sporadically among
filaments. (Glutaraldehyde perfusion,
× 35,000)

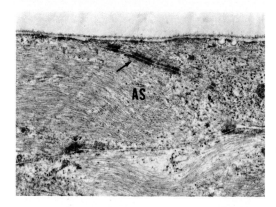

FIG. 12–13. Fibrous astrocytes (**AS**) adherent to each other by puncta adherentes (**arrow**) (desmosome-like attachments) at free (inner) surface of optic cup. (× 18,000)

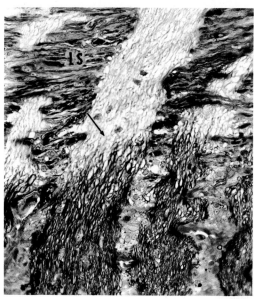

FIG. 12–14. Transition between myelination and nonmyelination (**arrow**) within single bundle of nerve fibers (axons). Collagenous vascular septa of lamina scleralis (**LS**) are prominent. (Epon, PD, × 360) (AFIP Neg. 69-10516)

FIG. 12–15. Bulbar portion of optic nerve in cross-section at three levels. A. Retinal layer. B. Choroidal layer. C. Scleral layer. D. Cross-section of retrobulbar optic nerve lying posterior to the sclera. Note heavy reticular pattern of collagenous septa within scleral layer. (Masson × 13) (AFIP Neg. 74-7769) (Courtesy Dr. D. Minckler)

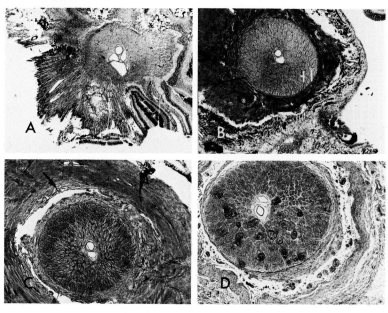

The fibrous astrocytes commonly attach to one another by desmosome-like attachments generally termed puncta adherentes in tissue of the central nervous system (Fig. 12–13). The septa contain the small vascular branches derived from the adjacent scleral vascular complex known as the **circle of Zinn-Haller,** which in turn is derived from the adjacent penetrating branches of the short posterior ciliary arteries.

ORBITAL (RETROBULBAR) PORTION

The orbital portion of the optic nerve extends from the lamina cribrosa to the apex of the orbit in a sinuous manner, permitting freedom of movement of the eye.

Myelination of the retinal ganglion cell axons appears rather abruptly (Fig. 12–14), immediately behind the scleral lamina cribrosa and, therefore, actually slightly within the scleral canal. Myelination doubles the cross-sectional thickness of the nerve so that it rapidly reaches its maximum diameter of ~3 mm at the posterior surface of the sclera (inset 2, Fig. 12–3).

In the embryo, myelination (14, 28) begins centrally within the brain and proceeds peripherally to cease abruptly at the lamina cribrosa. Myelination may occasionally be observed in portions of the nerve fiber layer of the retina, but even in such instances the region of the lamina cribrosa is typically nonmyelinated (see Ch. 6), even though myelin may be seen on either side.

Recent analysis of the total fiber count in the human optic nerve gives a count lying between 1.1 and 1.3 million axons while the corresponding figure for the rhesus monkey is 1.5–1.8 million axons (25).

As the axonal bundles pass posteriorly from the region of the optic disc toward the optic nerve, they acquire progressively more interaxonal glial tissue (Fig. 12–15), thus enlarging the cross-sectional diameter of the intraocular portion of the optic nerve posterior to the plane of Bruch's membrane. Mitochondria also increase in number within each axon in the region of the lamina choroidalis and scleralis. Some focal expansions and contractions of the axons are also present in these areas (19).

Flow of neuronal cytoplasm from the cell body (perikaryon) along the axon is called **axoplasmic flow** or transport (13, 18, 20, 30). The flowing proteins can be labeled by incorporating injected radioactive amino acids. At least five groups of labeled proteins have been found to be transported along the axon, each group being characterized by its polypeptide composition and by its transport velocity (31), *i.e.,* group I, > 240 mm/day; group II, 34–68 mm/day; group III, 4–8 mm/day; group IV, 2–4 mm/day; and group V, 0.7–1.1 mm/day. The retinal ganglion cell is said to export as much as 12% of its protein content to the axon terminals per day. A form of retrograde transport also occurs.

SHEATHS AND THEIR SPACES

The optic nerve is surrounded by the continuation of the three connective tissue meningeal sheaths that line the cranial cavity and encase the brain (Fig. 12–16): externally, the thick **dura mater,** which fuses distally with the outer layers of the sclera; internally, the thin, vascularized, tightly applied connective tissue sheath, the **pia mater,** covering the nerve proper; and in between, the delicate cellular connective tissue network, the **arachnoid.**

The narrow space between the arachnoid and the dura is but a potential continuation of the subdural space from the cranial cavity, whereas the wide, easily enlarged space between the arachnoid and pia is a true continuation of the subarachnoid space covering the brain. The central retinal artery and vein cross the spaces to enter the optic nerve. Before entering the

FIG. 12–16. Sheaths of optic nerve. Dura (**D**) and arachnoid (**A**) continue from cranial cavity to envelop optic nerve within orbit. **P,** pia mater; **S,** pial septum. (H&E, × 70) (AFIP Neg. 70-7288)

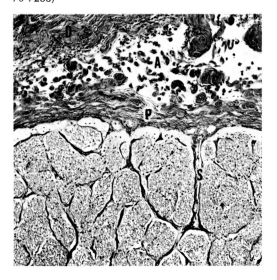

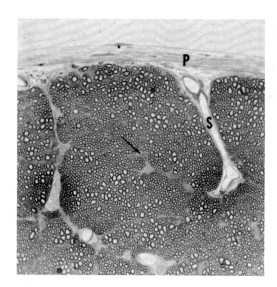

FIG. 12–17. Septum (**S**) carrying blood vessels into optic nerve from pia (**P**). Myelinated nerve tissue is separated into nerve fiber bundles. Nucleus and perikaryon of a glial cell (**arrow**) can be seen among myelinated axons. Rhesus monkey. (Epon section, PD, × 300) (AFIP Neg. 66-8676)

FIG. 12–18. Astrocytic glial processes (**G***)* resting on thin basement membrane (**arrow**) separating myelinated nerve fibers (**MF**) from collagenous pia. Rhesus monkey. (× 16,500)

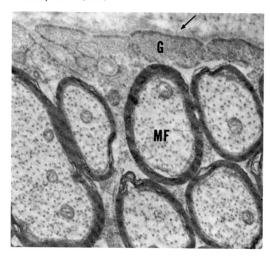

nerve, the vein frequently travels for some distance between arachnoid and pia in the subarachnoid space, whereas the artery generally takes a shorter and more direct route.

At the optic canal the dural sheath splits into two layers. One layer becomes continuous with the periosteum of the orbit, and the other adheres closely to and follows the optic nerve itself, finally becoming indistinguishable from the outer layers of the sclera.

The arachnoid sheath is composed of collagenous tissue and typical meningothelial cells. Delicate fibrous septa cross the subarachnoid space from the arachnoid sheath to the pial sheath, dividing the subarachnoid space into many interconnecting compartments. With aging, laminated calcareous bodies, **corpora arenacea,** may be produced by the meningothelial cells.

INTRANEURAL COMPONENTS

The collagenous pial sheath (Fig. 12–17, 12–18) enters the nerve, and vascularized *pial septa* subdivide the now myelinated nerve fiber bundles into columns. The pial septa blend with the lamina cribrosa (scleralis) anteriorly and with the central connective tissue axially around the central vessels of the optic nerve until the latter exit from the nerve inferiorly about 8–15 mm behind the globe.

As in the central nervous system, the pial septa are always isolated from the neural elements by a continuous layer of fibrous astrocytes.

In longitudinal section (Fig. 12–19) the myelinated nerve fiber bundles appear to be interrupted. Because the myelinated nerve fibers (axons) continue to their termination in the lateral geniculate body, the apparent interruptions are due to the variability in plane of section and to incomplete encirclement by the collagenous pial septa in any single plane.

The pial septum is separated from the nerve fiber bundles, by a layer of astrocytes (2, 6, 27). In both cross and longitudinal section many nuclei are seen. Those in intimate association with pial septa are probably astrocytic. Those

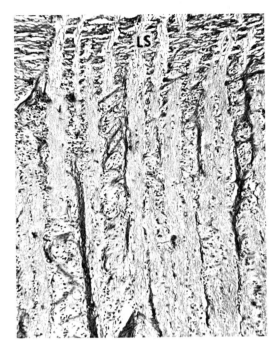

FIG. 12–19. Longitudinal section of orbital portion of optic nerve near lamina scleralis (**LS**). (H&E, × 80) (AFIP Neg. 70-7291)

unassociated with pial septa may be either astrocytic or oligodendrocytic.* Distinction between these glia cannot be made from a single conventional microscopic section. It is highly probable that very few of the nuclei observed in any single section belong to oligodendrocytes.

---

* In recent years electron microscopic identification and the nomenclature of the various types of glial cells (astrocytes, oligodendroglia, and all their variations) have elicited considerable controversy (21, 23). Characterization of these cells in the past has depended upon special "coatings" or "staining" with metallic salts (e.g., silver, gold), either positive or negative, and the subsequent appearance by light microscopy. Attempts to correlate these silver-salt impregnations for light microscopy with observations made by electron microscopy generally have been unsatisfactory. At present there is considerable agreement that a glial cell (i.e., nonneuronal cell) containing a *large* number of intracytoplasmic filaments should be designated a **fibrous astrocyte** and that one with a *few* such filaments, but with a large quantity of ribosomes and a dense cytoplasmic ground substance, should be designated an **oligodendrocyte**. Other criteria, such as the presence of glycogen, also assist in identifying an astrocyte. With initial glutaraldehyde fixation, the oligodendrocytic cytoplasm develops microtubules, but most of the cytoplasmic filaments of the astrocyte remain essentially unaltered (see Fig. 12–12). Microglia are currently believed to be monocytes that wander in from the bloodstream.

VASCULAR SUPPLY

The central retinal artery and vein penetrate the optic nerve from 8–15 mm behind the globe to assume an axial position within the nerve (Fig. 12–20A). The artery generally penetrates into the nerve at the same level or anterior to the vein. In its course through optic nerve, the artery may give off small branches to supply the adjacent nerve fibers, a supply that is exceedingly small at best. The precise arrangement of the blood supply to the optic nerve head remains somewhat controversial (4, 7, 11, 12, 16, 17, 33) (Fig. 12–20B). Much of the blood supply comes from the short posterior ciliary arteries, which also supply the posterior half of the uveal tract. The posterior ciliary arteries entering the sclera closest to the dura form a circle of anastamoses within the adjacent sclera, the arterial circle of Zinn-Haller. The vessels from this circle provide most of the capillaries lying within the lamina cribrosa as well as the adjacent pial vasculature, which nourishes much of the adjacent optic nerve. There is some variability in the form of the circle and its relationship to adjacent vasculature.

Retinal capillaries nourish much of the retinal layers of the optic nerve head while a small peripheral portion of the lamina choroidalis receives some nutrition by diffusion from the adjacent choroidal vasculature (9). There is no apparent connection between retinal and ciliary systems except for the cilioretinal arteries, which arise as branches of the circle of Zinn-Haller, and the much more rare cilioretinal veins, which drain either directly into the uveal tract or more directly into and through the sclera. The venous drainage of the intraocular portion of the optic nerve is mostly via the central retinal vein.

The structure of the nerve head capillaries is similar to that of capillaries in the retina, i.e., they have nonfenestrated endothelia with a small apical zonula occludens, producing a blood–nerve barrier analogous to that of the blood–retina barrier of the retinal capillaries. The vessels here, as in the retina, are separated

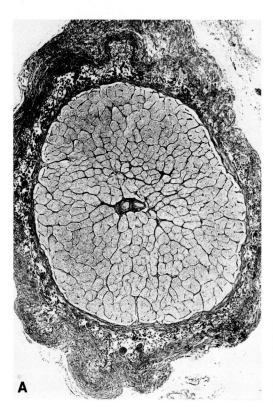

from the adjacent neurites (here axons) by glial cells (here astrocytes), which presumably act as agents in the transfer of nutrients and metabolic products between the nerve tissue and the bloodstream.

The central retinal artery has a fenestrated internal elastic lamina (Fig. 12–21, 12–22). The intima (*i.e.*, all tissue on the luminal side of the internal elastic lamina) frequently contains a number of muscle-like cells or "myointimal" cells (5) (Fig. 12–22).

Smooth muscle cells not only project through the fenestrated internal elastic lamina of larger arteries such as the aorta, but are also found wholly internal to the membrane (*i.e.*, in the subendothelial space). There is some evidence that these myointimal cells are of importance not only as a possible source for

FIG. 12–20. Optic nerve. A. Cross-section of orbital portion of optic nerve within 8–15 mm of globe (before exit of central vessels). (H&E, × 20) (AFIP Neg. 70-7290) B. Schematic drawing of blood supply to bulbar and retrobulbar portions of optic nerve.

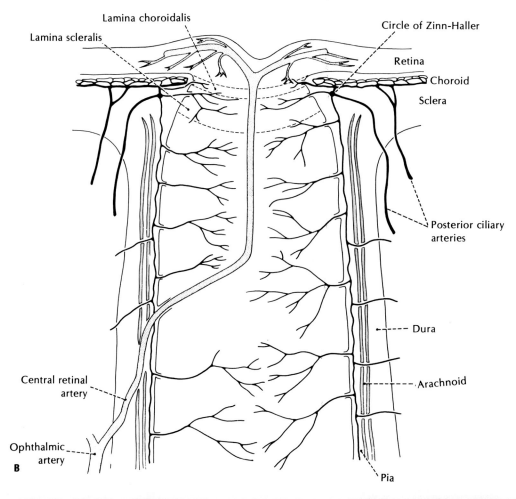

regeneration of endothelial cells (29) but also in the development of atherosclerosis of the vessel wall (22), in which the smooth muscle cells become lipid-laden "foam" cells (34).

Shortly after the vessels enter the retina, the internal elastic lamina is lost entirely (see Fig. 6–78) and the vessels are no longer considered arteries but rather arterioles.

The thin-walled central retinal vein is separated from the surface layer of astrocytes by a thick adventitial layer of collagen (Fig. 12–23). Only a few scattered cells are present within this collagenous layer, and the cells associated with the endothelium are discontinuous and few in number.

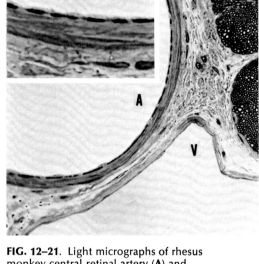

FIG. 12–21. Light micrographs of rhesus monkey central retinal artery (A) and vein (V) in nerve head just behind lamina scleralis. Internal elastic lamina of artery is fenestrated. (Epon, PD, × 300) (AFIP Neg. 66-8671) Inset. Discontinuous internal elastic lamina beneath endothelial lining. (× 900) (AFIP Neg. 66-8670)

FIG. 12–22. Electron micrograph of portion of artery illustrated in Figure 12–21. Intermittency of internal elastic lamina (arrows) beneath endothelium (EN) is apparent. Fragment of muscle-like cell (M) is seen here in plane of elastica. Typical smooth muscle cells (SM) surrounded by their thin basement membranes make up remainder of wall of artery. L, lumen. (× 4700)

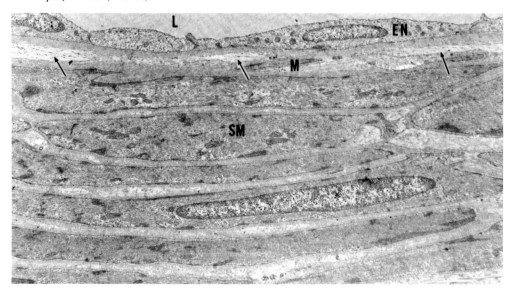

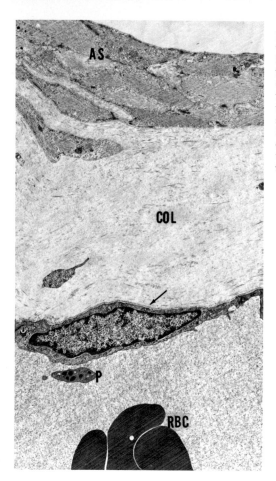

FIG. 12–23. Thin-walled central retinal vein (see Fig. 12–3), containing red blood cells (**RBC**) and a platelet or fragment of leukocyte (**P**). The vein endothelial cell is separated by its thin basement membrane (**arrow**) and a thick collagenous adventitia (**COL**) from surface layer of astrocytes(**AS**). Thin basement membrane lining free surface of optic cup is almost imperceptible at this magnification. (Glutaraldehyde fixation, × 4800)

REFERENCES

1. Anderson DR: Ultrastructure of human and monkey lamina cribrosa and optic nerve head. Arch Ophthalmol 82:800, 1969
2. Anderson DR, Hoyt WF: Ultrastructure of intra-orbital portion of human and monkey optic nerve. Arch Ophthalmol 82:506, 1969
3. Anderson DR: Ultrastructure of the optic nerve head. Arch Ophthalmol 83:63, 1970
4. Anderson DR: Vascular supply to the optic nerve or primates. Am J Ophthalmol 70:341, 1970
5. Buck RC: Intimal thickening after ligature of arteries: an electron microscopic study. Circ Res 9:409, 1961
6. Cohen AI: Ultrastructural aspects of the human optic nerve. Invest Ophthalmol 6:294, 1967
7. Cohen AI: Is there a potential defect in the blood-retinal barrier at the choroidal level of the optic nerve canal? Invest Ophthalmol 12:513, 1973
8. Fine BS: Observations on the axoplasm of neural elements in the human retina. In Titlback M (ed): Proceedings, Third European Regional Conference on Electron Microscopy. Prague, Czechoslovak Academy of Sciences, 1964, p 319
9. Grayson MC, Laties AM: Ocular localization of sodium fluorescein. Arch Ophthalmol 85:600, 1971
10. Hayreh SS: Blood supply of the optic nerve head and its role in optic atrophy: glaucoma and oedema of the optic disc. Brit J Ophthal 53:721, 1969
11. Hayreh SS: Anatomy and physiology of the optic nerve head. Trans Am Acad Ophthalmol Otolaryngol 78:240, 1974
12. Henkind P, Levitzsky M: Angioarchitecture of the optic nerve. I. The papilla. Am J Ophthalmol 68:979, 1969
13. Karlsson JO, Sjöstrand JO: Axonal transport of proteins in retinal ganglion cells. Characterization of the transport to the superior colliculus. Brain Res 47:185, 1972
14. Kuwabara T: Development of the optic nerve of the rat. Invest Ophthalmol 14:732, 1975
15. Lampert PW, Vogel MH, Zimmerman LE: Pathology of the optic nerve in experimental acute glaucoma: electron microscopic studies. Invest Ophthalmol 7:199, 1968
16. Levitzky M, Henkind P: Angioarchitecture of the optic nerve. II. Lamina cribrosa. Am J Ophthalmol 68:986, 1969
17. Lieberman MF, Maumenee AE, Green WR: Histologic studies of the vasculature of the anterior optic nerve. Am J Ophthalmol 82:405, 1976

18. McEwen BS, Grafstein B: Fast and slow components in axonal transport of protein. J Cell Biol 38:494, 1968
19. Minckler DS, McLean IW, Tso MOM: Distribution of axonal and glial elements in the rhesus optic nerve head studied by electron microscopy. Am J Ophthalmol 82:179, 1976
20. Minckler DS, Tso MOM: A light microscopic, auto-radiographic study of axoplasmic transport in the normal rhesus optic nerve head. Am J Ophthalmol 82:1, 1976
21. Mugnaini E, Walberg F: Ultrastructure of neuroglia. In Reviews of Anatomy, Embryology and Cell Biology, No. 37. Berlin, Springer, 1964
22. Parker F, Odland GF: A correlative histochemical, biochemical and electron microscopic study of experimental atherosclerosis in the rabbit aorta with special reference to the myointimal cell. Am J Path 48:197, 1966
23. Peters A, Palay S, Webster H DeF: The Fine Structure of the Nervous System: The Neurons and Supporting Cells. Philadelphia, WB Saunders, 1976
24. Peters A, Vaughn JE: Microtubules and filaments in the axons and astrocytes of early postnatal rat optic nerves. J Cell Biol 32:113, 1967
25. Potts AM, Hodges D, Shelman CB, et al.: Morphology of the primate optic nerve. I. Method and total fiber count. Invest Ophthalmol 11:980, 1972
26. Quigley HA: Gap junctions between optic nerve head astrocytes. Invest Ophthalmol 16:582, 1977
27. Salzmann M: The Anatomy and Histology of the Human Eyeball in the Normal State: Its Development and Senescence. Brown EVL (trans). Chicago, University of Chicago Press, 1912
28. Tennekoon GI, Cohen SR, Price DL, McKhann GM: Myelogenesis in optic nerve: a morphological, auto-radiographic and biochemical analysis. J Cell Biol 72:604, 1977
29. Ts'ao CH: Myo-intimal cells as a possible source of replacement for endothelial cells in the rabbit. Circ Res 23:671, 1968
30. Weiss P, Hiscoe HB: Experiments on the mechanism of nerve growth. J Exp Zool 107:315, 1948
31. Willard M: The identification of two intra-axonally transported polypeptides resembling myosin in some respects in the rabbit visual system. J Cell Biol 75:1, 1977
32. Williams V: Intercellular relationships in the external glial limiting membrane of the neocortex of the cat and rat. Amer J Anat 144:421, 1975
33. Wise GN, Dollery CT, Henkind P (eds): The retinal circulation. New York, Harper & Row, 1971
34. Wolinsky H: A new look at atherosclerosis. Cardiovasc Med 1:41, 1976

chapter **13**

THE OCULAR ADNEXA: LIDS, CONJUNCTIVA, AND ORBIT

Frederick A. Jakobiec, Takeo Iwamoto

EMBRYOLOGY   290
THE EYELIDS   292
  GENERAL ANATOMY   292
  MICROSCOPIC ANATOMY   294
    THE EPIDERMIS AND ORBICULARIS MUSCLE
    THE GLAND OF ZEISS
    THE GLAND OF MOLL
    THE TARSUS AND MEIBOMIAN GLAND
    THE CANALICULI AND LACRIMAL SAC
THE CONJUNCTIVA AND MÜLLER'S MUSCLE   308
THE ORBIT   317
  GENERAL ANATOMY   317
  MICROSCOPIC ANATOMY   325
    THE LACRIMAL GLAND   325
    THE EXTRAOCULAR MUSCLES   327
    THE PERIPHERAL NERVES   334
    ORBITAL FAT   335

The ocular adnexa are those structures which support, assist the function of, and protect the globe: the lids, the conjunctiva, and the orbital bones and soft tissues (Fig. 13–1).

EMBRYOLOGY

The surface of the embryo is covered by a delicate ectodermal membrane of two to three cells called the periderm (3). With progressive differentiation, the periderm develops into a fully keratinizing surface epidermis. In focal areas of the embryonic ectoderm, basal cells proliferate to form buds that burrow into the subjacent mesenchyme; these primary epithelial germs are called either the primary hair germ (giving rise to the hair follicles, sebaceous glands, and apocrine glands, in particular to glands of Moll) or the primary germs, the latter being unassociated with the prospective pilosebaceous apparatus. The meibomian sebaceous glands of the tarsus also derive from surface epithelial germs that are distinct from the hair germs. Lastly, the canaliculi, lacrimal sac, and nasolacrimal duct are surface ectodermal outgrowths. At birth almost three quarters of the nasolacrimal ducts, solid tubes at first, have not completely canalized, and approximately a third of the ducts have imperforate nasal meatuses (19).

The conjunctival epithelium is of surface ectoderm origin, but its definitive differentiation leads to a nonkeratinizing squamous epithelium with focal goblet cell (mucinous) differentiation. Both the major lacrimal gland and the minor ectopic lacrimal glands of Krause (fornices) and Wolfring (within or above the tarsi) represent end-stage differentiations of conjunctival buds or anlagen that grow into the mesenchyme. The hairs and sebaceous glands of the caruncle indicate that the surface epithelium of the conjunctiva retains many of the same differentiation capabilities as the keratinizing surface epidermis.

The formation of **cystic dermoids** in the orbit, brow, and lids, consisting of a lining of keratinizing epidermis and pilosebaceous units in the wall, is the result of surface epidermis being pinched off by embryonic soft tissue processes of the upper face or by the fusion of bony sutures which entrap invaginated surface elements. The embryonic conjunctiva may also become sequestered to produce lid and orbital dermoids lined by mucus-producing conjunctival type epithelium, which may also recapitulate skin appendages in the wall (9).

According to classical embryologic teaching, all of the connective tissues of the body are of mesodermal or middle embryonic layer origin. However, based on experimental embryologic studies in animals, it appears that the neural crest contributes most of the connective tissues in the head and neck, due to the absence of mesodermal somites in the cephalic region (13–18, 25). In the earliest stages of embryogenesis, the forebrain comes very close to the ectoderm because of the dearth of mesenchymal tissue. The neural crest-derived mesenchyme or connective tissue has been termed "mesectoderm" or "ectomesenchyme." Neural crest cells originating in the dorsal-lateral lips of the invaginating cephalic neural tube delaminate and migrate ventrally to supply practically all of the connective tissues of the frontonasal processes, maxillary processes, and first and second visceral arches (Fig. 13–2, 13–3), which ultimately are responsible for the definitive connective tissues of the face, lids, conjunctiva, orbit, and much of the orbital bones (Fig. 13–4). It is felt that only vascular endothelial cells and striated muscle cells are of mesodermal origin, originating from the preotic somites as well as from paraxial mesoderm that grows into the head and neck region. Even the muscle satellite cells and pericytes of blood vessels are now suspected of being of neural crest origin.

Unusual mesectodermal smooth muscle tumors in

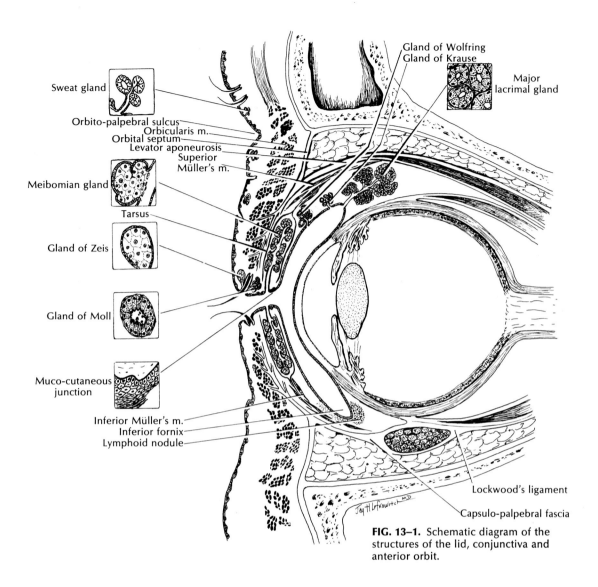

Sweat gland

Orbito-palpebral sulcus
Orbicularis m.
Orbital septum
Levator aponeurosis
Superior
Müller's m.

Meibomian gland

Tarsus

Gland of Zeis

Gland of Moll

Muco-cutaneous
junction

Inferior Müller's m.
Inferior fornix
Lymphoid nodule

Gland of Wolfring
Gland of Krause

Major
lacrimal gland

Lockwood's ligament

Capsulo-palpebral fascia

FIG. 13–1. Schematic diagram of the structures of the lid, conjunctiva and anterior orbit.

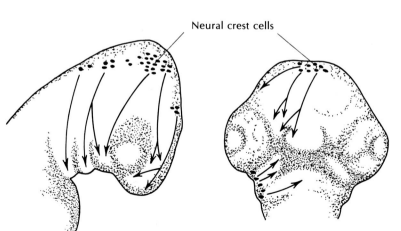

Neural crest cells

FIG. 13–2. Neural crest cells arise along the dorsolateral part of the neural tube and migrate ventrally to fill in the upper facial process (frontonasal and maxillary) and visceral arches. (From Johnston MD: Anat Rec 156:143–156, 1966)

THE OCULAR ADNEXA: LIDS, CONJUNCTIVA, AND ORBIT   **291**

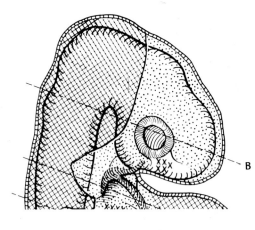

FIG. 13–3. Section (**B**) through the head of an embryo to show the eventual ventral location of the migrated neural crests in relationship to the paraxial mesoderm around the forebrain. (From Johnston, MC, Bhakdinaronk A, Reid YC: An expanded role of the neural crest in oral and pharyngeal development. In Bosma JF (ed): The Fourth Symposium on Oral Sensation and Perception, HEW Pub. No. 73-546. Bethesda, National Institutes of Health, 1973, pp 37–52)

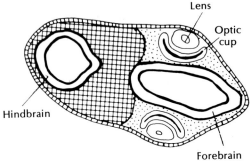

FIG. 13–4. Stippled areas indicate the tissues of the face and bones of the base of the skull that are contributed by neural crest cells. (From Johnston MD, Bhakdinaronk A, Reid YC: An expanded role of the neural crest in oral and pharyngeal development. In Bosma JF (ed): The Fourth Symposium on Oral Sensation and Perception, HEW Pub. No. 73-546. Bethesda, National Institutes of Health, 1973, pp 37–52)

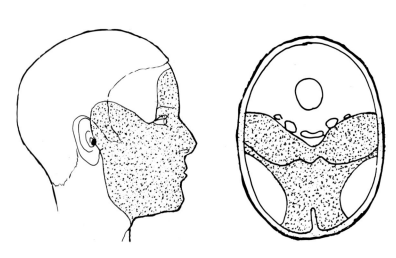

both the orbit and globe may display neurogenic features that reflect the origin of the tumor cells from the neural crest (10–12).

THE EYELIDS

GENERAL ANATOMY

The eyelids are specialized motile skin folds covered on the outside by keratinizing surface epidermis with associated adnexal structures and on the inside by nonkeratinizing conjunctival epithelium (Fig. 13–1, 13–5). The lids contain four layers: 1) the outermost skin with scant subcutaneous tissue, 2) the circularly oriented orbicularis striated muscle, 3) the densely fibrous tarsus and enclosed meibomian glands, and 4) an innermost layer of tightly adherent tarsal conjunctiva.

The orbitopalpebral sulcus or the superior palpebral furrow subdivides the upper lids into a preorbital portion and a lower pretarsal portion (Fig. 13–1). The skin is looser above than in front of the tarsus. The skin of the lids is more delicate than that elsewhere in the body and has a greater elasticity, allowing the collection of edema fluid and inflammatory exudates.

Laxity of this delicate tissue with ageing in the upper lids creates "baggy lids" called **blepharochalasis.** Multiple inflammatory episodes will often accelerate this change. Weakening of the orbital septum with ageing allows herniation of anterior orbital fat into the lids.

As with other facial muscles that insert into the skin, in no place else in the body does striated muscle come so close to the surface epidermis as does the orbicularis. Orbicularis muscle fibers are present all the way to the lid margin, where a small bundle of myofibers is sometimes called the muscle of Riolan (Fig. 13–5). At the lid margin there are as many as 150 cilia in the upper lid and 75 in the lower. Behind the cilia is the mucocutaneous junction (close to the gray line, which is a useful clinical landmark for surgically halving the pretarsal portion of the lid); just in front of the mucocutaneous junction are the orifices of 30–40 sebaceous meibomian glands in the upper tarsus and 20–30 in the lower. The lacrimal puncta, which remove tears from the lacus lacrimalis, are located in the medial aspects of the upper and lower lids; these drain via the canaliculi into the lacrimal sac and thence through the nasolacrimal duct into the nose. The medial heads of the pretarsal orbicularis muscle bundles insert onto the fascia of the sac and provide a pumping mechanism (19).

The pretarsal part of the lids derives its arterial blood supply from the superficial temporal and facial arteries, branches of the external carotid system, while the posttarsal part obtains its blood supply from terminal branches of the ophthalmic artery, a branch of the internal carotid. The anterior facial and superior temporal veins drain the pretarsal lids into the internal and external jugular systems, respectively; the posttarsal venous drainage is via the ophthalmic (orbital) veins into the cavernous sinus and pterygoid plexus. The lymphatic drainage of the lateral portion of the lids goes to the preauricular and intraparotid lymph nodes; the medial lymphatic drainage is to the submental and submandibular nodes. The sensory inner-

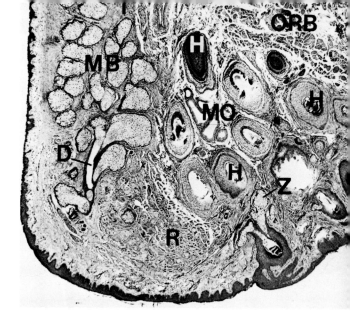

FIG. 13–5. Section through the lower part of the upper lid. The conjunctiva is present on the left, the skin on the right, and the lid margin at the bottom. Immediately beneath the skin of the lids is the orbicularis muscle (**ORB**), a small portion of which is present near the lid margin as the muscle of Riolan (**R**). The marginal cilia are shown in cross sections as hair shafts (**H**). Both the gland of Moll (**MO**) and the sebaceous gland of Zeis (**Z**) are related to the cilia. The posterior part of the lid is composed of the dense collagen of the tarsus (**T**) in which are embedded the alveoli of the meibomian glands (**MB**). The alveoli empty into a vertical duct (**D**) that will open onto the posterior aspect of the lid margin. (H&E, ×27)

vation of the upper lids is provided by terminal skin branches of the ophthalmic division of the trigeminal nerve; the skin of the lower lid receives its sensory innervation from the infraorbital nerve, a branch of the second or maxillary division of the trigeminal. The orbicularis muscle is innervated by the seventh (facial) cranial nerve.

A clinically and surgically important feature of the upper lid anatomy is the insertion of the levator palpebrae superioris aponeurosis (Fig. 13–1). This structure attaches to the lateral and medial orbital rims and terminates broadly throughout the upper lid as slits or strips that penetrate the orbital septum to commingle with the connective tissues of the orbicularis and skin. Many causes of lid droop or ptosis (senile dehiscences of the aponeurosis, myasthenia gravis, partial oculomotor nerve palsies) can

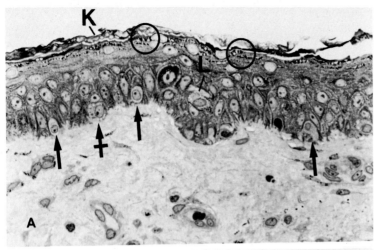

FIG. 13–6. A. The skin of the lids is composed of a keratinizing epidermis that sits on a poorly defined papillary dermis. The **arrows** point to clear cells at the dermo-epidermal junction; these are melanocytes, and the **crossed arrow** indicates a cell containing cytoplasmic pigment granules. A higher level clear cell is a Langerhans cell (**L**). The **circles** identify keratohyalin granules in the superficial granular layer, above which is the anuclear surface keratinizing layer (**K**). B. Transition (**arrow**) at the lid margin between keratinizing surface epidermis on the right and non-keratinizing squamous epithelium of the conjunctiva on the left. (1.0μ Araldite section, methylene blue; A, ×375; B, ×240)

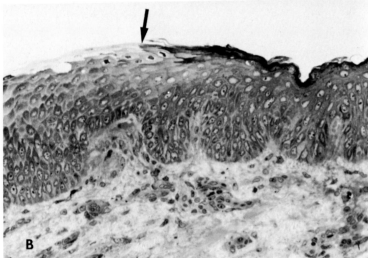

be surgically corrected by performing a resection of part of the aponeurosis, either transconjunctivally or transcutaneously. The amount of the resection can be estimated from measurements of the extent of the remaining levator muscle function. This can be gauged by observing how much the ptotic lid moves on having the patient look upward, while at the same time preventing the frontalis muscle from being called into play.

The stability and overall conformation of the lids are guaranteed by the medial and lateral palpebral (canthal) ligaments. These are condensations of fibrous tissue representing the insertions of the tendons of the orbicularis muscle into the midlateral and medial orbital rims. The posterior aspect of these ligaments is reinforced by contributions from the orbital fibrous connective tissue system, in particular, the transverse (suspensory) superior and in-

ferior orbital fascial expansions related to their respective extraocular muscles, the check ligaments of the horizontal rectus muscles, and the insertion of the levator aponeurosis. The function of the anterior orbital tissues is thereby integrated with that of the lids.

MICROSCOPIC ANATOMY

The **epidermis** of the skin of the lids (Fig. 13–6A) is formed by multilaminar keratinocytes consisting of a basal or germinal layer of quasi-columnar cells, suprabasilar (malpighiian) layers of polygonal prickle or squamous cells, a granular cell layer of more flattened cells, and finally a fully cornified superficial layer of anuclear keratin lamellas (30). At the mucocu-

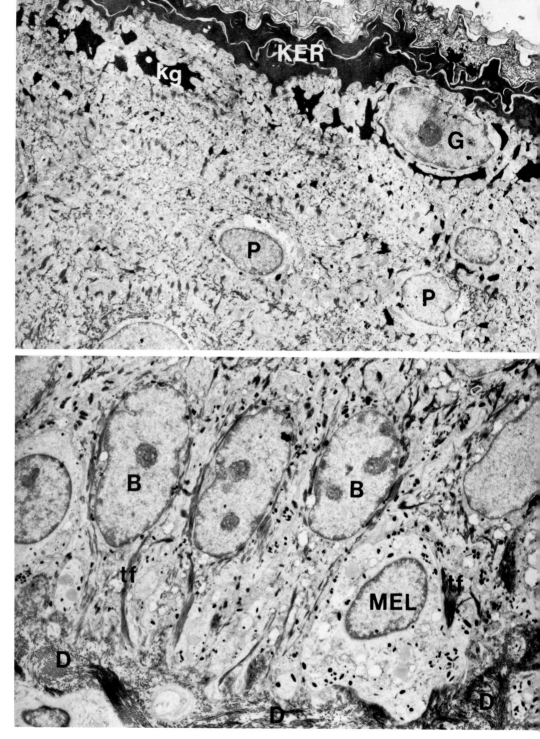

FIG. 13–7. Composite electron micrograph of the lid epidermis showing in the panel below columnar basal cells (**B**) with tonofilaments (**tf**). More superficial prickle (**P**) and granular cells (**G**) are present in the panel above. A melanocyte (**MEL**) is present among the basal cells lying against the collagenous dermis (**D**). Keratohyalin granules (**kg**) transform the granular cells into keratin (**KER**). (Top, ×4400; Bottom, ×4600)

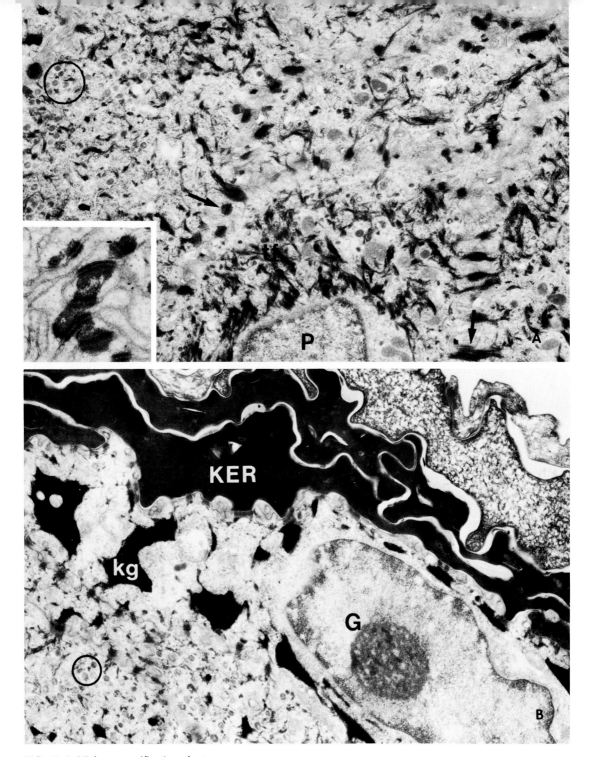

FIG. 13–8. Higher magnification electron micrographs showing upper level prickle cells (**P**) with tonofilaments (**tf**) in A and granular cells (**G**) with electron-dense keratohyalin granules (**kg**) in B. The **arrows** point to desmosomes between the prickle cells, shown more clearly in the inset; the **circles** highlight spherical keratinosomes in both the upper prickle and granular layers. Surface keratinization (**KER**) is brought about by fusion of tonofilaments with keratohyalin. (A, ×12,700; B, ×12,000; inset, ×23,300)

FIG. 13–9. A. The basal epidermal cells contain tonofilaments (**tf**) and are separated from the underlying papillary dermis by a basement membrane (**bm**). Banded special fibrils (**af**) ("anchoring" fibrils) extend from the thin basement membrane into the adjacent dermis. **ICS,** intercellular space between the basal cells; **free white arrows,** hemidesmosomes along the basal plasmalemma of the basal cells; **C,** thick collagen fibrils of the reticular dermis. B. A melanocyte (**MEL**) with melanosomes (**m**) but without tonofilaments is located among the basal cells containing tonofilaments (**tf**) and lies against the thin basement membrane (**arrows**). **g,** Golgi apparatus; **p,** small process of the melanocyte insinuated among the basilar epidermal cells. (A, ×26,100; B, ×12,200)

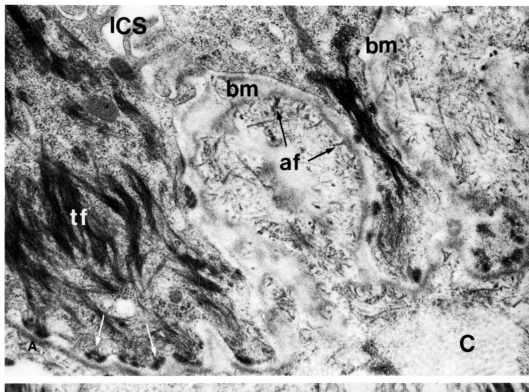

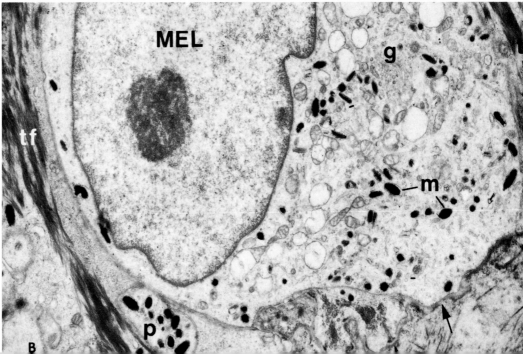

taneous junction on the lid margin, the granular and keratin layers disappear (Fig. 13–6B). Tonofilaments are present in the basilar cells but become far more numerous in the suprabasilar prickle or squamous cells (Fig. 13–7, 13–8). The tonofilaments insert into the desmosomes that join the cells together. The function of the keratinocytes is to generate protective and comparatively impermeable keratin on the surface of the epidermis. This occurs as the tonofilaments of the higher level keratinocytes become glued together by keratinohyalin granules. The intercellular compaction of the surface cells is also aided by small spherical inclusions in the superficial layers called keratinosomes or membrane-coating vesicles.

The basal cells rest on a basement membrane that separates the epidermis from the papillary dermis (Fig. 13–9A). Delicate, vertically oriented, and terminally branching anchoring fibrils of papillary collagen project from the undersurface of the basement membrane. Besides having cytoplasmic tonofilaments, the basilar cells possess hemidesmosomes which attach their basal plasmalemmas to the basement membrane. Scattered among the basilar cells are "clear cells," which in actuality are dendritic melanocytes that lack tonofilaments and desmosomes and that supply melanin to the surrounding keratinocytes (epidermal-melanin unit) (Fig. 13–9B). Higher level clear cells in the epidermis are called Langerhans' cells (29); once believed to be effete or worn out melanocytes, they are now considered to be a species of histiocyte.

Racial pigmentary differences are not caused by variations in the number of melanocytes within the epidermis, but rather by different kinds of melanin granules which upon transfer to the surrounding keratinocytes adopt various forms of dispersion within the keratinocytic cytoplasm. Suntanning involves increased production of melanin granules instead of cellular proliferation. Flat macules of hyperpigmentation that occur idiopathically are called freckles or ephelides; they represent increased production of melanin granules that are once again taken up by the basilar keratinocytes. Another form of impalpable hyperpigmentation is the lentigo; in this condition there are increased numbers of basilar melanocytes, usually without conspicuous nest formation. In nevi, there is benign proliferation of intraepithelial melanocytes forming nests; with the passage of time the melanocytes drop off into the upper dermis, accounting for the progressive nodularity and thickness of these lesions. Extensive congenital "kissing" nevi are the result of increased numbers of melanocytes migrating from the neural crest into the skin of the upper and lower lids while they are fused *in utero*. Malignant melanomas are progressive nodular growths with ulceration, irregular pigmentation, and bleeding; they are much rarer in the lids than in the conjunctiva, where intraepithelial melanocytes also occur and are capable of undergoing malignant transformation.

Langerhans' cells have been found in the connective tissues and are presumed to give origin to the histiocytosis X group of tumors which can produce eczematoid-papular lesions of the lids along with multisystem involvement. Langerhans' granules have been found in the cytoplasm of the proliferating histiocytes comprising the lesions.

The **papillary dermis** is not well developed in the lids because of the absence of prominent epidermal rete ridges (Fig. 13–6A), so that there is an imperceptible merging of the papillary with the reticular dermis. Small vellus hairs and sweat glands have their roots deep in the dermis of the lids. The sweat glands are composed of clear and dark cells surrounded by a myoepithelium. Their clear secretion is formed without loss of cell cytoplasm. The double-layered ducts of the sweat glands have a PAS-positive cuticulum on the luminal surface. The sweat glands of the lid share a heat regulating role with those of the rest of the body.

At the **lid margin,** the roots of the cilia lie deep against the tarsus. The cilia probably play a sensory role, because they are generously endowed with nerve endings; they also have their own sebaceous glands (glands of Zeiss) and apocrine glands (glands of Moll) (Fig. 13–10). The unilobular **Zeiss glands** are made up of cells with frothy vacuolated cytoplasm, due to the presence of myriad lipid droplets (Fig. 13–11). Separating these lipid vacuoles are profiles of rough surfaced and, especially, smooth surfaced endoplasmic reticulum. The Zeiss glands empty their secretion, which is produced by decomposition of the entire cell (holocrine secretion), into the follicles of the cilia. The cilia differ from other strong hairs in the body in not possessing erectores pilorum smooth muscle attached to the follicular wall.

Inflammations or infections of the glands of Zeiss are called a **hordeolum.**

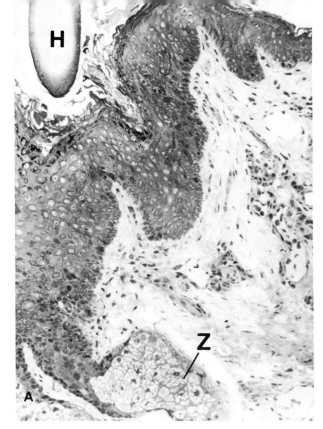

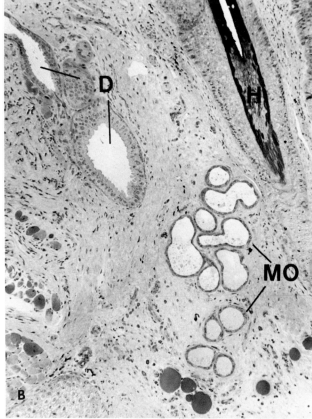

The **glands of Moll** (Fig. 13–12) are apocrine glands that also empty their secretion into the follicles of the cilia, but they differ from eccrine glands (sweat glands) in that they produce their secretion by decapitation of apical cytoplasmic processes (27). The cytoplasm of the Moll gland cells is deeply eosinophilic on light microscopic staining, and the lumens formed by the secretory cells are large compared with those of eccrine glands and contain cellular debris. The secretory cells manifest various stages of metabolic activity, some being flat to cuboidal, others being more columnar with apical granules and apical caps or snouts of decapitation secretion (Fig. 13–12). Tonofilaments are dispersed singly rather than in bundles in the cytoplasm, and there is a well-developed Golgi apparatus. Two types of secretory granules are synthesized: dark granules resembling lysosomes morphologically and histochemically and light granules with a filamentous and membranous character resembling the cristae of mitochondria (Fig. 13–13). Myoepithelial cells possessing filaments with fusiform densities surround the inner secretory cells. The thick basement membrane of the epithelium is unusual in that it lies outside of the myoepithelial cell layer. No clear ocular function has been ascribed to the apocrine glands of Moll; apocrine glands elsewhere in the body (axilla and anogenital region) are essentially scent organs.

The **tarsus** is composed of highly regimented collagen fibrils of uniform diameter (600–700A) that run horizontally and vertically, surrounding the alveolar units of the meibomian glands (Fig. 13–14 to 13–16). Elastic tissue is scattered among the collagen fibers of the tarsus. The ducts of the **meibomian glands** within the tarsus are vertically oriented with respect to the lid

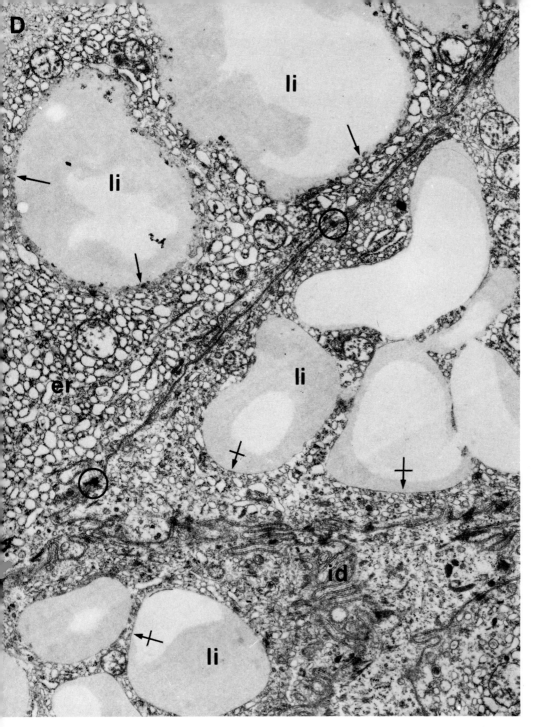

FIG. 13–11. Sebaceous cells of the gland of Zeis associated with a hair follicle display intracytoplasmic lipid droplets (**li**). The lipid droplets below have well delimited cytoplasmic outlines (**crossed arrows**), while the droplet outlines in the cells above are indistinct and manifest cytoplasmic blebs (**arrows**), indicative of early cytoplasmic dissolution. The glandular secretion is formed by progressive decomposition of the cytoplasm (**D**), which is entirely shed into the duct of the gland. **Circles,** small desmosomes; **id,** interdigitations of adjacent cytoplasmic processes; **er,** smooth-surfaced endoplasmic reticulum. (×15,900)

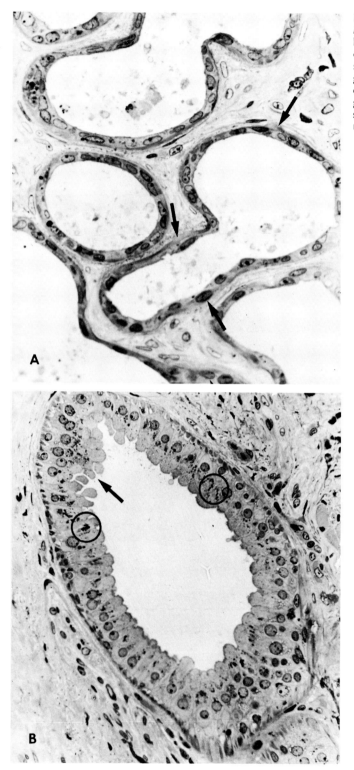

FIG. 13–12. A. The ectatic glands of Moll have cytoplasmic debris in their lumens. An outer row of myoepithelial cells **(arrows)** surrounds the inner secretory cells. B. Cells in the duct of the gland of Moll also show secretory characteristics, consisting of apical granules **(circles)** and apical cytoplasmic snouts **(arrow)**. (1.0μ Araldite section, methylene blue stain, ×350)

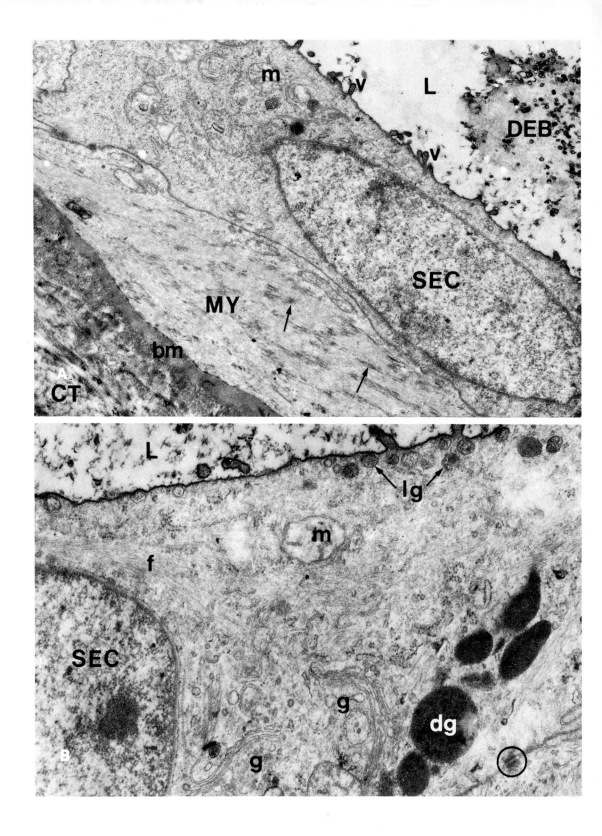

◀ **FIG. 13–13.** A. Secretory portion of the gland of Moll is composed of inner secretory cells (**SEC**) bordering the lumen (**L**) and an outer layer of myoepithelial cells (**MY**) possessing filaments with fusiform densities (**arrows**). Apical villi (**v**) project into the lumen which contains cytoplasmic debris (**DEB**) from the apocrine type secretion. A thick basement membrane (**bm**) separates the myoepithelial cells from the interstitial connective tissue (**CT**). **m,** mitochondria. B. Secretory cell (**SEC**) displays cytoplasmic filaments (**f**) and well-defined lamellas of the Golgi apparatus (**g**). Light secretory granules (**lg**) are found close to the lumen (**L**), while denser (**dg**) granules are present lower in the cell. Mitochondria (**m**) frequently appear degenerated in aprocrine cells. **Circle,** a desmosome between two secretory cells. (A, ×12,700; B, ×24,700)

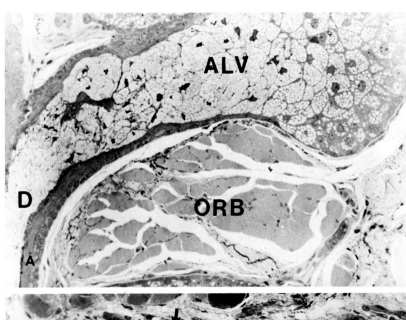

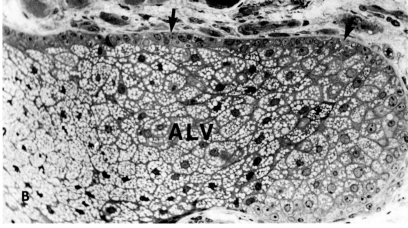

FIG. 13–14. A. The sebaceous cells of an alveolus (**ALV**) of a meibomian gland undergo total degeneration and shed into the duct (**D**). **ORB,** surrounding orbicularis muscle fibers of Riolan. B. A single layer of nonlipidized germinal cells (**arrows**) undergoes rapid differentiation into vacuolated sebaceous cells forming the alveolus (**ALV**).(1.0μ Araldite section, methylene blue stain, A ×208; B, ×250)

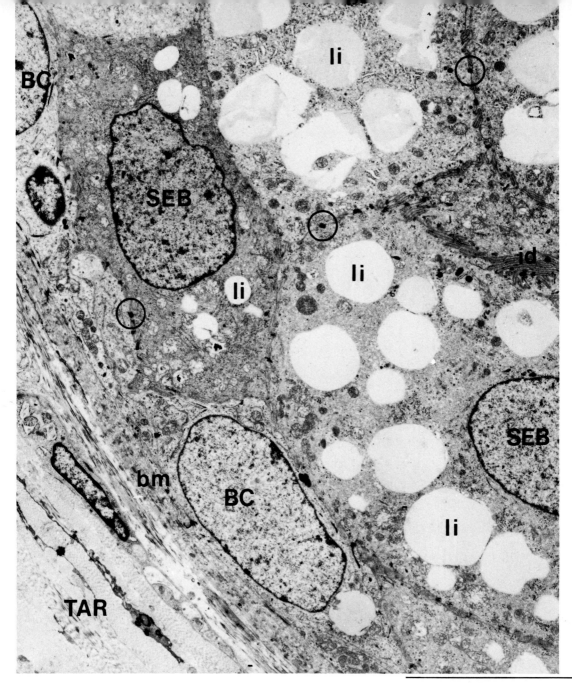

FIG. 13–15. Periphery of a meibomian sebaceous lobule embedded in the tarsus (**TAR**). Nonlipidized basal or reserve cells (**BC**) are separated from the tarsus by a basement membrane zone (**bm**). Inner cells manifest progressive lipidization (**li**) of the cytoplasm with conversion into sebaceous cells (**SEB**). Numerous desmosomes (**circles**) interconnect the lobular elements; cytoplasmic interdigitations (**id**) are also frequently seen. (×6000)

FIG. 13–16. A. Pale basal cells (**BC**) are connected with darker sebaceous cells (**SEB**) by numerous desmosomes (**d**). Thin bundles of tonofilament (**arrow**) are scattered within the cytoplasm of the basal cells. Hemidesmosomes (**circles**) fasten the basal cells to the underlying multilaminar basement membrane (**m-bm**). A fibroblast (**F**) and tarsal collagen (**TAR**) are present below. B. The tarsus is composed of highly regimented collagen fibrils separating slender fibroblasts (**F**) with attenuated cytoplasmic processes (**P**). The inset demonstrates the regularity and uniform diameter of the tarsal collagen as well as occasional elastic tissue (**arrow**). (A, ×12,000; B, ×5300; inset, ×40,000)

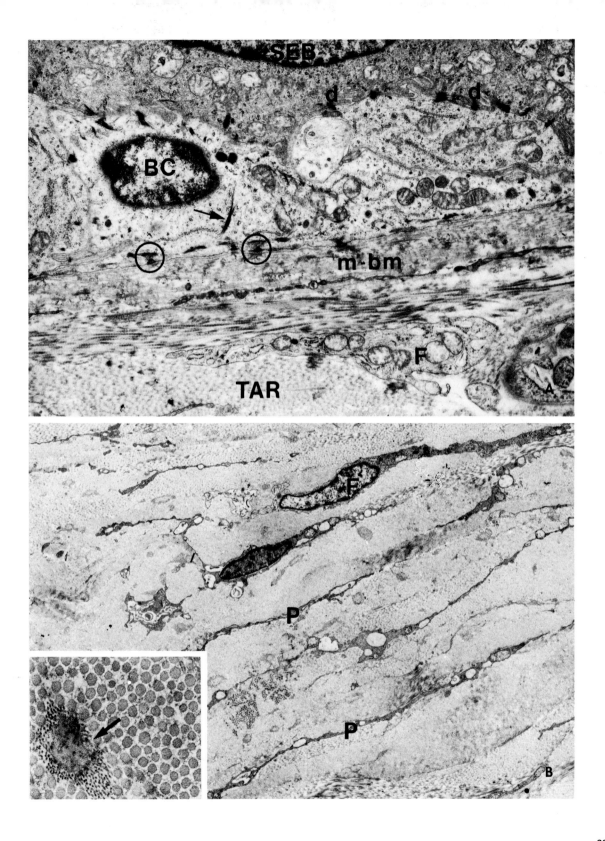

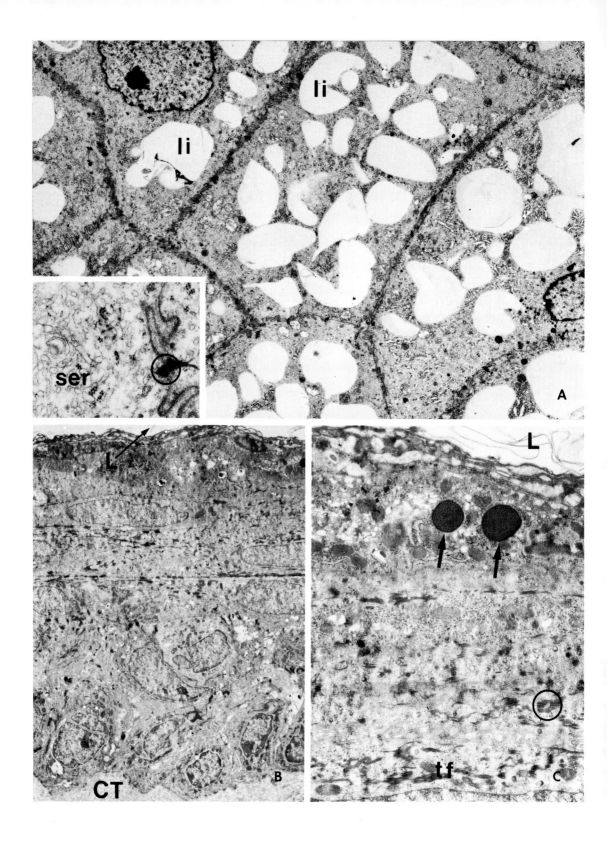

FIG. 13–17. A. Intralobular sebaceous cells of the meibomian gland display cytoplasmic lipid vacuoles (**li**) and profiles of smooth-surfaced endoplasmic reticulum (**ser**), shown in the inset. **Circle,** a desmosome. B. Meibomian gland duct is composed entirely of partially keratinizing squamous cells extending from the connective tissue (**CT**) to the lumen (**arrow**). C. The innermost cells of the duct wall exhibit tonofilaments (**tf**), desmosomes (**circle**), and incomplete cornification near the lumen (**L**). The **arrows** point to laminated trichohyalin globules in the most superficial cells. (A, ×4600; inset, ×23,800; B, ×2300; C, ×11,200)

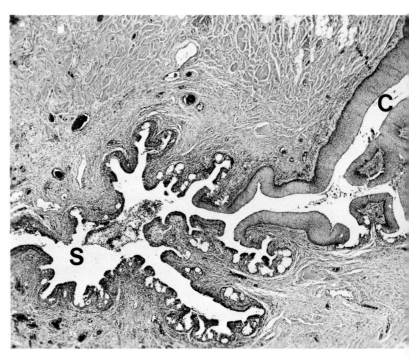

FIG. 13–18. The canaliculus (**C**) is lined by nonkeratinizing squamous epithelium and the lacrimal sac (**S**) by columnar and mucinous epithelium. (H&E, ×38) (From Ryan S, Font R: Am J Ophthalmol 76:73–88, 1973)

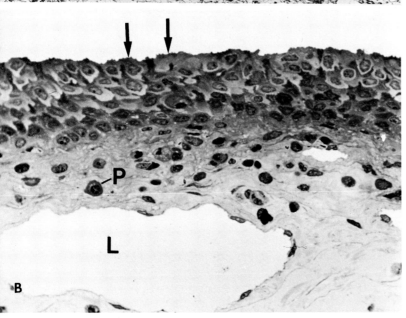

FIG. 13–19. A. Conjunctiva from the epibulbar surface shows clear mucus-producing goblet cells (**arrows**) within the nonkeratinizing surface epithelium. An invagination (**EV**) of the surface epithelium is seen in the loose collagen of the substantia propria (**SP**). B. The surface epithelium shows no evidence of keratinization and the most superficial cells possess villi or plicae (**arrows**). A lymphatic channel (**L**) is found in the substantia propria, which includes a scattering of mononuclear cells and plasma cells (**P**). (A, H&E, ×80; 1.0μ Araldite section, methylene blue stain, ×375)

margin; lateral lobules or alveoli of secretory cells empty into the duct. As with all sebaceous glands, including the Zeiss glands, their secretion is formed by decomposition of the cells which are shed into the ducts (27). A single outside layer of nonlipidized germinal basal cells with scattered tonofilaments is found in each lobule and sits on a multilaminar basement membrane without a myoepithelial layer. The sebaceous cells in the center of the alveoli contain abundant smooth-surfaced endoplasmic reticulum (Fig. 13–17A). The duct cells display keratinizing features without a granular layer (tricholemmal keratinization) (Fig. 13–17B). Besides lubricating the lids, the function of the oily secretion of the meibomian glands is to provide the outermost layer of the trilaminar precorneal tear film. The oily layer retards tear loss by evaporation.

Inflammations of the meibomian glands produce the common clinical entity known as a **chalazion.** When the damaged sebaceous cells release their content of lipid, a granulomatous response ensues featuring multinucleated giant cells and epithelioid cells. A highly malignant epithelial tumor of sebaceous cells—a **sebaceous carcinoma**—can arise from the meibomian glands and is more common in the lids than anywhere else in the body. It is often confused clinically and pathologically with basal cell epithelioma, the most frequent form of lid malignancy, which, however, is only locally infiltrating and nonmetastasizing.

The canaliculi of the nasolacrimal drainage apparatus are lined by multilaminar nonkeratinizing squamous cells (Fig. 13–18). The lacrimal sac combines both mucus-secreting goblet cells and columnar and occasionally ciliated cells; the latter are sometimes confusingly called transitional epithelium.

CONJUNCTIVA AND MÜLLER'S MUSCLE

The conjunctiva is a mucous membrane (26). Its surface is composed of nonkeratinizing

FIG. 13–20. A. The conjunctiva of the superior fornix (**SF**) contains accessory lacrimal glands of Krause (**K**); the **arrows** indicate the duct of the gland. B. Beneath the conjunctival epithelium of the inferior fornix (**IF**) are aggregates of lymphoid tissue (**arrows**). Deep to the substantia propria are fascicles of smooth muscle cells (**M**), which constitute the inferior tarsal muscle of Müller. (H&E, A, ×60, B, ×30)

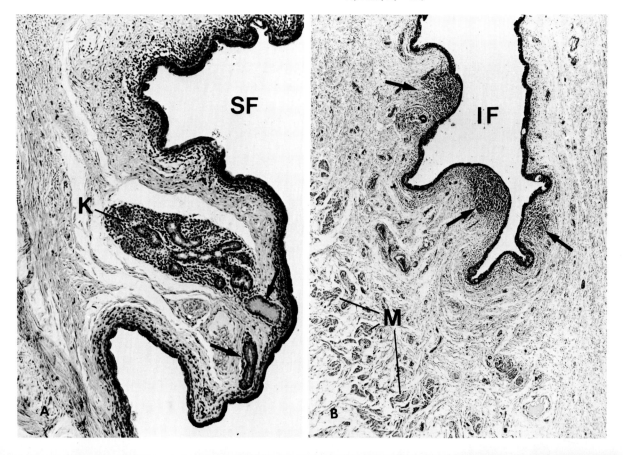

squamous epithelium with intermixed goblet cells, which rest on a connective tissue substantia propria. The conjunctiva receives its blood supply from the anterior ciliary arteries, branches of the ophthalmic artery. Its sensory innervation derives from the first or ophthalmic division of the trigeminal nerve.

Three geographic zones of the conjunctiva are easily recognized: the tarsal, forniceal-orbital, and bulbar. The tarsal conjunctiva (Fig. 13–5) originates at the mucocutaneous junction of the lid margin. Its substantia propria is densely adherent to the tarsus, and therefore the tarsal conjunctiva is not freely movable. By contrast, the substantia propria of the bulbar conjunctiva is freely movable and very delicate (Fig. 13–19), but toward the limbus it fuses with Tenon's capsule. In the fornices (Fig. 13–20) the substantia propria is redundant. In the upper fornix it is augmented by the fibrous expansion of the levator aponeurosis and Müller's muscle and in the lower by the fibrous expansion of the inferior rectus muscle sheath (capsulopalpebral fascia) and the inferior tarsal muscle. Small ectopic lacrimal glands of Krause are found in the fornices (Fig. 13–20A) and, together with the glands of Wolfring (Fig. 13–21) within or above the tarsus, provide the baseline secretion of tears under sympathetic nervous system control. Lymphocytes and plasma cells as well as lymphoid aggregates are also found in the substantia propria of the fornices, particularly in the inferior fornix (Fig. 13–20B).

Because of the standing population of lymphoid cells in the substantia propria, the conjunctival sac has been likened to an opened up lymph node. Some of the lymphocytes produce IgA in common with the production of this immunoglobulin at other mucosal interfaces (tracheobronchial tree and gut). The antibody crosses the conjunctival epithelium after the latter has added a "secretory piece." Hyperplasia of this lymphoid tissue produces the clinical appearance of a folliculosis or follicular conjunctivitis. Virus infections, trachoma, and allergic reactions to drugs (pilocarpine and iododeoxyuridine—IDU) are possible causes of follicular hyperplasia.

The **conjunctival epithelium** ranges from two to five cells in thickness, depending on topography (Fig. 13–22A); we have not been impressed that there is any consistent difference in thickness from site to site. Mucus cells (gob-

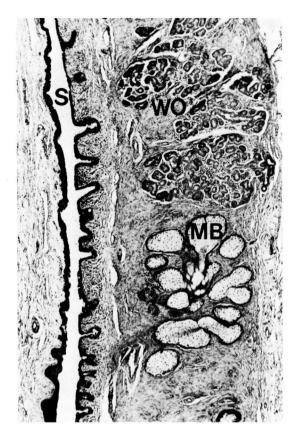

FIG. 13–21. An accessory gland of Wolfring (**WO**) is located in the tarsus above the meibomian gland (**MB**). **S,** conjunctival sac. (H&E, ×38)

let cells) are most concentrated in the caruncle, semilunar fold, and fornices; they are also seen in the epibulbar conjunctiva, but they are virtually absent from the limbal conjunctiva. The mucous secretion serves as a wetting agent that permits adherence of the precorneal tear film.

The basal layer is composed of cuboidal cells; the suprabasilar layers are somewhat polyhedral; and on the surface there are more flattened nonkeratinizing squamous cells with apical villi. At times the most superficial layer of cells may adopt a cuboidal or columnar apocrine appearance with apical snouts and somewhat more eosinophilic cytoplasm than normal, particularly when there are only two layers or when there are invaginations of the conjunctival epithelium into the substantia propria (Fig. 13–19A). These invaginations lead to the formation of the clear cysts that are so often encountered in the fornices.

Inclusion cysts may continue to secrete mucoid material, which ultimately can become calcific concretions. These may be visualized clinically in the fornices and above the tarsus as hard white nodules and can create a foreign body sensation necessitating removal.

Whereas the conjunctiva is for the most part flat, there are papillary arrangements at the limbus (palisades of Vogt) as well as above the tarsus, the so-called crypts of Henle. In these crypts one may see mucus cells or cells with the apocrine type transformation mentioned above.

Marked edema of the conjunctival substantia propria due to vasodilatation, as in bacterial conjunctivitis or vernal catarrh, can throw any part of the conjunctiva into exaggerated papillary folds. These papillae can be seen on biomicroscopy to have central dilated vessels; follicles, in contrast, display peripheral vessels that diminish toward the dome of the follicles.

The conjunctival epithelium can convert into a fully keratinizing epithelium, so-called epidermalization. Chronic exposure from poor lid function, postradiation damage, extensive scarring, and vitamin A deficiency are among the factors that may bring this transformation about. Focal areas of conjunctival keratinization are nonspecifically referred to as **leukoplakia.** The Bitot spot is a patch of hyperkeratosis acted upon by *Corynebacterium xerosis* in hypovitaminosis A.

The basilar epithelium displays hemidesmosomes and tonofilaments (Fig. 13–22B); it is separated from the substantia propria by a thin basement membrane, beneath which lie the collagen fibrils of the connective tissue. Dispersed within the basilar cell region one may also find melanocytes and Langerhans' cells (Fig. 13–23). Intercellular processes and the intercellular space are more prominent in the conjunctival epithelium compared with the corneal epithelium (see Ch. 9). Numerous desmosomes with inserting tonofilaments attach the cells to each other. The conjunctival tonofilamentary bundles are stouter than those of the corneal cells, and there are also more numerous mitochondria compared with the latter. The uppermost cells exhibit microvilli with a glycocalyx type coating (Fig. 13–24A), as well as small univacuolar collections of mucinous material (24) (Fig. 13–24, inset). Most of the conjunctival mucosubstance, however, comes from unicellular mucus glands, the goblet cells, in which the cytoplasm is honeycombed by cord-

FIG. 13–22. A. The conjunctival epithelium is separated from the connective tissue of the substantia propria (**SP**) by a thin basement membrane (**arrows**). The cells possess numerous tonofilaments (**tf**) and mitochondria (**m**); a wide intercellular space (**ICS**) displays digitate cytoplasmic processes. B. Higher power electron micrograph of the basilar cells which have tonofilaments (**tf**), desmosomes (**circle**), and plasmalemmal hemidesmosomes (**white arrowheads**) distributed along the basilar plasmalemma next to the thin basement membrane (**arrows**). ICS, intercellular space with villous cellular processes; **F,** attenuated process of a stromal fibroblast; **C,** collagen of the substantia propria. (A, ×5000; B, ×12,200)

like collections of ropy mucin (Fig. 13–24B). These cells do not manifest advanced tonofilamentary differentiation yet are connected to the surrounding keratinocytes by desmosomes. The Langerhans cells and melanocytes are also bereft of tonofilaments and, additionally, do not form desmosomes. In the substantia propria, capillaries and lymphatic channels can be identified (Fig. 13–25).

The juxtalimbal collagen of the substantia propria along the interpalpebral fissure undergoes an ageing change called *elastotic degeneration,* producing a **pingueculum.** If this change coexists with tissue overgrowing the limbus onto the cornea, it is called a **pterygium.**

Specialized areas of the conjunctiva are the medially situated **plica semilunaris** and **caruncle** (Fig. 13–26). The plica is a fold of conjunctiva representing a vestigial remnant of the nictitating membrane of animals. Its surface epithelium is very rich in goblet cells, and occasionally in the substantia propria smooth muscle bundles may be found. The caruncle is a fleshier mass of tissue found toward the medial interpalpebral commissure. It mirrors a microcosm of differentiations of which the conjunctiva is capable. There are approximately 15–20 hairs with associated sebaceous glands, acini of lacrimal gland tissue, lobules of fat, and occasionally smooth muscle fibers. Very rarely foci of cartilage may be discovered. The surface epithelium is very rich in goblet cells, and there are frequent adenoidal invaginations of the epithelium into the substantia propria.

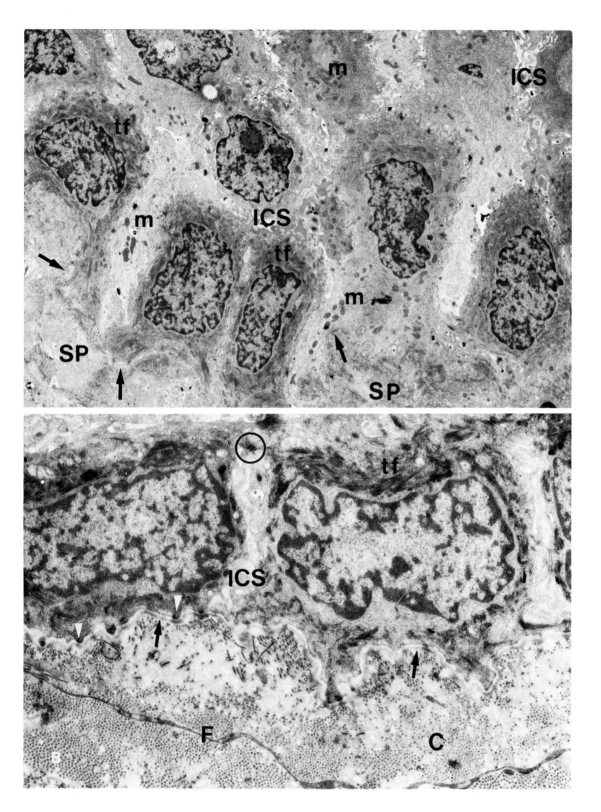

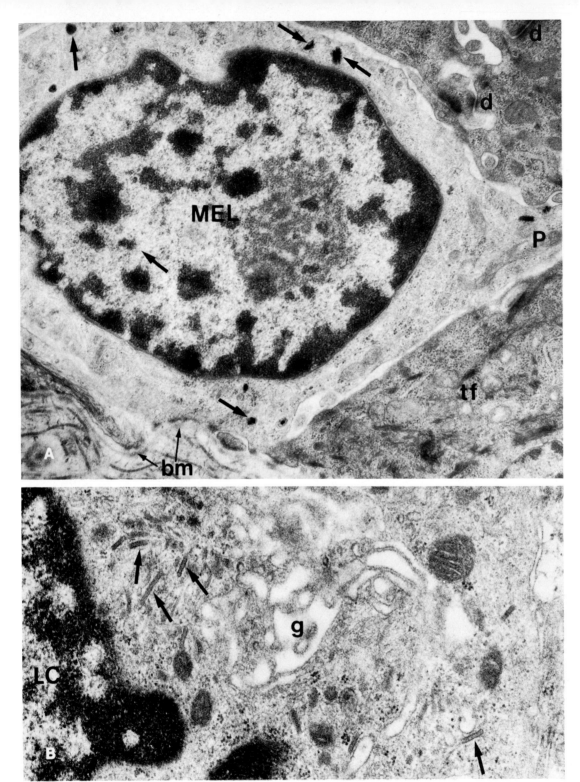

FIG. 13–23. A. A melanocyte (**MEL**) containing melanosomes (**arrows**) and extending a cytoplasmic process (**P**) is located along the basement membrane zone (**bm**). It stands out among the surrounding keratinocytes, which are darker and contain numerous tonofilaments (**tf**) and form desmosomes (**d**). B. A Langerhans cell (**LC**) within the conjunctival epithelium displays a dilated Golgi zone (**g**) and numerous striated cytoplasmic rodlets referred to as Langerhans' granules (**arrows**). This cell, like the melanocyte, does not have tonofilaments nor does it form desmosomes; it is probably a histiocyte. (A, ×34,200; B, ×23,800)

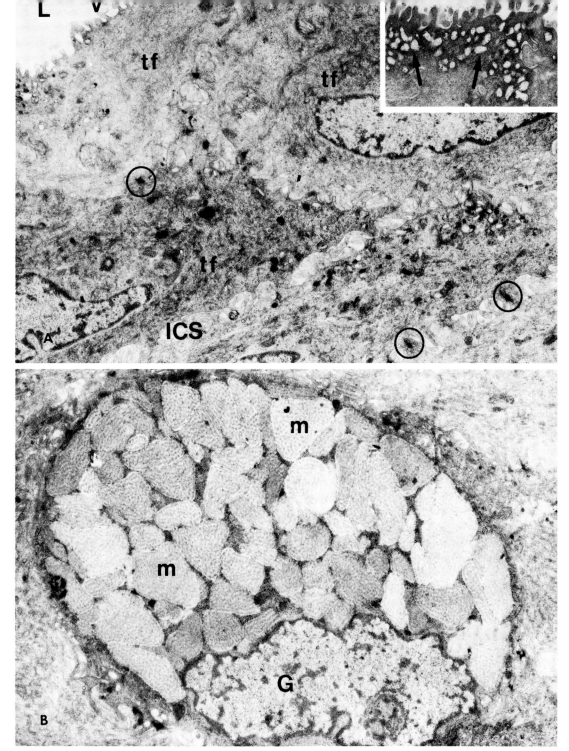

FIG. 13–24. A. Conjunctival keratinocytes toward the surface of the conjunctiva (**L**) display cytoplasmic tonofilaments (**tf**) and form desmosomes (**circles**) but remain viable and do not undergo cornification. There is a wide intercellular space (**ICS**) that contains villous cytoplasmic processes. The surface cells display microvilli (**v**) or microplicae. Inset. Microvilli have a fine spiculated coating, probably corresponding to mucous material, and the apical cytoplasm possesses vacuoles (**arrows**), which histochemically stain positively for mucus. B. A goblet cell (**G**) is distended by ropy or filamentous mucus granules (**m**). (A, ×12,200; inset, ×17,100; B, ×12,200)

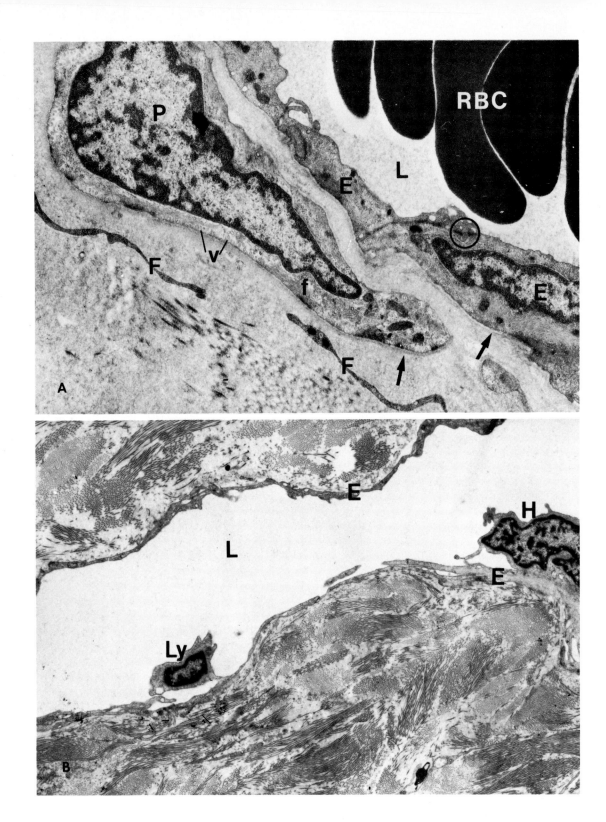

FIG. 13–25. A. A capillary in the conjunctival substantia propria has erythrocytes (**RBC**) in its lumen (**L**). The endothelial cells (**E**) are joined by dense junctions (**circle**). An adjacent pericyte (**P**) displays scattered cytoplasmic filaments (**F**) and plasmalemmal vesicles (**v**); both it and the endothelial cells are surrounded by thin basement membranes (**arrows**). The surrounding stroma contains delicate processes of fibroblasts (**F**). B. A lymphatic channel in the substantia propria has both a lymphocyte (**Ly**) and a histiocyte (**H**) in its bloodless lumen (**L**). The endothelial cells (**E**) are highly attenuated, nonfenestrated, and lack a continuous basement membrane (A, ×12,200; B, ×4600)

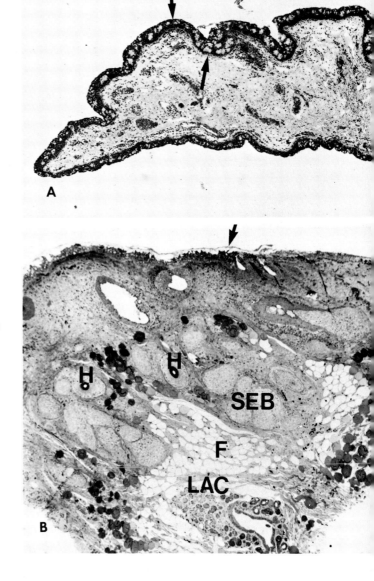

FIG. 13–26. A. The plica semilunaris is composed of a fold of fibrovascular connective tissue covered by goblet cell-rich (**arrows**) conjunctival epithelium. B. The caruncle contains hair shafts (**H**) and associated sebaceous glands (**SEB**), lobules of fat (**F**), and lacrimal gland tissue (**LAC**). A thin layer of mucus coats the epithelium (**arrow**). (A, H&E, ×50; B, 1.0μ Araldite section, methylene blue, ×38)

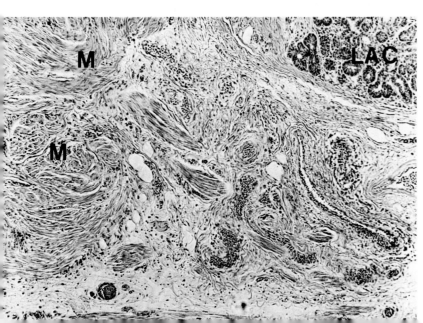

FIG. 13–27. The smooth muscle cells (**M**) of the superior tarsal muscle of Müller are more numerous than in the lower fornix. The muscle is closely related to the lacrimal gland (**LAC**). (H&E, ×69)

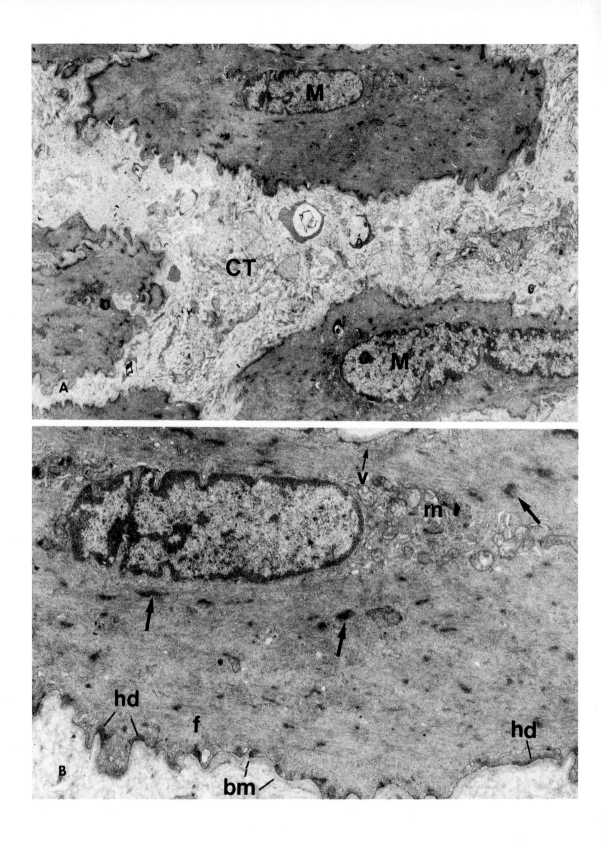

A. Smooth muscle cells (**M**) of the tarsal muscle of Müller are separated from each other by connective tissue (**CT**). B. The cytoplasm is filled with filaments (**f**) possessing fusiform densities (**arrows**). Pinocytotic vesicles (**v**) and hemidesmosomes (**hd**) are present along the plasma membrane. The cytoplasmic organelles consisting mostly of mitochondria (**m**) are aggregated near the pole of the nucleus. Thin basement membranes (**bm**) separate the cells from the connective tissue. (A, ×5500; B, ×13,700)

Müllers muscle (tarsal muscle) is better developed in the upper fornix (Fig. 13–27) than in the lower (see Fig. 13–20 B); it is innervated by the sympathetic fibers following branches of the ophthalmic artery. The fascicles of smooth muscle lie deep to the substantia propria of the forniceal conjunctiva and underneath the levator aponeurosis in the upper lid. Posteriorly the fascicles of smooth muscle interdigitate with the striated muscle of the levator palpebrae, practically the only place in the body where such an arrangement exists between these disparate muscle types. Anteriorly the muscle cells insert into the upper border of the tarsus. The smooth muscle cells have centrally located, ellipsoidal or cigar-shaped nuclei with rounded or blunt ends. The cytoplasm stains brightly on routine hematoxylin and eosin staining because of the presence of longitudinal cytoplasmic filaments, which are brought out most vividly with various trichrome stains. The cytologic features (Fig. 13–28) are those characteristic of smooth muscle cells, *viz*, cytoplasmic filaments (60 A in diameter, actin filaments) with fusiform densities, pinocytotic vesicles, plasmalemmal hemidesmosomes, and an enveloping basement membrane.

Horner's syndrome is caused by interruption of the sympathetic fibers to Müller's muscle, causing a lid droop or ptosis. The pupil is miotic due to sympathetic denervation of the dilator muscle of the iris. Lung or neck tumors that interrupt the sympathetic axons can cause an acquired Horner's syndrome.

THE ORBIT

The orbit presents a complex anatomy (5, 20, 22, 28) (Fig. 13–29 to 13–34). It contains a wide variety of tissue types: epithelial tissue in the form of the lacrimal gland, the optic nerve (a fiber tract of the central nervous system), peripheral motor, sensory, and autonomic nerves, the ciliary ganglion, striated muscle (the six extraocular muscles), smooth muscle (Müller's muscles, present not only in the superior and inferior fornices as the tarsal muscles but also as a separate bundle, of unknown function, bridging the inferior orbital fissure), arteries and veins, a complicated network of fibroadipose tissue enveloping all the other orbital contents and also related to the extraocular muscle sheaths, Tenon's capsule and the periorbita (the periosteum of the orbital bones), and finally cartilage in the form of the trochlea of the superior oblique tendon. The optic nerve is discussed in Chapter 12, and Müller's muscle is described earlier in this chapter because of its close anatomic and functional relationship with the conjunctiva and lids.

GENERAL ANATOMY

The orbital contents are bounded by seven bones (Fig. 13–29) (frontal, sphenoidal, maxillary, zygomatic, lacrimal, palatine, and ethmoidal—including the thin, medial lamina papyracea) that create a quadrangular, pear-shaped structure whose stem is the optic canal located medially in the depths of the orbit. The orbit has a volume of about 30 cu ml. The anterior limit of the orbit is formed by the orbital septa in the upper and lower lids, which reflect from the periorbita as a membrane that blends into the connective tissues of the lids.

The **orbital walls** are interrupted by three major apertures (Fig. 13–29 to 13–32) besides the anterior aditus: 1) The optic canal (5–10 mm in length) transmits the optic nerve, sympathetic fibers, and the ophthalmic artery, the last being the first branch of the internal carotid artery after it leaves the dura of the cavernous sinus. 2) The superior orbital fissure, formed by the greater and lesser wings of the sphenoid bone and separated from the more medial optic canal by a thin strip of bone, the optic strut, transmits the superior ophthalmic vein to the cavernous sinus and the third, fourth, fifth and sixth cranial nerves as well as some sympathetic fibers. 3) The inferior orbital fissure in the orbital floor permits the inferior ophthalmic vein to empty into the pterygoid plexus and ascending branches of the sphenopalatine ganglion to reach their orbital destinations. There are several vascular foramina as well, the most important being the openings for the anterior and posterior ethmoidal arteries. The infraorbital nerve, a branch of the maxillary (second) division of the trigeminal, travels in the infraorbital groove to emerge through the infraorbital foramen onto the skin of the lower lid and cheek. Fractures of the orbital floor can cause hypesthesia of the skin of the cheek.

The **lacrimal gland** is housed in a shallow fossa in the anterosuperolateral orbit (Fig. 13–29 to 13–34). Whitnall (28) has estimated that the lacrimal gland weighs approximately 78 g and on the average measures 20 × 12 × 5 mm. Its largest dimension is in the anteroposterior direction. It is pancaked in a concave fashion against the globe, from which it is separated by Tenon's capsule and the fibroadipose tissue of the orbit (Fig. 13–33). The lateral expansion of the levator aponeurosis separates the gland into a larger orbital lobe and a smaller palpebral lobe, which can be observed in the superolateral conjunctival fornix upon everting the upper lid; a small isthmus of parenchymal tissue may connect the two lobes. The ducts of the orbital portion pass through the substance of the palpebral lobe, creating a total of 12 ducts that empty into the superolateral fornix about 5 mm above the lateral convex margin of the tarsus.

The blood supply to the lacrimal gland comes from the lacrimal artery, an early branch of the

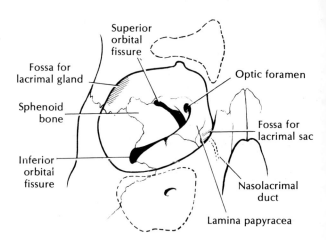

FIG. 13–29. View of right orbit from front. Major posterior openings are the optic foramen which transmits optic nerve, ophthalmic artery, and sympathetic fibers; the superior orbital fissure which transmits central retinal and superior ophthalmic veins, cranial nerves III, IV, V-1, and VI, some sympathetic fibers, and anastomotic artery from the middle meningeal to the ophthalmic or lacrimal artery; and the inferior orbital fissure which transmits inferior ophthalmic vein. Sphenoid bone contributes to lateral and posterior orbital walls and provides optic strut. **Dotted lines** delimit the frontal sinus (above) and maxillary sinus (below). (From Jones I, Jakobiec F, Nolan B: Patient examination and introduction to orbital disease. In Duane TD (ed): Clinical Ophthalmology, vol 2. Hagerstown, Harper & Row, 1976)

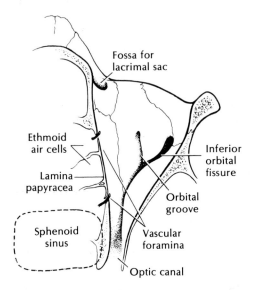

FIG. 13–30. View of floor of right orbit from above. Ethmoidal air cells are separated from orbit by thin lamina papyracea. Anterior and posterior ethmoidal arteries (branches of ophthalmic artery) pass through foramens in the medial wall. Sphenoidal sinus is situated posterior to ethmoidal air cells, and pathologic processes in sphenoidal sinus usually involve posterior ethmoidal cells as well. (From Jones I, Jakobiec F, Nolan B: Patient examination and introduction to orbital disease. In Duane TD (ed): Clinical Ophthalmology, vol 2. Hagerstown, Harper & Row, 1976)

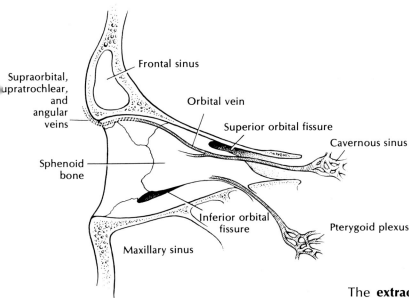

Supraorbital, supratrochlear, and angular veins

Frontal sinus

Orbital vein

Superior orbital fissure

Cavernous sinus

Sphenoid bone

Inferior orbital fissure

Pterygoid plexus

Maxillary sinus

FIG. 13–31. View of lateral aspect of right orbit from nasal side. Most of the orbital venous blood travels through the superior orbital fissure to the cavernous sinus. Anastomoses are shown between superior orbital (ophthalmic) vein and supraorbital, supratrochlear, nasofrontal, and angular veins of forehead and medial face and nose. Inferior orbital (ophthalmic) vein passes through the inferior orbital fissure to the pterygoid plexus. (From Jones I, Jakobiec F, Nolan B: Patient examination and introduction to orbital disease. In Duane TD (ed): Clinical Ophthalmology, vol. 2. Hagerstown, Harper & Row, 1976)

ophthalmic; its sensory innervation is from the lacrimal nerve, a branch of the ophthalmic division of the trigeminal; and its autonomic innervation is provided by parasympathetic branches that synapse in the sphenopalatine ganglion, postsynaptically joining the zygomatic nerve, a branch of the maxillary division of the trigeminal, and terminating around the lobules of the lacrimal gland parenchyma.

In addition to the main bilobed lacrimal gland, there are also the **accessory lacrimal glands** of Krause, numbering 20 in the upper fornix and 6–8 in the lower, as well as the accessory glands of Wolfring, usually three separate lobules in the superior aspect of the upper tarsus. These accessory glands appear to be under sympathetic control and furnish the baseline tear secretion, whereas the secretion of the main lacrimal gland is called into play during reflex or psychogenic stimulation.

Diffuse scarring of the conjunctiva after lye injury or in the Stevens-Johnson syndrome causes obstruction of the ducts of the major and ectopic lacrimal glands. This produces a dry eye syndrome (keratoconjunctivitis sicca), which can cause corneal damage from breakup of the precorneal tear film. In the dry eye syndrome there is a secondary, conpensatory increase in the number of mucus-producing goblet cells. Systemic autoimmune collagen diseases like rheumatoid arthritis may also be associated with inflammatory involution of the major and minor lacrimal glands (Sjögren's syndrome).

The **extraocular muscles** (Fig. 13–33, 13–34) consist of four rectus muscles and two oblique muscles. The four recti share a common origin from the annulus of Zinn at the optic foramen, where the dural sheath of the optic nerve fuses with the periorbita of the bony rim of the canal to provide a thickening for the shared tendinous origin of the recti. The four recti are variable in length but average around 20 mm and insert on the globe from 5–8 mm behind the limbus (the so-called spiral of Tillaux). The levator palpebrae arises above the superior rectus to end as a broad aponeurotic expansion in the anterior orbit with insertions into the medial and lateral palpebral ligaments as well as into the substance of the upper lid. The superior oblique has a separate origin medial to the annulus of Zinn and travels along the superomedial aspect of the orbit, converting into a long tendon that passes through the cartilaginous trochlea behind the superonasal orbital rim and reflecting obliquely and posteriorly to insert on the midsuperior aspect of the globe under the superior rectus muscle. The inferior oblique takes origin along the anterior-inferomedial portion of the orbital wall and traverses the inferior orbit obliquely to cross beneath the inferior rectus muscle (to which it is joined by Lockwood's ligament) and insert on the globe in the vicinity of the fovea (macula).

Strabismus is an imbalance in the extraocular muscle coordination resulting in a "turn" in the eyes. To date no reproducible muscle changes have been identified, and the abnormality may have a

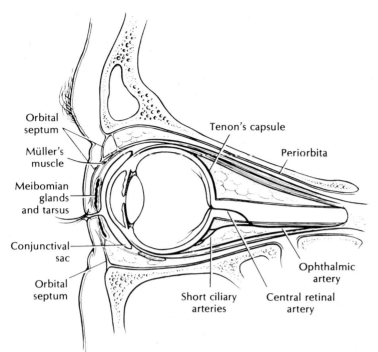

FIG. 13–32. Sagittal section through lids, globe, and orbit. Lids are separated from the orbit by the orbital septum, a continuation of the periorbita (orbital periosteum). Müller's muscle is composed of smooth muscle and is interposed between the levator palpebrae muscle and the tarsus. Meibomian glands are embedded in dense fibrous plaques (tarsus) in the lids. Tenon's capsule is an outer fibrous tunic that loosely adheres to sclera and blends posteriorly with dura of the optic nerve and anteriorly with muscular fascia. Ophthalmic artery enters the orbit from the optic foramen and divides into the central retinal artery and posterior ciliary arteries among many others. (From Jones I, Jakobiec F, Nolan B: Patient examination and introduction to orbital disease. In Duane TD (ed): Clinical Ophthalmology, vol 2. Hagerstown, Harper & Row, 1976)

central or a complex peripheral neuromuscular cause. In the progressive external ophthalmoplegias a similar combined neuromuscular derangement has been indicted, and in these diseases there is fibrosis and atrophy of the muscles. Myasthenia gravis can cause motility disturbances, due to antibodies directed against receptors in the postsynaptic membrane. Inflammations directed against the extraocular muscles are seen in Graves' disease and in idiopathic inflammatory pseudotumor of the orbit. Rhabdomyosarcoma, an embryonal tumor showing striated muscle differentiation and the most common primary orbital malignancy of childhood, appears not to develop in the preformed extraocular muscle tissue but rather from orbital mesenchyme.

The **intermuscular fibrous membrane** appears to connect the four rectus muscles in the neighborhood of the globe separating the so-called central or intraconal space from the peripheral space that goes to the periorbita, but recent anatomic investigations employing macrosections of intact orbits indicate that such a clear-cut compartmentalization of the orbital spaces does not really exist behind the globe (21) (Fig. 13–35). Due to the retention in these studies of the relationship between the orbital fibroadipose tissue and the orbital walls, it has emerged that there is a highly organized architecture to the orbital alveolar tissues that is bi-

laterally symmetric for each individual and that the fundamental patterns are preserved from individual to individual. The superior ophthalmic vein, for example, is suspended by a fibrous band containing smooth muscle cells, and most of the extraocular muscles have predictable fascial arrangements to the periorbita of the orbital walls, to the other muscles, and to the globe (i.e., Tenon's capsule).

These studies have helped to explain one of the anomalous features of fractures of the orbital floor. Restrictions of upward gaze are frequently seen after traumatic floor fractures, but during surgical explorations the inferior rectus and oblique muscles are virtually never found to be trapped in the fracture. Instead, it appears that the restrictions result from herniations of the orbital fibroadipose tissue, including entrapment of the fibrous strands extending from the muscles to the periorbita of the orbital floor. Cases have also occurred where manipulation of the orbital fat through an anterior orbitotomy or during the course of a blepharoplasty has caused an occlusion of or hemorrhage from the central retinal artery or ophthalmic artery. In such cases it can be postulated that tugging on the fat is transmitted to the posterior vasculature through the highly ordered fibrous retinacula of the orbital connective tissue system.

The **arterial vascular system** of the orbit derives from the ophthalmic artery which carries

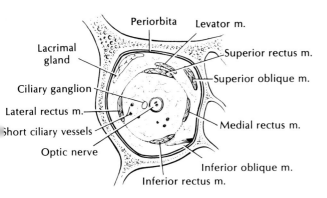

Periorbita Levator m.

Lacrimal
gland

Ciliary ganglion

Lateral rectus m.

Short ciliary vessels

Optic nerve

Superior rectus m.

Superior oblique m.

Medial rectus m.

Inferior oblique m.

Inferior rectus m.

FIG. 13–33. Coronal section behind globe. The four rectus muscles are connected by an intermuscular membrane that separates the central (intraconal) space from the peripheral orbital space. Ciliary ganglion is located lateral to the optic nerve in the posterior orbit. (From Jones I, Jakobiec F, Nolan B: Patient examination and introduction to orbital disease. In Duane TD (ed): Clinical Ophthalmology, vol 2. Hagerstown, Harper & Row, 1976)

sympathetic fibers off the pericarotid sympathetic plexus. In the optic canal the artery lies inferolateral to the optic nerve within a split layer of dura. At the orbital optic foramen the artery curves over the lateral margin of the optic nerve to run superomedially. The first intraorbital branch is the comparatively small central retinal artery, which perforates the dural sheath of the optic nerve approximately 10 mm from the optic foramen and 8–10 mm behind the globe (Fig. 13-32). As it passes superomedially above the nerve the ophthalmic artery gives off two long posterior ciliary arteries, six to eight short posterior ciliary arteries, the lacrimal artery, the anterior and posterior ethmoidal arteries, and the supraorbital artery. The extraocular muscles are supplied by two small branches of the ophthalmic artery which enter their bellies near the annulus of Zinn. The terminal or distal branches of the ophthalmic artery penetrate the orbital septum and emerge beneath the orbital rim as the dorsonasal and frontal arteries. The supraorbital artery passes through the supraorbital foramen above the orbital rim. Major anastomoses occur between branches of the ophthalmic artery and those of the external carotid system, including a branch of the middle meningeal artery which enters the orbit through a lateral foramen or the superior orbital fissure. These anastomoses may save vision if the ophthalmic artery is occluded, but the central retinal artery can still be furnished with blood from the external carotid system.

Vascular tumors are a common cause of proptosis. These tumors include the comparatively rare lymphangioma, which is a choristoma in the orbit because lymphatic channels have never been convincingly demonstrated in normal orbital connective tissues.

FIG. 13–34. View of orbital contents from above. Rectus muscles originate from a fibrous ring at the optic foramen, the annulus of Zinn. Superior oblique muscle has a separate origin medially in the posterior orbit, and its anterior tendinous portion passes through a cartilaginous pulley (trochlea) in the superonasal aspect of the anterior orbit. Tenon's capsule fuses with sclera anteriorly near the limbus. (From Jones I, Jakobiec F, Nolan B: Patient examination and introduction to orbital disease. In Duane TD (ed): Clinical Ophthalmology, vol 2. Hagerstown, Harper & Row, 1976)

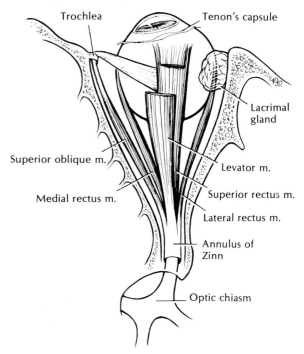

Trochlea

Tenon's capsule

Lacrimal
gland

Superior oblique m.

Levator m.

Medial rectus m.

Superior rectus m.

Lateral rectus m.

Annulus of
Zinn

Optic chiasm

The **orbital veins** (Fig. 13–31), in common with those of the head and neck, contain no valves and readily communicate with the veins of the face and lids. The superior ophthalmic (orbital) vein is formed by a confluence of the angular, nasofrontal, and supraorbital veins. The superior ophthalmic vein initially runs posterior-laterally in the superior orbit, penetrates the muscle cone in the midorbit, receives venous drainage from the globe, and leaves the orbit outside of the annulus of Zinn through the superior orbital fissure to empty into the cavernous sinus. The inferior ophthalmic vein drains the tissues over the floor of the orbit as well as a network of channels in the inferomedial area, including the region of the lacrimal sac. An anastomosis to the superior ophthalmic vein occurs before the inferior vein exits through the inferior orbital fissure into the pterygoid plexus. The majority of the orbital venous effluent is accommodated by the superior ophthalmic vein.

Infections on the face and lids, and in particular in the skin around the nares, can rarely produce a catastrophic retrograde septic cavernous sinus thrombosis because of the free interanastomoses between the valveless facial and orbital veins. Furthermore cavernous sinus thromboses and arteriovenous malformations or fistulas produce exophthalmos and episcleral corkscrew venous dilatations because of unrestricted retrograde flow through these valve free veins.

The **orbital nerves** enter the orbit through the superior orbital fissure (Fig. 13–36). The entrance of these nerves into the orbit can be conveniently analyzed if the annulus of Zinn is used as the reference point. The bifid origin of the lateral rectus muscle from the annulus describes an inner space sometimes called the oculomotor foramen. Outside of this foramen, the superior orbital fissure transmits the two major branches of the ophthalmic division of the trigeminal, namely, the lacrimal and frontal nerves (the later eventually emerges onto the forehead), and the trochlear (fourth cranial) nerve. Within the oculomotor foramen, the fissure transmits the inferior and superior branches of the oculomotor (third cranial) nerve, the abducent (sixth cranial) nerve, and the nasociliary nerve, another branch of the ophthalmic division of the trigeminal. Once in the orbit these latter nerves travel within the muscle cone, whereas the former group travel

FIG. 13–35. Fibromuscular system in the posterior orbit is shown on the left and at the level of the globe on the right. A highly reproducible architecture exists between the fibrous strands of the orbital connective tissue and the extraocular muscles. In the anterior orbit radial septa subdivide the orbital fat and connect Tenon's capsule to the periorbita. (Modified from Koorneef L: Spatial Aspects of Orbital Musculofibrous Tissue in Man, Amsterdam. Swets and Zeitlinger, BV, 1977, p 129)

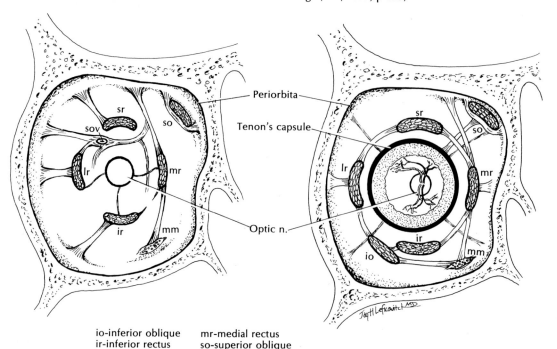

io-inferior oblique   mr-medial rectus
ir-inferior rectus   so-superior oblique
lr-lateral rectus   sr-superior rectus
mm-Müller's m.   sov-superior ophthalmic vein

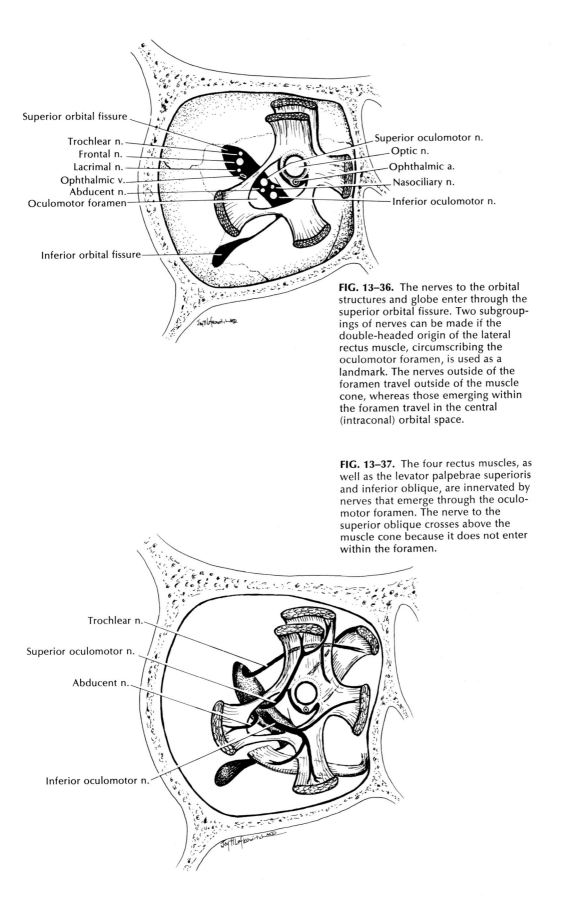

Superior orbital fissure
Trochlear n.
Frontal n.
Lacrimal n.
Ophthalmic v.
Abducent n.
Oculomotor foramen

Inferior orbital fissure

Superior oculomotor n.
Optic n.
Ophthalmic a.
Nasociliary n.
Inferior oculomotor n.

FIG. 13–36. The nerves to the orbital structures and globe enter through the superior orbital fissure. Two subgroupings of nerves can be made if the double-headed origin of the lateral rectus muscle, circumscribing the oculomotor foramen, is used as a landmark. The nerves outside of the foramen travel outside of the muscle cone, whereas those emerging within the foramen travel in the central (intraconal) orbital space.

FIG. 13–37. The four rectus muscles, as well as the levator palpebrae superioris and inferior oblique, are innervated by nerves that emerge through the oculomotor foramen. The nerve to the superior oblique crosses above the muscle cone because it does not enter within the foramen.

Trochlear n.
Superior oculomotor n.
Abducent n.
Inferior oculomotor n.

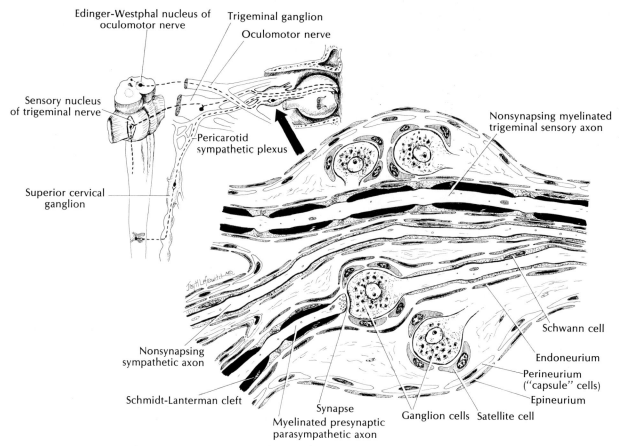

Edinger-Westphal nucleus of oculomotor nerve

Trigeminal ganglion

Oculomotor nerve

Sensory nucleus of trigeminal nerve

Pericarotid sympathetic plexus

Superior cervical ganglion

Nonsynapsing myelinated trigeminal sensory axon

Schwann cell

Endoneurium

Perineurium ("capsule" cells)

Epineurium

Nonsynapsing sympathetic axon

Schmidt-Lanterman cleft

Synapse

Myelinated presynaptic parasympathetic axon

Ganglion cells   Satellite cell

FIG. 13–38. The ciliary ganglion receives sensory (trigeminal) and sympathetic axons, with central connections shown on the upper left. These axons pass through the ganglion without synapsing. Myelinated presynaptic parasympathetic axons, arising from the Edinger-Westphal nucleus of the oculomotor nuclear complex and destined for the ciliary body and iris, synapse on the ciliary ganglion cells. The posterior ciliary nerves are formed by a confluence of these sympathetic, sensory, and postsynaptic parasympathetic axons.

in the superior orbit in a plane immediately beneath the periorbita and above the levator palpebrae and superior rectus muscle sheaths. The superior branch of the oculomotor nerve supplies the superior rectus and levator muscles; the inferior branch passes beneath the optic nerve to innervate the medial and inferior rectus muscles as well as the inferior oblique (Fig. 13–37). The nerves to the various extraocular muscles enter their bellies at the junction of the posterior and middle thirds.

The **ciliary gangion** (Fig. 13–33, 13–38) is located on the temporal aspect of the optic nerve toward the orbital apex. It measures 2 mm in length and 11 mm in width. It receives parasympathetic fibers traveling in the inferior branch of the oculomotor nerve and sends out postsynaptic fibers destined for the ciliary body and iris. A twig from the nasociliary nerve passes through the ganglion without synapsing to provide sensory fibers for the 8–10 short posterior ciliary nerves emanating from the gan-

glion that pierce the posterior sclera. Sympathetic fibers also traverse the ganglion to join the ciliary nerves but also do not synapse in the ganglion.

Loss of the ganglion cells can occur idiopathically or after viral infections (herpes zoster). Disturbances of pupillary reaction and of accommodation are functional correlates. **Adie's syndrome** combines decreased tendon reflexes with a pupil that responds minimally to light or the near vision reflex (tonic

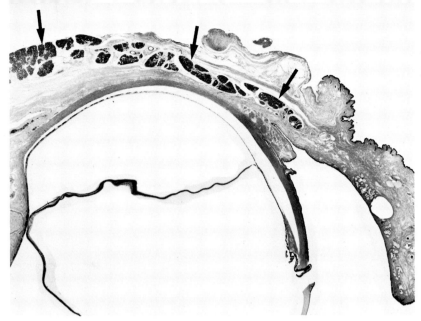

FIG. 13–39. Lobules of lacrimal gland tissue (**arrows**) extend across the superolateral aspect of the globe from the fornix to behind the globe. (H&E, ×8)

pupil). Due to hypersensitivity of the denervated iris secondary to loss of the postsynaptic axons from degeneration of the ciliary ganglion cells, very dilute solutions of parasympathomimetics (e.g., mecholyl) cause constriction of the pupil.

MICROSCOPIC ANATOMY

The Lacrimal Gland

From the terminal ducts of the lacrimal gland, tubuloracemose branchings create the acini of the lobules of the lacrimal gland tissue. These lobules are loose and separated by adipose tissue or interstitial fibrovascular septa; they can extend behind the globe (Fig. 13–39). Within the lobules one can identify intralobular ducts among the predominant secretory parenchymal elements (Fig. 13–40). The lacrimal gland is wholly composed of serous cells, lacking the mucinous cells which are also present in the parotid gland. In light microscopic sections, the cytoplasm of the acinar cells stains basophilic due to the presence of zymogenic secretory granules (Fig. 13–41) and rough-surfaced endoplasmic reticulum. A myoepithelial layer surrounds the secretory cells of the acini. The intralobular ducts empty into larger interlobular ducts, and finally the latter converge to create the main excretory ducts that empty into the superolateral fornix.

Electron microscopy (Fig. 13–42) reveals that the outside rim of myoepithelial cells is joined to the inner secretory cells by desmosomes and that the myoepithelial cells are covered by a basement membrane which may be multilaminar in places. The secretory cells have considerable rough-surfaced endoplasmic reticulum concentrated in the basilar part of the cells and sometimes oriented in a parallel array. In the apical supranuclear region, there is an active Golgi apparatus with the formation of either dense or light secretory (zymogenic) granules (5, 7, 20–22, 26–28). The secretory granules are synthesized on the ribosomes of the rough-surfaced endoplasmic reticulum and are channeled through the membranous profiles to the Golgi zone for packaging. Lipid droplets, glycogen, and polyribosomes may be scattered throughout the cytoplasm. The luminal borders of the glandular cells (Fig. 13–43) display villous processes; the zymogenic granules fuse with the apical plasmalemma to be discharged into the lumens (emeiocytosis). Movement of the granules to the luminal surface is probably effected by means of cytoplasmic filaments and microtubules. The intercellular arrangements at the apex consist of a junctional complex, with an adluminal zonula occludens, beneath which is a zonula adherens, and lastly a desmosome. The zonula occludens and zonula adherens run completely around the cells through 360 degrees, while the desmosomes occur only at focal points. The nature of the zymogenic granules has not been satisfactorily elucidated.

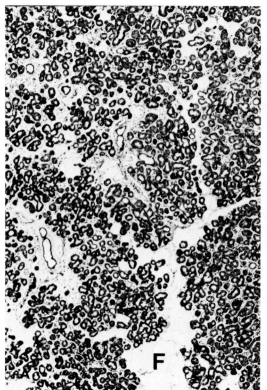

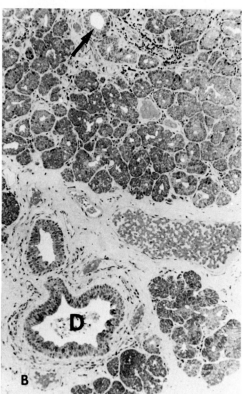

FIG. 13–40. A. Acini of lacrimal gland parenchyma are loosely set in a fibrous stroma and are occasionally separated by bands of fat (**F**). B. The **arrow** points to an intralobular duct within a lobule of acinar tissue; a larger interlobular duct (**D**) is shown below. (A, H&E, ×40; B, 1.0μ Araldite section methylene blue, ×80)

Lysozyme in the tears acts as a bacteriostatic agent and is produced by the lacrimal gland (8).

The duct system (Fig. 13–44) exhibits pseudo-stratification of two to three cells in the intra-lobular portion and three to four cells in the interlobular segments. The cytoplasm of the duct cells (Fig. 13–45, 13–46) is furnished with short profiles of rough-surfaced endoplasmic reticulum, scattered mitochondria, and oc-casional lipid droplets. A thin basement mem-brane separates the basal cells from the con-nective tissue without the interposition of a myoepithelial layer. The lateral margins of the cells are relatively straight, except at the base of the duct, where the intercellular space is widened. Poorly developed desmosomes are found along the lateral borders of the cells. Cytoplasmic filaments are present, but they are not grouped together in the manner of epi-dermal tonofilaments. At the luminal surface small apical villi are present, and there is a junctional complex. The duct cells may help to maintain the proper tonicity of the tears, which is important for corneal function and comfort (7b).

Unlike the parotid gland, the lacrimal gland does not possess its own lymph nodes. The lacrimal gland, however, does contain a light dispersal of lymphocytes and plasma cells in the interstitium of its lobules (1, 2). These immuno-cytes produce a disproportionate amount of the immunoglobulin IgA, similar to the production of this species by the conjunctival lymphoid elements. While exceptionally sparse in the young, the lacrimal gland lymphoid cells in-crease in number as an individual ages, *pari passu* with the deposition of increasing amounts of collagen within the lobules and cir-cumferentially around the ducts.

Epithelial tumors of the lacrimal gland (e.g., be-nign mixed tumors) appear to arise only from the terminal duct cells, rather than from the acinar cell.

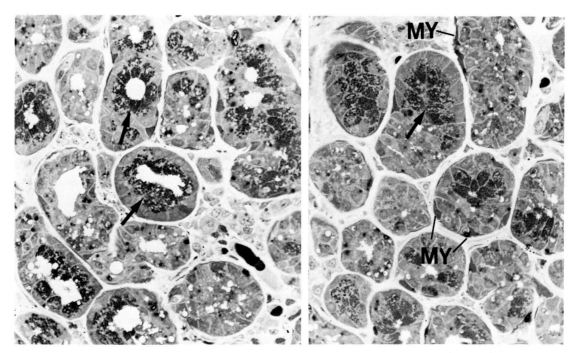

FIG. 13–41. Two fields of acinar tissue which contain prominent cytoplasmic zymogenic granules (**arrows**). Occasional dark-staining myoepithelial cells (**MY**) are applied against the basal region of the acinar units. (1.0μ Araldite section, methylene blue, ×350)

Lymphoid lesions (inflammatory pseudotumors, pseudolymphomas, and true lymphomas) have a propensity to develop in the lacrimal gland. Some of these lesions may represent hyperplasias of the normally scant lymphoid cells of the gland or else the proliferation of initially exogenous lymphocytes that have receptors that allow them to seek out or "home in" specifically to the lacrimal gland parenchyma, where they subsequently proliferate *in situ*, a phenomenon termed ecotaxis (7a). Benign ductular proliferation within a lymphoid process replacing the acinar elements is called the benign lymphoepithelial lesion and is typical of, but not exclusively seen in, Sjögren's syndrome. All chronic lymphocytic inflammations of the lacrimal gland are accompanied by increased levels of immunoglobulins in the tears, particularly IgA and IgG, and decreased lysozyme.

The Extraocular Muscles

The extraocular muscles are composed of striated muscle cells (myofibers), which are elongated tubular cells with multiple, widely spaced nuclei present along the cell membrane (sarcolemma) (Fig. 13–47, 13–48). There has been some debate as to whether each individual muscle cell extends completely from the origin to the insertion or only part way, albeit a considerable distance. In addition to the nuclei of

the muscle cells themselves, there are also satellite cells approximated to their sarcolemmas and enclosed by the same basement membrane. These satellite cells may play a role in the regeneration of damaged muscle cells (22a).

The primary bundles of extraocular muscles are surrounded by a thin connective tissue sheath referred to as the perimysium, while the outermost mantle of the cortical connective tissue sheath is called the epimysium. Small septa of connective tissue (the endomysium) further segregate some of the muscle cells into smaller units. Abundant blood vessels and elastic fibers are present within the extraocular muscles, and their proximal third is also furnished with large numbers of nerve endings. The muscle cells vary in thickness from 10μ–50μ in diameter. The thinner muscle fibers tend to be collected as an outer rim of each muscle mass, and the thicker fibers are concentrated in the center. In addition to the contractile "extrafusal" muscle

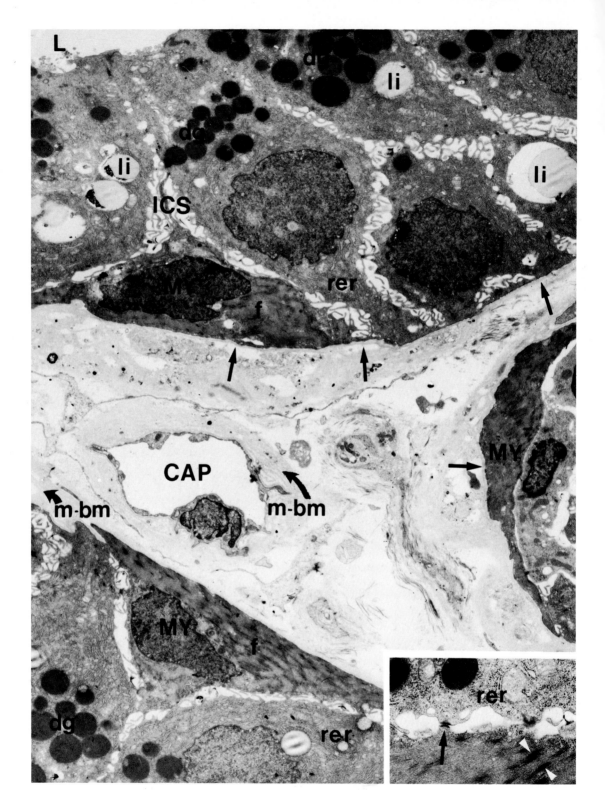

FIG. 13–42. Three acini of lacrimal gland tissue are separated by a collagenized septum containing a capillary (**CAP**). The acini have an outer myoepithelial layer (**MY**) containing cytoplasmic filaments (**f**) with fusiform densities. A thin basement membrane (**arrows**) separates the myoepithelial cells from the stroma, but in one focus there is some multilaminar basement membrane (**m-bm**), resembling that around the capillary. The inner secretory cells bordering the glandular lumens (**L**) contain dense granules (**dg**). Lipid droplets (**li**) are scattered throughout many cells, and the rough-surfaced endoplasmic reticulum (**rer**) is well developed. The intercellular space (**ICS**) is widely dilated with delicate finger-like processes. Inset. Desmosome connecting an inner secretory cell with an outer myoepithelial cell; **rer,** rough-surfaced endoplasmic reticulum in the secretory cell; **arrowheads,** fusiform densities among the myofilaments. (Main figures, ×6100; inset, ×16,100)

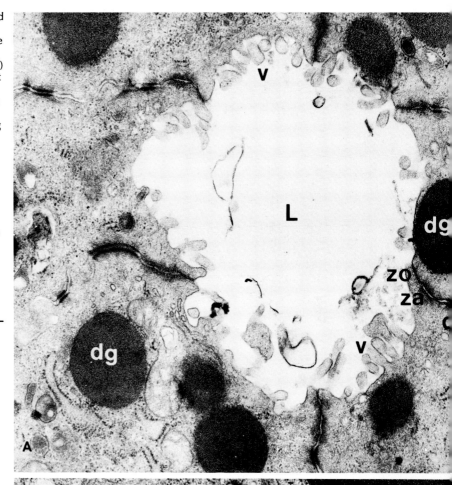

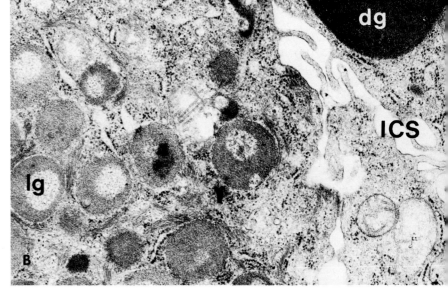

FIG. 13–43. A. Electron dense granular inclusions (**dg**) border the lumen (**L**) of an acinus. Small villi (**v**) project into the lumen. The lateral apical plasmalemma of the secretory cells displays a junctional complex consisting of a zonula occludens (**zo**), zonula adherens (**za**), and a desmosome (**d**). B. Besides typical dense granules (**dg**), light granules (**lg**) with a rarefied central zone are also seen. **ICS,** intercellular space. (A, ×23,300; B, ×26,600)

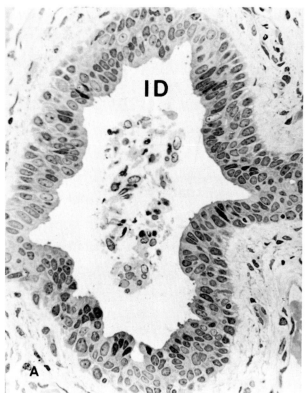

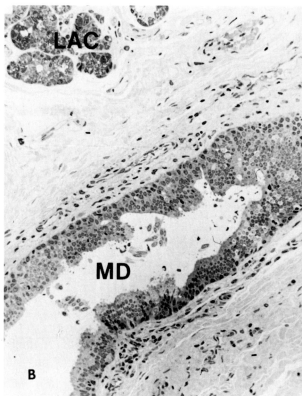

FIG. 13–44. A. An interlobular duct **(ID)** displays stratification of the nonkeratinizing lining cells. B. A main duct **(MD)** drains into the superior fornix. **LAC,** adjacent lacrimal gland tissue. (1.0μ Araldite section, methylene blue stain, A, ×350; B, ×180)

fibers, there are also sensory or proprioceptive muscle spindles located proximally in the muscle bellies: these muscle spindles have a thin capsule within which are separately innervated "intrafusal" muscle fibers supplying feedback information to the central oculomotor regulatory centers.

The contractile system of striated muscle cells (Fig. 13–49) is built up of repeating units of myofibrils, called sarcomeres, delimited by regularly spaced transverse Z lines. Within each myofibrillary compartment created by two transverse Z lines, there are interdigitating myofilaments of thick myosin (150 A in diameter) and thin actin (60 A in diameter) filaments. Contraction is effected as the thin and thick filaments slide upon each other, thereby shortening the distance between the anchoring Z lines. Energy for contraction is provided by ATPase, which is an essential part of the myofilaments. The myofibrils are separated from each other by variable amounts of sarcoplasm (muscle cell cytoplasm) containing mitochondria. Transverse tubules representing invaginations of the sarco-

FIG. 13–45. Interlobular duct consists of ▶ pseudostratified cells resting on a thin basement membrane **(arrow)** against the connective tissue **(CT)** without an interposed myoepithelial layer. The intercellular space **(ICS)** is wide in the basilar region but is narrow above. The cytoplasm contains scattered profiles of rough-surfaced endoplasmic reticulum **(rer)**, mitochondria **(m)**, and lipid droplets **(li)**. Small surface villi project into the lumen **(L)**. (×6600)

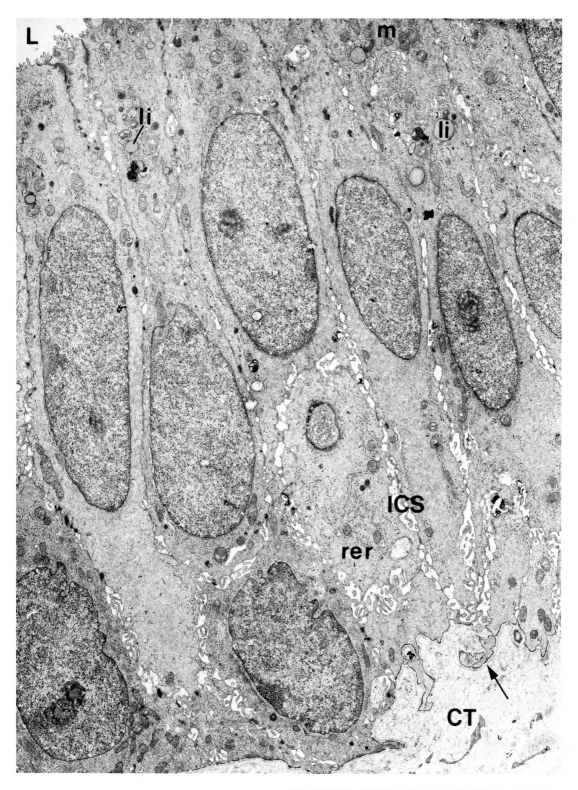

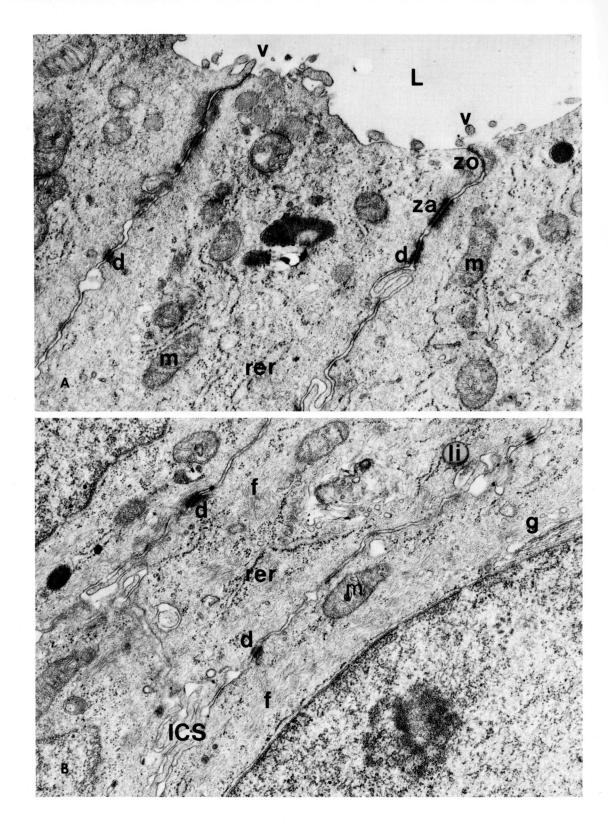

lemma extend across the muscle cell and allow the intracellular penetration of ions during the spread of the action potential or graded postsynaptic potentials. An elaborate smooth-surfaced endoplasmic reticulum (sarcoplasmic reticulum) surrounds the myofibrils and becomes organized into "triads" with the transverse tubule near the A-I junction of the sarcomere. Changes in the membrane potential are reflected along the transverse tubules and coupled to the sarcoplasmic reticulum at the sites of the triads; calcium fluxes in and out of the sarcoplasmic reticulum are an integral part of excitation-contraction.

Two polar types of extraocular muscle cells have been identified (Fig. 13–50, 13–51), although muscle cells combining morphologic features of both also exist (4). These two major types are referred to as felderstruktur and fibrillenstruktur, based upon the appearance of the myofibrils within the sarcoplasm. In the felderstruktur cells the myofibrils literally fuse; in the fibrillenstruktur cells the myofibrils are more distinct and better separated in their longitudinal course. The fibrillenstruktur cells are larger and have more abundant sarcoplasm and smooth-surfaced endoplasmic reticulum (sarcoplasmic reticulum) separating the myofibrils. These cells have an aerobic metabolism and are analogous to the twitch or white muscle fibers of the peripheral musculature. It is believed that these muscle fibers subserve rapid or saccadic movements of the eye. The felderstruktur cells, besides displaying a blending together of their fibrils, also have more numerous mitochondria (anaerobic metabolism), less well-regimented Z lines, and less sarcoplasmic reticulum with few or no triads. These muscle cells are felt to subserve tonic slow movements (vergences) of the eyes and are distinctive to the extraocular muscles, not being present in the peripheral or limb musculature. Muscle cells of similar structure, however, are present in the stapedius muscle of the inner ear. The fibrillenstruktur cells are innervated by *en plaque* types of motor end-plates, whereas the felderstruktur cells are innervated by *en grappe* motor end-plates. The twitch or fibrillenstruktur cells generate an "all or none" action potential, whereas the felderstruktur cells generate graded, nonpropagated postsynaptic potentials underlying tonic contraction.

While heuristically valuable, the division of the extraocular muscle cells into two classes is undoubtedly an oversimplification. The trichrome stain and enzymologic studies (6, 22b) utilizing NADH (for mitochondrial) and ATPase (for myofilaments) as markers for cell type have produced a tripartite light microscopic classification—fine, coarse, and granular fibers—based upon the stippled appearance of the sarcoplasmic contents in cross section. The fine fiber corresponds to type I twitch fibers of peripheral skeletal muscle, and the granular fibers to type II twitch fibers; both are singly innervated. The fine fibers stain moderately for NADH, whereas the granular fibers are very positive for ATP (pH 9.4). These two muscle fibers therefore appear to be subtypes of fibrillenstruktur cells.

FIG. 13–47. Striated extraocular muscle near the apex of the orbit showing rich innervation (**arrows**). (H&E, ×69)

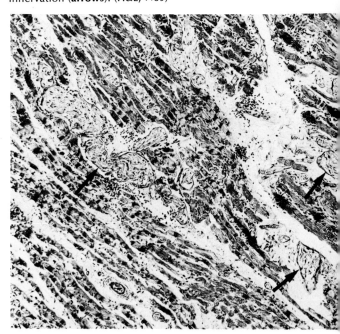

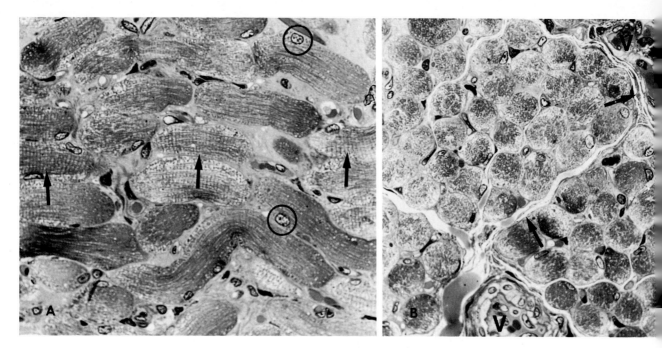

FIG. 13–48. A. Longitudinal section of extraocular muscle cells shows cross striations (**arrows**) of the cytoplasmic filaments. The circled nuclei are typically vesicular and are located eccentrically at the sarcolemma of the muscle fiber. B. Cross section of the muscle cells displays relative uniformity of the diameter of the myofibers and variable granularity of the cytoplasm. The **arrows** point to the delicate connective tissue endomysium; **V**, vessels present within the connective tissue. (1.0μ Araldite section, methylene blue stain; A, ×375; B, ×340)

The coarsely staining fibers stain positively for ATP and NADH and probably represent tonic or felderstruktur cells; these fibers are multiply innervated. It is of interest that the coarse fibers are aggregated at the periphery or cortex of the muscle mass, correlating with the known localization of the small diameter felderstruktur cells to this region. The central zone of the muscles is composed predominantly of granular fibers (55%), followed by coarse fibers, and least numerously by fine fibers. The correlation of muscle function with enzymologic-histochemical, morphologic (light and electron microscopic), and innervational patterns awaits further research, but one can expect the characterization of more than two or three types of muscle cells.

The Peripheral Nerves

In contrast to the optic nerve, which is a fiber tract of the central nervous system, the orbital cranial nerves are peripheral nerves (Fig. 13–52). This distinction means that the Schwann cell envelops the axons of the peripheral orbital nerves and provides myelin by the spiraling of its cell membrane around the axon —a role assumed by the oligodendrocyte for the myelination of central nervous system

(optic nerve) axons (see Figs. 12–1, 12–2). Whereas the oliogodendrocyte may wrap around several different axons, the Schwann cell wraps around only one axon. Nodes of Ranvier define where one Schwann cell ends and another picks up; the clefts of Schmidt-Lantermann represent separations in the plane of the myelin sheath where there are entrapments of Schwann cell cytoplasm. The peripheral nerves have endoneural fibroblasts between the myelinated axons which may produce small amounts of mucosubstance and fibrillar material. The axons are bundled into subunits by a perineurium, and the entire nerve is clothed by an outer capsule or epineurium (Fig. 13–38). It is an anatomic curiosity that perineural cells have some smooth muscle characteristics ultrastructurally (23).

Orbital Fat

Few tissues are more uninteresting than adipose tissue. New insight into the highly ordered arrangements of the fibroadipose tissue of the orbit has been gleaned from 0.5-cm macrosections of intact orbits (21) (Fig. 13–53). Microscopically, the fibrovascular septa contain fibroblasts and highly permeable capillaries (Fig. 13–54). The latter probably allow the escape of antigens and other noxious moieties that may localize in the fat and be conducive to the development of lipogranulomatous inflammatory pseudotumors. Smooth muscle cells have also been identified in the larger septa of the orbital fat. The fat cells themselves are dominated by a large lipid vacuole that indents the nucleus and displaces it against the plasma membrane (Fig. 13–55). Only thin remnants of cytoplasm can be observed next to the plasmalemma. The lipid vacuole is not membrane bound. Short profiles of rough-surfaced endoplasmic reticulum and occasional mitochondria are dispersed in the outer rim of cytoplasm. Orbital fat cells are metabolically rather inert; during active lipogenesis, however, more abundant profiles of smooth-surfaced endoplasmic reticulum are present.

The inactivity of the orbital fat is exemplified by the fact that changes in weight with thickening or thinning of the panniculus adiposus are not accompanied by fluctuations in the volume of the orbital fat. Only under extraordinary circumstances of extreme starvation, cachexia, or marasmus is there depletion of the orbital fat with resulting enophthalmos, which might also be due in part to dehydration and loss of intravascular venous volume within the orbit.

FIG. 13–49. The extraocular muscle cell (myofiber) is an extended tube containing evenly spaced nuclei along the sarcolemma and scattered satellite cells approximated to the outside of the sarcolemma. The myofibrils are composed of a highly ordered system of thick (myosin) and thin (actin) myofilaments, subdivided by transverse Z lines. Invaginations of the surface membrane create the transverse tubular system, which comes into intimate relationship with elements of the smooth-surfaced sarcoplasmic reticulum (triads). At the myoneuronal junction, vesicles of acetylcholine are released which depolarize the postsynaptic sarcolemma. The resultant membrane depolarization spreads along the transverse tubule and becomes coupled with the sarcoplasmic reticulum at the triads. Calcium fluxes across the sarcoplasmic reticulum are essential for bringing about actinomyosin complexing and contraction.

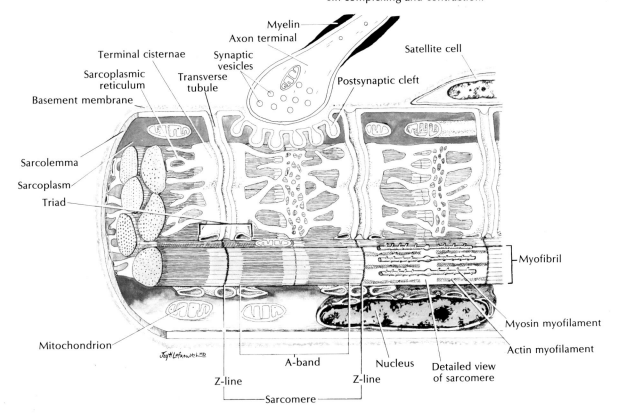

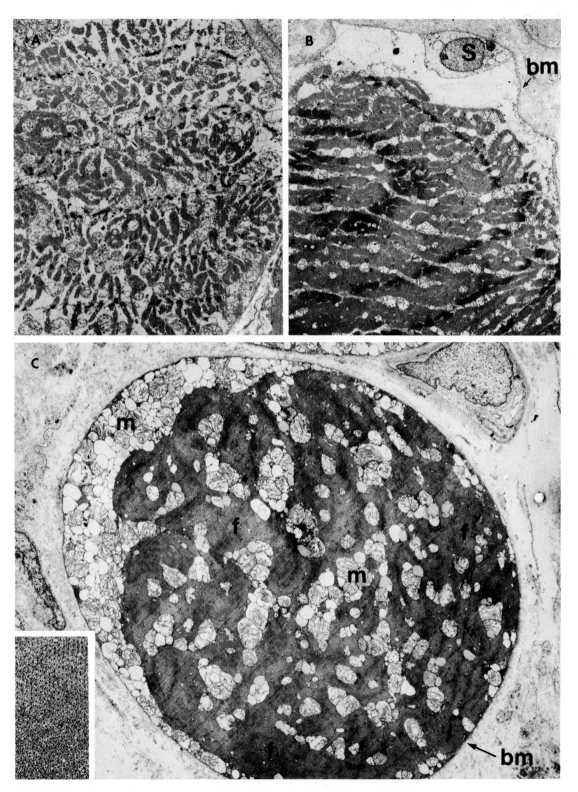

FIG. 13–50. A and B. The upper electron micrographs demonstrate so-called fibrillenstruktur type of extraocular striated muscle cells, in which the cytoplasmic myofibrils are distinct from each other. In B a muscle satellite cell (**S**) is enclosed within the thin basement membrane (**bm**) of the striated cell to which it belongs. C. A felderstruktur type of extraocular muscle cell has myofibrils (**f**) that blend and fuse together. Numerous mitochondria (**m**) are trapped between the coalesced myofibrils. A thin basement membrane (**bm**) ensheaths the cell. The inset displays a hexagonal array of the felderstruktur myofilaments cut in cross section. (A, ×4800; B, ×3900; C, ×4500; inset, ×38,000)

FIG. 13–51. A fibrillenstruktur muscle cell (**FIB**) is shown on the left and a felderstruktur cell (**FEL**) on the right. Individual myofibrils are more clearly defined within the generous sarcoplasm of the fibrillenstruktur cell, whereas there is coalescence of the fibrils in the cell on the right. Large numbers of mitochondria (**m**) are present in both cell types. The inset in the upper left shows the smooth-surfaced sarcoplasmic reticulum (**ser**) as well as the transverse tubules (**T**), both of which are better developed in the fibrillenstruktur cell. **CAP,** an interstitial capillary with an erythrocyte (**RBC**); **bm,** muscle cell basement membrane. (Main figure, ×5100; inset, ×21,400)

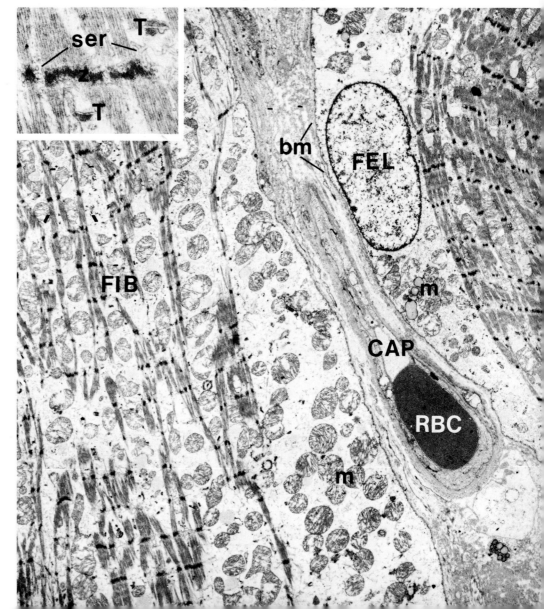

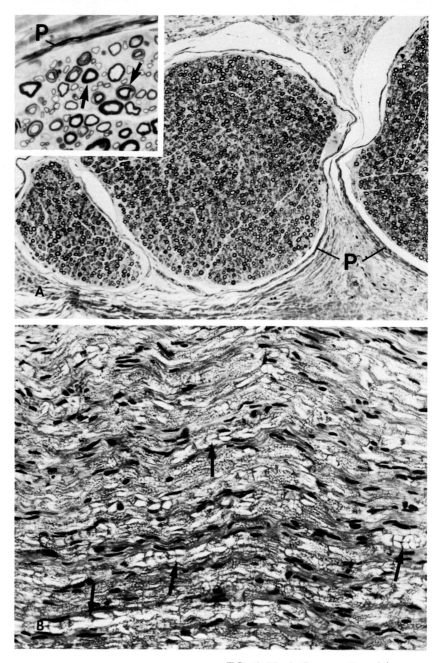

FIG. 13–52. A. Cross section of the supraorbital nerve shows bundles of nerve fibers surrounded by a perineurium (**P**). The inset displays the myelinated axons (**arrows**) present within the endoneural space adjacent to the perineurium. B. A longitudinal section of an orbital nerve near the orbital apex displays the typical wavy fasciculation of the Schwann cells surrounding the axons. The **arrows** indicate artifactual separation of the clefts of Schmidt-Lantermann in the myelin sheath surrounding central axons (**arrows**). (A, 1.0μ Araldite section, methylene blue stain, ×80; inset ×350; H&E, ×280)

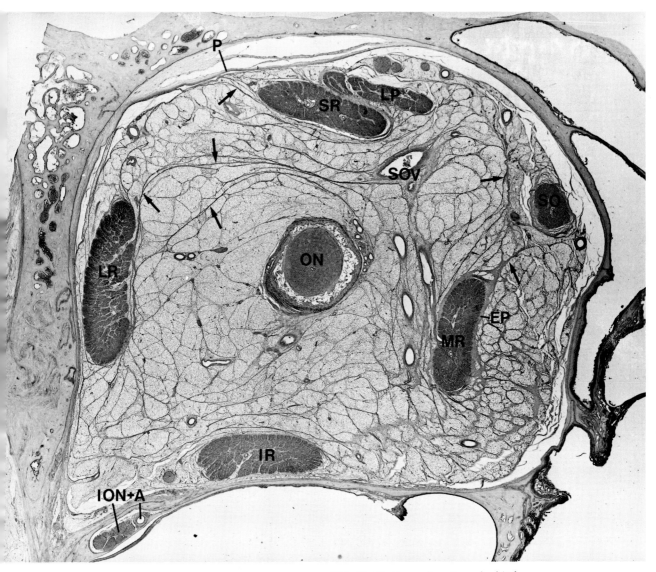

FIG. 13–53. Coronal section of orbital contents just behind the right globe. The orbital anatomy in this preparation is displayed intact and without collapsing away from the periosteum (**P**). Fat invests all of the orbital tissues. A fine lacework of highly ordered fibrous septa subdivides the fat into lobules and interrelates the orbital tissues to each other. Major septa (**arrows**) support the superior ophthalmic vein (**SOV**) and connect the extraocular muscles to the periosteum. Note the absence of a continuous intermuscular membrane. **SR,** superior rectus; **LP,** levator palpebrae superioris; **SO,** superior oblique; **MR,** medial rectus; **IR,** inferior rectus; **LR,** lateral rectus; **EP,** epimysium of the medial rectus; **ON,** optic nerve; **ION** & **A,** infraorbital nerve and artery. (Courtesy of Dr. L. Koornneef)

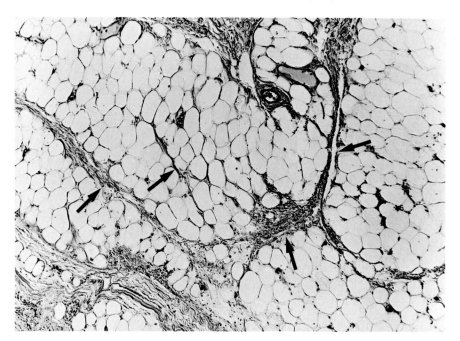

FIG. 13–54. Retrobulbar orbital fat containing various sized collagenous septa (**arrows**). (H&E, ×69)

FIG. 13–55. A. Two fat cells (**F**) are dominated by large lipid vacuoles (**li**). A smaller lipid vacuole (**va**) is also present in the upper cell. There is a delicate extracellular connective tissue (**CT**) separating the cells. B. The large lipid vacuole (**li**) is not membrane bound and compresses the cytoplasm, which contains short profiles of rough-surfaced endoplasmic reticulum (**rer**) and mitochondria (**m**). C. Only a thin rim of cytoplasm (**arrows**) separates the lipid vacuoles (**li**) from the plasma membranes of these two cells. **CT**, collagen fibrils in the narrow connective tissue space between the lipocytes. (A, ×29,000; B, ×29,000; C, ×29,000)

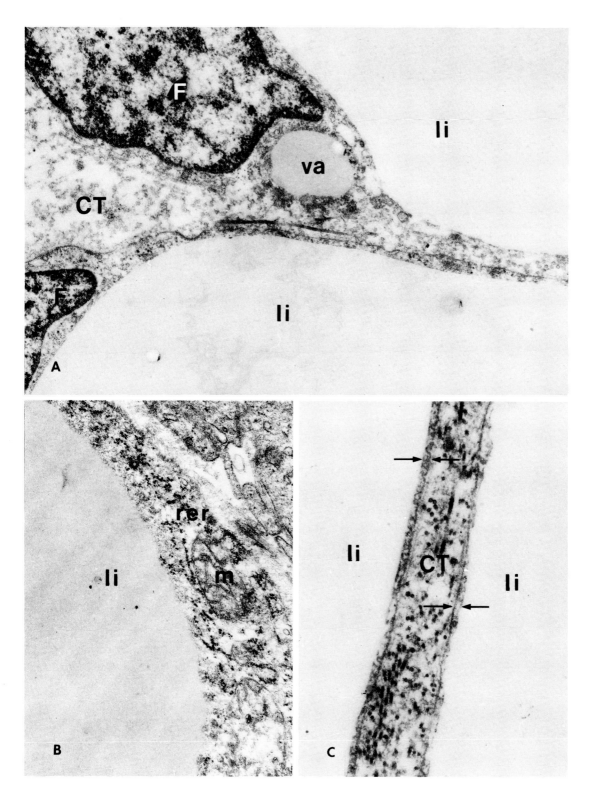

REFERENCES

1. Allansmith M: Immunology of the tears. Int Ophthalmol Clin 13:47, 1973
2. Allansmith M, Kajujama G, Abelson M, Simm M: Plasma cell content of main and accessory lacrimal glands and conjunctiva. Am J Ophthalmol 82:819, 1976
3. Anderson H, Ehlers N, Matthiessen M, Claesson M: Histochemistry and development of the human eyelids. II. A cytochemical and electron microscopic study. Acta Ophthalmol (Kbh) 54:288, 1967
4. Breinin G: The structure and function of extraocular muscle—an appraisal of the duality concept. Am J Ophthalmol 72:1, 1971
5. Duke-Elder S, Wybar K: The Anatomy of the Visual System. In Duke-Elder S (ed): System of Ophthalmology, vol II. St. Louis, C. V. Mosby Co., 1961
6. Durston JH: Histochemistry of primate extraocular muscles and the changes of denervation. Brit J Ophthalmol 58:193, 1974
7. Egeberg J, Jensen O: The ultrastructure of the acini of the human lacrimal gland. Acta Ophthalmol (Kbh) 47:400, 1969
7a. Goudie R, MacFarlane F, Lindsay M: Homing of lymphocytes to nonlymphoid tissues. Lancet 1:292, 1974
7b. Gilbard J, Farris L, Santamaria J: Osmolarity of tear microvolumes in keratoconjunctivitis sicca. Arch Ophthalmol 96:677, 1978
8. Iwata S: Chemical composition of the aqueous phase. Int Ophthalmol Clin 13:29, 1973
9. Jakobiec FA, Bonnano P, Sigelman J: Adnexal conjunctival cysts and dermoids. Arch Ophthalmol (in press)
10. Jakobiec FA, Font RL, Tso MOM, et al.: Mesectodermal leiomyoma of the ciliary body: A tumor of presumed neural crest origin. Cancer 39:2102, 1977
11. Jakobiec FA, Iwamoto T: Mesectodermal leiomyoma of the ciliary body associated with a nevus. Arch Ophthalmol 96:692, 1978
12. Jakobiec FA, Mitchell J, Chauhan P, Iwamoto T: Mesectodermal leiomyosarcoma of the antrum and orbit. Am J Ophthalmol 85:51, 1978
13. Jakobiec FA, Tannenbaum M: Embryological perspectives in the fine structure of orbital tumors. Int Ophthalmol Clin 15:85, 1975
14. Johnston MC: The neural crest abnormalities of the face and brain. In Bergsma B (ed): Brain and Face Malformations. New York, Liss, 1974, pp 1–18
15. Johnston MC: A radioautographic study of the migration and fate of cranial neural crest cells in the chick embryo. Anat Rec 156:143, 1966
16. Johnston MC, Bhakdinaronk A, Reid YC: An expanded role of the neural crest in oral and pharyngeal development. In Bosma JF (ed): The Fourth Symposium on Oral Sensation and Perception, HEW Pub. No. 73-546. Bethesda, National Institutes of Health, 1973, pp 37–52
17. Johnston MC, Listgarten MA: Observations on the migration, interaction and early differentiation of orofacial tissues. In Slavkin HC, Bavetta LA (eds): Developmental Aspects of Oral Biology. New York, Academic Press, 1972, pp 53–80
18. Johnston MC, Morriss GM, Kushner DC, Bingle GJ: Abnormal organogenesis of facial structures. In Wilson JG, Fraser FC (eds): Handbook of Teratology. New York, Plenum, 1977, pp 421–452
19. Jones LT. Anatomy of the tear system. Int Ophthalmol Clin 13:3, 1973
20. Jones IS, Jakobiec FA, Nolan B: Patient examination and introduction to orbital disease. In Duane TD (ed): Clinical Ophthalmology, vol 2, Ch. 21. Hagerstown, Harper & Row, 1976
21. Koornneef L: Spatial Aspects of Orbital Musculo-Fibrous Tissue in Man. Amsterdam, Swets and Zeitlinger, B.V., 1977
22. Last RJ: Wolff's Anatomy of the Eye and Orbit. Philadelphia, W. B. Saunders, 1968
22a. Moss R, Leblond C: Satellite cells as the source of nuclei in muscles of growing rats. Anat Rec 170:421, 1971
22b. Ringel S, Wilson B, Kaiser K: Histochemistry of human extraocular muscle. Arch Ophthalmol 96:1067, 1978
23. Ross M, Reith E: Perineurium: Evidence for contractile elements. Science 165:604, 1969
24. Srinivasan B, Worgul B, Iwamoto T, Merriam G: The conjunctival epithelium. II. Histochemical and ultrastructural studies on human and rat conjunctiva. Ophthalmic Res 9:55, 1977
25. Torczynski E, Jakobiec F, Johnston M, et al.: Synophthalmia and cyclopia: A histopathologic, radiographic and organogenetic analysis. Doc Ophthalmol 44:311, 1977
26. Weingeist T: The conjunctiva. Int Ophthalmol Clin 13:85, 1973
27. Weingeist TA: The glands of the ocular adnexa. Int Ophthalmol Clin 13:243–261, 1973
28. Whitnall SE: The Anatomy of the Human Orbit and Accessory Organs of Vision. New York, Oxford University Press, 1932
29. Wolff K: The fine structure of the Langerhans cell. J Cell Biol 35:468, 1967
30. Zelickson A: Ultrastructure of human epidermis. In Graham J, Johnston W, Helwig E (eds): Dermal Pathology. Hagerstown, Harper & Row, 1972, pp 25–46

Abducent nerve, 322, 323
Acid mucopolysaccharides, 41–42. *See also* Mucopoly-
    saccharides
Acini, of lacrimal gland, 325, 326, 328
Actin filaments, 26, 330, 335
   in retinal pigment epithelium, 64
Adenosine diphosphate, 23
Adenosine triphosphate, 23
Adie's syndrome, 324–325
Aging
   and arteriolar sclerosis, 111
   and basement membrane changes, 47
     in corneal epithelium, 189
     thin basement membrane, 99
   and blepharochalasis, 293
   and Bruch's membrane changes, 64, 220
   and collagen aggregation, 136
   and conjunctival changes, 310
   and corpora amylacea formation, 276
   and cystoid degeneration of peripheral retina, 124
   and drusen formation, 220
   and lacrimal gland lymphoid cell increase, 326
   and macular degeneration, 219
   and Schlemm's canal changes, 258, 259
Air cells, ethmoid, 318
Alcian blue, 42
Amacrine cells, 71, 73, 89, 91, 92
Amino acids
   in collagen, 39
   in elastic tissue, 41
   in elastin, 41
Anatomy
   of eyelids, 292–294
   of orbit, 317–324
   and orientation of eye, 56–57
Angiography, fluorescein, 68–69, 112, 203, 216, 218
Angle
   drainage, of anterior chamber, 251, 252, 254, 266–267
   iridocorneoscleral, 251
Annular reflex, 120
Annulus of Zinn, 319, 321, 322
Anterior chamber of eye, 251, 252
   drainage angle of, 251, 252, 254, 266–267
Apocrine glands, of eyelids, 299
Aponeurosis, levator palpebrae superioris, 291, 293, 318,
     319, 339
Aqueous, 251
   transport of, 258–259
Aqueous compartment, 251, 252
   anterior chamber of, 171, 198, 200, 251, 252
   posterior chamber of, 251, 252
Aqueous tubes, 266
Aqueous veins of Ascher, 191, 261, 263

Arachnoid, 281
Arciform density, 87
Area centralis, 111, 121
Area Martegiani, 137
Arterioles, 106, 107–111
Artery(ies)
   central retinal, 107, 278, 281–282, 283, 284, 285, 320, 321
   ciliary, 56, 57. *See also* Ciliary arteries
   cilioretinal, 111, 283
   dorsonasal, 321
   end arteries, 111
   ethmoidal, 321
   facial, 293
   frontal, 321
   hyaloid, 131
   infraorbital, 339
   lacrimal, 318, 321
   nasal, 107
   ophthalmic, 293, 317, 320–321, 323
   orbital, 320–321
   supraorbital, 321
   temporal, 107, 293
Ascher, aqueous veins of, 191, 261, 263
Astrocytes, 73, 101
   attachments of puncta adherentes, 274, 280, 281
   cytoplasmic filaments and tubules of, 277, 278, 283
   fibrous, 276, 278, 280, 283
   in optic cup, 274, 275, 276
   perivascular, 108, 109
Autophagocytosis, 28
Autoradiography, 11–12
Avascular regions
   cornea, 163
   foveal, 111, 112, 113
   in foveola, 116
   Tenon's capsule, 191
Axenfeld nerve loop, 189, 191
Axons
   bipolar cell, 89
   of ganglion cells, 94–95
   photoreceptor, 82–83, 84
Axoplasmic flow or transport, 281

Banding, collagen, 39
   intraperiod, 39
Basal cells
   of corneal epithelium, 163–164
   of limbal epithelium, melanin granules in, 183, 185, 186

Basal lamina, 42
Basement membrane, 42–49
    aging affecting, 47
    of astrocytes in optic cup, 276
    calcification in, 42
    of canal of Schlemm, 259, 260
    of capillary endothelial cells, 104, 105
    of capillary pericytes, 104, 105
    of choriocapillaris, 216, 219
    conjunctival, 186
    of corneal epithelium, 178, 179, 180
    ciliary
        external, 239, 242, 243
        internal, 230
    Descemet's, 176
    excess, and Hassall-Henle warts, 176
    facets and Müller cells, 97, 99
    of fovea, 111
        transition from thick to thin, 113, 138
    of iris blood vessels, 202, 203
    of lacrimal gland duct cells, 326
    of lens, 153–154
    of lid epidermis, 297, 298
    multilaminar, 43, 46
    retinal
        peripheral, 230, 231
        in pigment epithelium, 61, 63–64
        posterior, 134
        thick, 99
        thin, 99
    of Schwann cell, 273
    thick, 43, 46
    thin, 42, 45
    of trabecular meshwork, 261, 264
Basement membrane-like material, adjacent to kera-
        tocytes, 171
Basophil(s), in connective tissue, 55
Basophilia, cytoplasmic, 26
Berger retrolental space, 140
Bergmeister's papilla, 274
Bipolar cells, retinal, 87–89
    amacrine, 71, 73
    dendrites of, 87–88
    dyad configuration of, 90, 91
    flat, 87, 89, 92
    horizontal, 71, 73
    midget, invaginating, 78, 92
    ribbon synapse of, 90, 91, 92
    synaptic expansions of, 90
Bitot spot, 310
Blepharochalasis, 293
Blood–retinal barriers, 65, 105
Blood supply
    of choroid, 216–219
    of iris, 201, 202–203
    of lacrimal gland, 318
    of optic nerve, 283–286
    of orbit, 320–321
    of retina, 70, 73, 103–111
        arterioles, 106, 107–111
        capillaries, 104–107, 110
        venules, 104, 107, 110, 111
Blue iris, 198, 199, 202, 205, 206
Bodies
    ciliary, 55, 225, 226–245. See also Ciliary body
    lipoidal, 27

Bodies, lipoidal (continued)
        in foveal cone inner segments, 118
        in photoreceptors, 74
    microbodies, 29
    residual, 28
    vitreous, 131–144. See also Vitreous body
Bones, orbital, 317
Bowman's layer, 169
Bowman's membrane, 168–169
Bruch's membrane, 61, 219–226
    calcification of, 42, 64
    changes in aging, 64
    connective tissue portion, 64
    cuticular portion, 61

Calcific spherule, in corneal basement membrane,
        178, 181
Calcification, 42
    of Bruch's membrane, 42, 64
Calyx, of photoreceptor inner segment, 74, 79
Canal
    of Cloquet, 131, 134, 139, 140, 274
    of Hanover, 144
    optic, 282, 317, 318
    of Petit, 144
    of Schlemm, 185, 191, 252–261. See also Schlemm's
        canal
    scleral, 187
    of Sondermann, 266
Canaliculi
    from canal of Schlemm, 266, 268
    of nasolacrimal drainage apparatus, 307, 308
Capillaries
    of choroid. See Choriocapillaris
    of ciliary crests, 241
    in conjunctival substantia propria, 310, 315
    endothelial cells of, 104–105
    micropinocytotic vesicles of, 105, 107
    pericytes of, 104, 105
    pore system of, 107
    retinal, 104–107, 283
Capsule, Tenon's, 191, 318, 320, 321, 322
Capsulopalpebral fascia, 291, 309
Carbohydrate, of membrane glycoprotein, 19
Carcinoma, of eyelids, 308
Carotid arteries, external, 321
Caruncle, 310, 315
Cataract, nuclear, 159
Cavernous sinus thrombosis, 322
Cell(s)
    columnar, of epithelium, 53
    cuboidal, of epithelium, 53
    cytoplasm of, 19. See also Cytoplasm
    endothelial, 53. See also Endothelial cells
    epithelial, 53. See also Epithelial cells
    of extraocular muscles, 333–334
    felderstruktur, 333, 334, 336
    fibrillenstruktur, 333, 336
    and intercellular space, 33–36
    lens, 149, 156
    membrane of. See Plasmalemma

Cell(s) (*continued*)
  mesothelial, 53
  Müller. *See* Müller's cell
  neural crest, 290, 291, 292
  nucleus of, 19. *See also* Nucleus
  Schwann, 273, 334, 338
  squamous, of epithelium, 53
Cellophane macula, 101
Centrioles, 24–25
  fixed, 24
  free, 25
  in photoreceptors, 76
Cement substance
  hemidesmosomal. *See* Hemidesmosomes
  intercellular, 33
    of ciliary body, 229–230
Chalazion, 308
Chamber of eye
  anterior, 251, 252
    drainage angle of, 251, 252, 254, 266–267
  posterior, 251, 252
Cherry-red spot, 116
Chondroitin, 44
Chondroitin sulfate, 44
Choriocapillaris, 48–49, 61, 64, 103, 216, 218–219, 220, 222
  fenestrated, 219, 220, 225
  at foveola, 115
Choristoma, orbital, 321
Choroid, 55, 215–226
  blood vessels of, 216–219
  Bruch's membrane of, 219–226
  pigmented cells in, 215, 216, 217
  stroma of, 216–226
  suprachoroidal space, 215–216
Choroidal layer, of optic nerve, 278, 280
Chromatin, nuclear, 22
Chrome-osmium fixative, 4, 14
Cilia, 24–25
  of lids, 293, 298
  motile, 25
  nonmotile, 25
  of photoreceptors, 74, 76, 77
    isthmus of, 76
    microtubules of, 74, 76
Ciliary arteries, 56, 57
  anterior, 309
  and circle of Zinn-Haller, 281, 283
  long, 321
  and major arterial circle of iris, 246
  passage in sclera, 191, 215
  posterior, 283
  short, 320, 321
  in suprachoroidal space, 216
Ciliary body, 55, 225, 226–245
  basement membrane of
    external, 239, 242, 243
    internal, 230
  components of, 226
  intercellular cement substance of, 229–230
  intercellular spaces in, 230
  nonpigmented epithelium of, 230–239
    union with pigmented epithelium, 228–230
  pars plana of, 225, 226
    anterior, 232–233, 234
    cysts of, 124, 226
    posterior, 141, 230–232

Ciliary body (*continued*)
  pars plicata of, 225, 226, 236, 237
    interciliary fibers in, 233
  pigment epithelium of, 68, 226, 229, 239, 240, 241, 242
  retinal (neuroepithelial) portion of, 226–239
  uveal (mesodermal) portion of, 239–246
  zones of, 226
  zonular fibers in, 232–233, 235
Ciliary crests, 226, 236, 237, 240
  capillaries of, 241
Ciliary ganglion, 321, 324–325
Ciliary muscle, 243, 245, 246
  attachment to scleral roll, 215
Ciliary nerves, 56, 57
  loop of Axenfeld, 189, 191
  posterior, 324
  in suprachoroidal space, 216
Ciliary veins
  anterior, 246
  passage in sclera, 191
Cilioretinal arteries, 111, 283
Cilioretinal veins, 283
Circle
  arterial, of iris, 246
  of Zinn-Haller, 281, 283
Cleavage planes
  natural, in foveomacula, 122
  submembranous, potential, 97
Cleft, Schmidt-Lantermann, 324, 334, 338
Clivus, of fovea, 111
Cloquet's canal, 131, 134, 139, 140, 274
Clump cells of Koganei, in iris, 206, 207
Collagen, 39–40
  aggregation with aging, 136
  banding of, 39
    intraperiod, 39
  embryonic, 39
  mature, 39
  staining of, 9
  types of, 40
Collagen fibrils, 39, 40
  in Bowman's membrane, 168
  in choroidal stroma, 215, 216, 217, 219
  in corneal stroma, 163, 169, 170, 172
  in iris anterior border layer, 199, 200
  in iris stroma, 201, 202
  in scleral stroma, 190–191
  in tarsus of eyelid, 299, 305
  in uveal trabecular meshwork, 261, 264, 265, 266
  in vitreous body, 132
Collarette, of iris, 197
Cones and rods. *See* Photoreceptors
Conjunctiva, 307, 308–317
  basement membrane of, 186
  bulbar, 309
  caruncle of, 310, 315
  corneal transition to, 183–186
  epithelium of, 309–310
    invagination into substantia propria, 307, 309
  forniceal-orbital, 309
  goblet cells of, 163, 164, 186, 187, 307, 309, 310, 313
  plica semilunaris of, 310, 315
  tarsal, 309
Conjunctival sac, 320
Connective tissue, 53, 55
  of extraocular muscles, 327

Connective tissue (*continued*)
  of iris anterior border layer, 198
  juxtacanalicular, at canal of Schlemm, 257, 258, 260, 268
  at lens basement membrane, 153
  of vitreous body, 131
Cornea, 55, 163–183
  adbasal cell layer of, 164
  anterior, 171
  basal cells of, 163–164
  Bowman's membrane of, 168–169
  Descemet's membrane of, 175, 176–177
  dystrophy of
    congenital hereditary, 171
    Fuchs' endothelial, 171, 183
  endothelium of, 171–176
    relation of Descemet's membrane, 178, 181, 182
  epithelium of, 163–167
    basement membrane of, 178, 179, 180
    transition to conjunctiva, 183–186
  fetal, 173
  guttata, 176, 179
  hemidesmosomes of, 163–164, 166
  limbus of, 251–252
  mesothelium of, 171
  peripheral, 171, 173
    compared to central portion, 178–183
  posterior, 171, 173
  stroma of, 169–171
    edema of, 171
    lamellas of, 169, 172
    zones of relucency, 171, 174
  surface cells of, 164, 166
  tear film of, 163
  verticillata, 164
  wing cell layer of, 164, 166
Corneoscleral coat, 253
Corona ciliaris, 225, 226
Corpora
  amylacea, 101, 103
    in astrocytes of optic cup, 276
  arenacea, 276, 282
Corpuscle
  Meissner, 72
  Pacini, 72
Coxtex, lens, 149, 156–159
Counterions, in acid mucopolysaccharides, 42
Cranial nerves, 322, 323, 334
Crests
  ciliary, 226, 236, 237, 240
  neural, 290, 291, 292
Cristae mitochondriales, 23
Crypts
  of Henle, 310
  in iris anterior border layer, 198, 200
Crystal(s), hydroxyapatite, 42
Crystalline material in ocular tissue, 42
Crystalloid, Kolmer, 91–92
Cul-de-sac, subretinal
  anterior, 123, 124
  posterior, 123, 124
Cup, optic, 274
Cyst(s)
  in fornices, 309–310
  in pars plana, 124, 126
  pigment, in iris, 210
Cystic dermoids, in orbit, 290

Cystoid degeneration, of peripheral retina, 123, 124
Cytochalasin B, 25–26
Cytoplasm, 19
  of Müller cell, 100
  of retinal pigment epithelial cells, 65–70
Cytoplasmic inclusions, 26–29
  glycogen particles, 26
  lipoidal bodies, 27
  lysosomes, 27–29
  microbodies, 29
  pigment granules, 26–27
  ribosomes, 26
  secretion granules or vacuoles, 29
Cytoplasmic organelles, 20–26
  centrioles and cilia, 24–25
  endoplasmic reticulum, 20–23
  filaments, 25–26
  Golgi complex, 23–24
  microtubules, 26
  mitochondria, 23
  nucleolus, 22
Cytosomes, 27–29

Dalton's chrome-osmium fixative, 4, 14
Dendrites
  bipolar cell, 87–88
  ganglion cell, 93, 94
  horizontal cell, 87
  melanocyte, in limbal region, 185, 186
Dense bodies, cytoplasmic, 27–29
Density
  arciform, 87
  synaptic, 87
Dermis of lids, 298
Dermoids, cystic, of orbit, 290
Descemet's membrane, 175, 176–177
  relation to corneal endothelium, 178, 181, 182
  Schwalbe's ring or line of, 183, 184
  termination of, variations in, 268, 269
Desmosine, in elastin, 41
Desmosome(s), 33
  in ciliary body, 230
  in corneal epithelium, 164, 166, 167
  in lacrimal gland acini, 325, 328
  in lacrimal gland duct cells, 326, 332
  in lid epidermis, 296, 298
  in limbal epithelium, 185, 186, 187
Desmosome-like densities, of bipolar cells, 88
Dextrans, as tracers for transport mechanisms, 10
Diabetes
  and basement membrane of ciliary epithelium, 241
  and loss of capillary pericytes, 104
Diaphragm, iris, 197
Diastase digestion, of glycogen particles, 9, 26, 42
Dilator muscle, of iris, 206, 208
Disc, optic, 70, 274
Dot
  Gunn, 97
  Mittendorf, 140
Drainage angle, 251, 252, 254, 266–267
Drusen, 220, 222, 224

Dry eye syndrome, 319
Duct, nasolacrimal, 318
Dura mater, 281
Dyad configuration, of bipolar cells, 90, 91

Ecotaxis, 327
Ectoderm, 53, 61
    surface, 61
Ectomesenchyme, 290
Ectoplasm, 19
Ectropion, 210
Edema
    of conjunctival substantia propria, 310
    of corneal stroma, 171
    of optic nerve head, 278
Edinger-Westphal nucleus, of oculomotor nerve, 324
Egger's line, 140
Elastic lamina
    of Bruch's membrane, 61, 64, 220, 225
    of retinal artery, 284, 285
Elastic tissue, 40–41
    in tarsus of eyelids, 299, 305
    in trabecular meshwork, 264, 265
Elastin, 41
    in choroid stroma, 217
    staining of, 9
Electron microscopy, 3–14
    and autoradiography, 11–12
    misinterpretations in, 13
    scanning, 7–8
    special examination techniques in, 4–12
        freeze-fracture etch in, 6
        shadow-casting in, 5
        surface replication in, 5
    tissue preparation for, 3–4
        for scanning electron micrograph, 7
        staining and histochemical methods in, 9
        thickness of sections in, 14
    and tracers for transport mechanisms, 10
Elschnig border tissue, 278
Elschnig inner limiting membrane, 274
Elschnig intercalary tissue, 275, 278
Embedding of ocular tissue, for electron microscopy, 3–4
Embryology
    of lens, 149–153
    of ocular adnexa, 290–292
    of retina, 61, 62
    of vitreous body, 131
Emeiocytosis, 325
End arteries, 110
End bulbs of Krause, 72
Endomysium, of extraocular muscles, 327, 334
Endoplasm, 19
Endoplasmic reticulum, 20–23
    agranular (smooth), 21
        of myofibrils, 333
        of photoreceptors, 74
        of retinal pigment epithelium, 65, 67
        of Zeis gland cells, 298, 300
    granular (rough), 21
        of ciliary nonpigmented epithelium, 230, 232, 234

Endoplasmic reticulum, granular (rough) (continued)
        of ganglion cells, 93, 94
        of lacrimal gland acini, 325, 328
        of lacrimal gland duct cells, 326, 332
        of retinal pigment epithelium, 68
Endothelial cells, 53
    of canal of Schlemm, 252, 256, 257, 258
    capillary, 104–105
    of choriocapillaris, 216, 219
    corneal, 171–176
        relation to Descemet's membrane, 178, 181, 182
    of iris blood vessels, 202, 203
    of trabecular meshwork, 261, 264, 265
Enzymes, of mitochondrial membrane, 23
Eosinophils, in connective tissue, 55
Ephelides, 298
Epidermalization, conjunctival, 310
Epidermis, of skin of lids, 294–298
Epimysium, of extraocular muscles, 327, 339
Epineurium, 334
Episclera, 191
Epithelial cells, 53
    of ciliary body, 226–229
    conjunctival, 309–310
    of cornea, 163–167
        basement membrane of, 178, 179, 180
        transition to conjunctiva, 183–186
    of iris pigment epithelium, 210, 214
    of lens, 155–156
    neural or medullary, 55
    pigment, 61–70. See also Pigment epithelium
Equatorial plane of eye, 56
Erythrocytes. See Red cells
Ethmoid air cells, 318
Ethmoid bone, 317
Ethmoidal arteries, 318, 321
Examination techniques, with electron microscopy, 4–12
Extracellular materials, 39–49
Eye
    anatomic orientation of, 56–57
    planes of, 56
    three-coat arrangement of, 55
    three-tissue arrangement of, 57
Eyelids, 292–308. See also Lids

Facial arteries, 293
Facial nerve, 293
Facial veins, 293
Fascia
    adherens, 36
        of ciliary body, 227, 229
    capsulopalpebral, 291, 309
    occludens, 36
        of ciliary body, 227, 229
Fat
    droplets in cells, 27
    orbital, 335, 339, 340, 341
Felderstruktur cells, 333, 334, 336
Fenestrated endothelia
    in capillaries of ciliary crests, 241
    in choriocapillaris, 219, 220, 225

Fenestrated membranes, 33
Ferritin, as tracer for transport mechanisms, 10
Fibers
  lens, 156
    primary, 149
    secondary, 149
    zonular, 40, 153
  Müller, 101
  zonular
    of lens, 40, 153
    of vitreous body, 141–144
Fibril(s)
  collagen, 39, 40. See also Collagen fibrils
  myofibrils, 330
  tonofibrils, 33
Fibrillenstruktur cells, 333, 336
Fibroblast, 55
Fibrous component, of vitreous body, 132
Fibrous materials, of ocular tissues, 39–41
Filaments
  actin, 330, 335
  in astrocytes, 101, 277, 278, 283
  collagen, 39, 40
  in corneal basal cells, 164
  cytoplasmic
    in extraocular muscle cells, 334
    in lacrimal gland acini, 325, 328
    in lacrimal gland duct cells, 326, 332
  intracellular, 25–26
  in lens capsule, 153
  in Müller cells, 100
  myosin, 330, 335
  tonofilaments, 33
  in vitreous body, 132
    aggregation into fibers, 141
    anterior, 140
    posterior, 134, 135
Fissure, orbital
  inferior, 317, 318, 323
  superior, 317, 318, 322, 323
Fixation of ocular tissue, for electron microscopy, 4
Fluorescein angiography, 68–69, 112, 203, 216, 218
Footplates, Müller cell, 94, 97, 107
Foramen
  infraorbital, 318
  oculomotor, 322, 323
  optic, 321
  vascular, in orbit, 318
Fornix, conjunctival, 308, 309
  cysts in, 309–310
Fossa
  for lacrimal gland, 318
  patellar, of lens, 134
Fovea, 56
  anatomic, 120
  avascular zone of, 111, 112, 113
  basement membrane of, 111
    transition from thick to thin, 113, 138
  centralis, 111–113, 114, 115
  clivus of, 111
  externa, 116
  photoreceptor in, 78
Foveola, 111, 113, 115, 116–118
Foveolar reflex, 113, 116, 120
Foveomacular region, pigment epithelium of, 68–69
Fracture, of orbital floor, 318–320

Freckles, 298
Freeze-fracture etch of tissue, 6
Frontal arteries, 321
Frontal bone, 317
Frontal nerve, 322, 323
Fuchs' endothelial dystrophy, of cornea, 171, 183
Fuchs' heterochromic iridocyclitis, 202
Fuchs' spurs, of iris, 204, 205
Furrows
  of iris
    circumferential, 210
    longitudinal, 210
    structural, 212
  palpebral, superior, 293
  of photoreceptors, longitudinal, 76, 79
  of sclera
    circumferential, 192
    inner, 251
    outer, 251

Ganglion
  cervical, superior, 324
  ciliary, 321, 324–325
  sphenopalatine, 318
  trigeminal, 324
Ganglion cells, 92, 93, 94
  dendrites of, 93, 94
  of macula lutea, 120–121
  Nissl substance of, 93, 94
  of retina, 72
Gap junction, 34–36
  in retinal pigment epithelium, 65, 66, 67
Gland
  lacrimal, 291, 318, 325–327
    accessory, of Krause, 291, 308, 309, 319
  meibomian, 163, 291, 299, 303–308, 320
  of Moll, 163, 291, 299, 301, 302
  of Wolfring, 291, 309, 319
  of Zeis, 163, 291, 298, 299, 300
Glial cells, 283
  and foveal basement membrane, 113
  retinal, 70, 73, 99–103
Glial plaque, of optic cup, 274
Globe. See Eye
Glutaraldehyde, cold, as fixative, 4
Glycocalyx, 19
Glycogen particles, 26
  in choroid cells, 217
  in cone pedicles, 87
  detection with diastase digestion, 9, 26, 42
  detection with thiosemicarbazide, 9, 26
  in glial cells, 103
  in Müller cells, 96, 100
  in photoreceptors, 74, 78
Glycoprotein, 42
  collagen, 39
  definition of, 41
  insoluble, in lens capsule and zonules, 132
Goblet cells, conjunctival, 163, 164, 186, 187, 307, 309, 310, 313
Golgi complex, 23–24

Golgi complex (*continued*)
  immature face of, 24
  in lacrimal gland acinar cells, 325
  in lens epithelial cells, 155
  mature face of, 24
  in Müller cells, 100
  in photoreceptors, 74
  in retinal pigment epithelium, 70, 71
Gonioscopy, 252, 268, 269
Granules
  of endoplasmic reticulum. *See* Endoplasmic reticulum, granular
  keratohyalin, in epidermis of lids, 295, 296, 298
  lipofuscin, 26. *See also* Lipofuscin granules
  melanin, 26. *See also* Melanin granules
  mitochondrial or matrix, 23
  Palade, 21
  pigment, 26–27
  secretion, 29
  zymogenic, in lacrimal gland acini, 325, 327
Graves' disease, extraocular muscles in, 320
Grids, in electron microscopy, 4
Ground substance
  cytoplasmic, 26
  mitochondrial, 23
Gunn's dots, 97

Haidinger brushes, 122
Hanover canal, 144
Hassall-Henle warts, 176, 179, 182
Heinrich-Müller reticulum, 239
Hemidesmosomes
  and conjunctival basement membrane, 186
  in conjunctival epithelium, 310, 311
  corneal, 163–164, 166
  in lid epidermis, 297, 298
Hemoglobin, in red cells, 27
Hemorrhage, 140, 197
  retinal, 97, 101
Henle crypts, 310
Henle fibers
  in foveomacula, 122
  retinal, 72, 82, 83, 84, 85
Heparin, 44
  in mast cells, 55
Heparin monosulfuric acid, 44
Heterochromia, of iris, 202
Heteropolysaccharides, 41
Histiocytes, 55
Histochemical methods, in electron microscopy, 9
Homopolysaccharide, 41
Hordeolum, 298
Horizontal cells, of retina, 71, 73, 87, 89, 92
  dendrites of, 87
Horner's syndrome, 317
Horseradish peroxidase, as tracer for transport mechanisms, 10
Hyalocytes, 141
Hyaloid artery, 131
Hyaloid of vitreous body
  anterior, 140
  posterior, 136, 137

Hyaloideocapsular ligament, 144
Hyaluronic acid, 44
  in vitreous body, 133
Hydroxyapatite crystals, 42
Hydroxylysine, in collagen, 39
Hydroxyproline
  in collagen, 39
  in elastic tissue, 41

Immunocytes, lacrimal gland, 326
Inclusions, cytoplasmic, 26–29
India ink, as tracer for transport mechanisms, 10
Infraorbital artery, 339
Infraorbital nerve, 293, 318
Intercellular space, 333
  desmosomes in, 33
  gap junction in, 34–36
  terminal bar region of, 33–34
Iridocorneoscleral angle, 251
Iridocyclitis, Fuch's heterochromic, 202
Iridodialysis, 197
Iridodonesis, 197
Iris, 55
  anterior border layer of, 198, 210
  blood vessels of, 202–203
  blue, 198, 199, 202, 205, 206
  clump cells of, 206, 207
  dilator muscle of, 206, 208
  pigment epithelium of, 68, 198, 209, 210–214
    anterior layer of, 214
    posterior layer of, 210, 214
  pigmentation of, 197, 198, 199, 200
    alterations in, 202
  retinal (neuroepithelial) portion of, 203–214
  sphincter muscle of, 203–206
  stroma of, 198, 202–203
  trabeculae of, 198, 200
  uveal (mesodermal) portion of, 198–203
Iris processes, 268
Isodesmosine, in elastin, 41

Jacoby, border tissue of, 278
Junctional complex, 34
  in iris blood vessel endothelium, 202, 203
  in lacrimal gland duct cells, 326, 332
  in retinal pigment epithelium, 67

Keratectomy, 170
Keratinocytes
  conjunctival, 310, 313
  in lid epidermis, 294, 298

Keratinosomes, in lid epidermis, 296, 298
Keratoconjunctivitis sicca, 319
Keratocytes, 55, 169–170
Keratohyalin granules, in epidermis of lids, 295, 296, 298
Keratopathy, calcific band, 178
Keratosulfate, 44
Koganei, clump cells of, 206
Kolmer crystalloid, 91, 92
Krause accessory lacrimal glands, 291, 308, 309, 319
Krause end bulbs, 72
Kuhnt central supporting tissue meniscus, 274, 275
Kuhnt intermediary tissue, 277, 278

Lacrimal artery, 318, 321
Lacrimal bone, 317
Lacrimal gland, 318, 325–327
  acini of, 325
  duct system of, 326, 330
  tumors of, 326–327
Lacrimal nerve, 319, 322, 323
Lacrimal sac, 307, 308
Lamellas
  of corneal stroma, 169, 172
  of lens, zonular, 154
  photoreceptor, 74, 76, 78, 79
    in outer segment of fovea, 118
  suprachoroidal, 215, 216, 217
  synaptic, 86, 87
Lamina
  cribrosa
    choroidalis, 278, 279
    scleralis, 274, 278, 279, 282
  elastica
    of Bruch's membrane, 61, 64, 220, 225
    of pars plana, 241, 242
  fusca, of sclera, 192
  papyracea, 317, 318
  vitrea, 61, 64, 219
Langerhans' cells
  in conjunctival epithelium, 310, 312
  in lid epidermis, 294, 298
  in limbal region, 186
Lens, 149–159
  basement membrane of, 153–154
  capsule of, 151, 152, 153–155
    exfoliation of, 154
    pseudoexfoliation of, 154
  cortex of, 149, 156–159
    microplicae of, 156, 158
  embryology of, 149–153
  epithelium of, 155–156
  fibers of, 156
    primary, 149
    secondary, 149
    zonular, 153, 252
  intercellular spaces in, 155
  lamella of, zonular, 154
  nuclear cataract of, 159
  patellar fossa of, 134
  shagreen, 154
  structure of, 153–159
  suspensory ligaments of, 141

Lens (continued)
  suture lines of, 149
  zones of relucency
    first, 154
    second, 156
Lens cells, 149, 156
  nuclei of, 149, 150, 156–159
    adult, 153
    embryonic, 149
Lentigo, 298
Leucofuchsin, 42
Leukocytes, polymorphonuclear, 55
Leukoplakia, conjunctival, 310
Levator palpebrae superioris, 291, 293, 318, 319, 339
Lids of eye, 292–308
  epidermis of, 294–298
  general anatomy of, 292–294
  papillary dermis of, 298
  pigmentation of, 298
  tarsus of, 299, 304, 305
Ligament
  hyaloideocapsular, 144
  Lockwood's, 291
  palpebral, 294
  suspensory, of lens, 141
  of Wieger, 140
Limbus of cornea, 183–186, 251–252
  surgical, 183
  transitional epithelium of, 186, 187
  true, 185
Limiting membrane
  inner, of Elschnig, 274
  retinal
    external, 72, 73, 74, 81
    internal, 72, 73, 107, 108, 109, 111
    middle, 72, 73, 88
Line
  limbal, 183
  Schwalbe, 183, 184
    anterior, 251, 268, 269
    posterior, 252
  suture, of lens, 149
Lipid droplets
  in lacrimal gland acini, 325, 328
  in lacrimal gland duct cells, 326, 332
  in Zeis glands, 298, 300
Lipid layers, of cell membrane, 19
Lipid vacuoles, in orbital fat cells, 341
Lipofuscin granules, 26
  in ciliary epithelium, 238, 240
  in corneal endothelial cells, 182
  in retinal pigment epithelium, 68–69
Lipoidal bodies, 27
  in foveal cone inner segments, 118
  in photoreceptors, 74
Lobules
  of choriocapillaris, 216, 218
  of lacrimal gland, 325
Lockwood's ligament, 291, 319
Lye injury, of conjunctiva, 319
Lymphangioma, orbital, 321
Lymphatic drainage, of eyelids, 293
Lymphocytes
  in conjunctival substantia propria, 309
  in connective tissue, 55
  in lacrimal gland, 326
Lysosomes, 27–29

Lysosomes (*continued*)
  primary, 28, 29
  secondary, 28
Lysozyme, in tears, 326, 327

Macrophages, 55, 103
Macropinocytotic transport mechanisms, 258
Macula
  adherentes. *See* Desmosomes
  cellophane, 101
  communicans, 34, 65
  histologic, 121
  lutea, 69, 118–124
    yellow substance of, 122
Macular ring reflex, 120
Macular stars, 122
Martegiani area, 137
Mast cells, 55
  in limbal subepithelial tissue, 186, 188
Maxillary bone, 317
Meibomian glands, 163, 291, 299, 303–308, 320
Meissner corpuscles, 72
Melanin granules, 26
  in ciliary epithelium, 238–240
  in ciliary pigment epithelium, 239
  in clump cells of Koganei, 206
  in iris dilator muscle, 206, 208
  in iris pigment epithelium, 212, 213–214
    transitional, 214
  in iris sphincter muscle cells, 205, 207
  in iris stromal cells, 198, 199, 212, 213
  in lid epidermis, 298
  in limbal epithelial basal cells, 183, 185, 186
  in retinal pigment epithelium, 68, 71
  uveal, 68
Melanocytes
  in choroid, 216, 217
  in conjunctival epithelium, 310, 312
  in lid epidermis, 295, 297, 298
  in limbal region, 185, 186
  in scleral lamina fusca, 192
Melanoma
  of eyelids, 298
  uveal, 187, 191, 202, 210
Melanosome, 68
Membrane
  basement. *See* Basement membrane
  Bowman's, 168–169
  Brunch's, 61, 219–226
  of cells. *See* Plasmalemma
  Descemet's, 175, 176–177
  fibrous, intermuscular, 320, 321
  limiting. *See* Limiting membrane
Meniscus, central supporting tissue, of Kuhnt, 274, 275
Meridional plane of eye, 56
Mesaxon, 273
Mesectoderm, 290
Mesenchyme
  primary, 54
  secondary, 54
Meshwork, trabecular, 261–269
  corneoscleral, 261, 265

Meshwork, trabecular (*continued*)
  intertrabecular spaces, 265–266
  transtrabecular spaces, 265
  uveal, 261, 264, 265
Mesoderm, 53–54
Mesothelial cells, 53
  corneal, 171
Metachromasia, 42
  in mast cells, 55
Michel's spurs, of iris, 205, 206
Microbodies, cytoplasmic, 29
Microfibrils, of elastic tissue, 41
Microfilaments, intracellular, 25–26
Microglia, 103, 283
Microperoxisomes, in retinal pigment epithelium, 70
Microphages, 55
Micropinocytotic vesicles
  of canal of Schlemm, 257, 258
  of capillary endothelial cells, 105, 107
Microplicae, of lens cortical cells, 156, 158
Microscopy. *See* Electron microscopy
Microtomes, 4
Microtubules
  in bipolar cell dendrites, 87
  in centrioles, 24–25
  in cilia of photoreceptors, 74, 76
  cytoplasmic
    in astrocytes, 277, 278, 283
    in lacrimal gland acini, 325
  in ganglion cells, 95, 96
  intracellular, 26
  Müller cell, 100
Minerals, in ocular tissue, 42
Mitochondria, 23
  in bipolar cell dendrites, 87
  in corneal endothelial cells, 176
  in Müller cells, 100
  in synaptic expansions, 87
Mittendorf dot, 140
Moll gland, 163, 291, 299, 301, 302
Monocytes, in connective tissue, 55
Mounting of ocular tissue, for electron microscopy, 3–4
Mucinous material, in ocular tissue, 41–42
  in vitreous body, 134
Mucoid, interreceptor, 70, 74, 78, 80, 81
Mucopolysaccharides, acid, 41–42
  characteristics of, 42, 44
  in ciliary nonpigmented epithelium, 232, 233
  in cornea, 163, 170
  intercellular
    in ciliary body, 230
    between photoreceptors, 77, 81
  in iris stroma, 201, 202
  in photoreceptors, 74
  polyanionic nature of, 42
  in vitreous body, 133, 232, 233
    cortical zone, 141
Müller cell, 73, 99–100, 276
  adhering to detached limiting membrane, 137, 138
  basement membrane facets of, 97, 99
  cytoplasm of, 100
    dense, 100
      in foveomacular, 124
    lucent, 78, 82, 84, 100, 102, 122
  footplates of, 94, 97, 107
  function as oligodendroglia, 95, 101
  intercellular spaces, 100

Müller cell (continued)
  intermediate or transitional zone of, 100, 103
  nuclei of, 89
  projections of, 80
Müller fibers, 101
Müller muscle, 291, 315, 316, 317, 320, 322
Muscle, 55, 319–320, 327–334
  ciliary, 243, 245, 246
    attachment to scleral roll, 215
  contractile system of, 330
  intermuscular fibrous membrane, 320, 321
  of iris
    dilator, 206, 208
    sphincter, 203–206
  Müller's, 291, 315, 316, 317, 320, 322
  oblique, 56, 319, 321, 322, 339
  orbicularis, 291, 293
  rectus, 56–57, 191, 319, 321, 322, 339
  of Riolan, 293, 303
  types of cells in, 333–334
Muscle stars, suprachoroid, 216
Myasthenia gravis, 293, 320
Myelin, 273–274
Myelinated retinal nerve fibers, 95, 96, 97
Myelination, 281
Myeloid bodies, in retinal pigment epithelium, 70
Myoepithelial cells
  of lacrimal gland, 325
  of Moll glands, 299, 303
Myofibers, of extraocular muscles, 327, 334, 335
Myofibrils, 330, 335
Myosin filaments, 330, 335

Nasal arteries, 107
Nasociliary nerve, 322, 323, 324
Nasolacrimal duct, 318
Neovascularization, retinal, 88
  at periphery, 220
  subretinal, 64
Nerve tissue, 55
  abducent, 322, 323
  ciliary, 56, 57. See also Ciliary nerve
  cranial, 322, 323, 334
  frontal, 322, 323
  infraorbital, 339
  lacrimal, 319, 322, 323
  nasociliary, 322, 323, 324
  oculomotor, 322, 323, 324
  optic, 273–286. See also Optic nerve
  orbital, 322–324
  peripheral, 334
  retinal systems
    glial, 70, 73, 99–103
    neuronal, 70, 71–99
  supraorbital, 338
  trochlear, 322, 323
  zygomatic, 319
Neural crest cells, 290, 291, 292
Neural retina, 70–124
Neuroectoderm, 53, 55, 61
  and pars optica retinae, 70
Neuroepithelium, melanin granules in, 26

Neurofilaments, in ganglion cells, 95, 96
Neuronal system, retinal, 70, 71–79
Neurotubules. See Microtubules
Nevi, 202, 298
Nissl substance, of ganglion cells, 93, 94
Nodes of Ranvier, 274, 334
Nuclear layers, retinal
  inner, 72, 87–90
  outer, 72, 81–82
Nucleoid, in microbodies, 29
Nucleolus, 22
Nucleus of cells, 19
  chromatin of, 22
  of lens cells, 149, 150, 156–159

Oblique muscles, 319, 321, 322, 339
  inferior, 56
  superior, 56
Oculomotor nerve, 322, 323, 324
  Edinger-Westphal nucleus of, 324
Oligodendrocyte(s), 273, 283, 334
  Müller cell functioning as, 95, 101
Oligodendrocyte-like cells in retina, 101
Ophthalmic artery, 293, 317, 320–321, 323
Ophthalmic nerve, 293, 309
Ophthalmic veins, 293, 317, 319, 323
  inferior, 322
  superior, 320, 322
Ophthalmoplegia, progressive external, 320
Optic canal, 317, 318, 321
Optic cup, 61, 274
Optic disc, 70, 274
Optic nerve, 56, 273–286, 322, 323, 339
  choroidal layer of, 278, 280
  intraneural components of, 282–283
  intraocular (bulbar) portion of, 274–281
  laminar part of, 274
  orbital (retrobulbar) portion of, 281–283, 284
  passage in sclera, 191
  prelaminar part of, 274
  retinal layer of, 274–278, 280
  scleral layer of, 278–281
  sheaths of, 281–282
  vascular supply of, 283–286
Optic papilla, 70
Optic stalk, 61
Optic strut, 317
Optic vesicle, 61
  lumen of, 226
    remnants of, 214
  secondary, 61
Ora serrata, 61, 122, 124
Orbicularis muscle, 291, 293
Orbiculus ciliaris, 225, 226
Orbit, 317–341
  fat cells of 335, 339, 340, 341
  fractures of floor, 318, 320
  general anatomy of, 317–324
  nerves in, 322–324
  vascular system of, 320–321
  walls of, apertures in, 317–318

Orbitopalpebral sulcus, 291, 293
Osmium tetroxide fixative, 4

Pacini corpuscles, 72
Palade granules, 21
Palatine bone, 317
Palisades of Vogt, 310
Papilla
    Bergmeister, 274
    optic, 70, 274
Papilledema, 278
Pars
    optica retinae, 70
    plana, of ciliary body, 225, 226
        anterior, 232–233, 234
        cysts of, 124, 226
        posterior, 141, 230–232
    plicata, of ciliary body, 225, 226, 236, 237
        interciliary fibers in, 233
PAS reaction, 42
Patellar fossa, of lens, 134
Pericytes
    of choriocapillaris, 216
    in iris, 202
    of retinal capillaries, 104, 105
Periderm, 290
Periganglion cells, 103
Perikarya, 72
    bipolar cell, 89
    cone cell, 82
Perimysium, 327
Perineurium, 334, 338
Periodic acid Schiff reaction, 42
Periorbita, 320, 322
Peroxidase, as tracer for transport mechanisms, 10
Peroxisome, 29
Petit canal, 144
Phagocytosis, 28
Phagosomes, in retinal pigment epithelium, 70
Phosphotungstic acid, for staining of tissue, 9
Photography, in electron microscopy, 12–14
Photoreceptors, 64, 70, 71–81
    acid mucopolysaccharides in, 74
    axonal extensions of, 82–83, 84, 122
    cilia of, 74, 76, 77
        isthmus of, 76
    connecting fibers of, 82
    endoplasmic reticulum in, agranular, 74
    extracellular space between, 81
    extrafoveolar cone, 76, 81
    in foveola, 115, 116
    glycogen in, 74, 78
    Golgi complex of, 74
    inner segment of, 72, 74, 76, 78
        calyx of, 74, 79
        in fovea, 116–118
    interreceptor mucoid, 70, 74, 78, 80, 81
    lamellas of, 74, 76, 78, 79
    lipoidal bodies in, 74
    longitudinal furrows of, 76, 79
    outer segment of, 74, 76, 77, 78
        in cone cell, 76

Photoreceptors, outer segment of (continued)
        in fovea, 118
        in rod cell, 74, 76
    pedicle of cone, 85, 86, 87
        synaptic arrangement with rod spherule, 92
    plasmalemma of, 74
    relation to retinal pigment epithelium, 76, 80
        in fovea, 118
    ribosomes in, 74
    rod spherule, 83, 85, 86, 87
        synaptic arrangement with cone pedicle, 92
    synaptic expansions of, 83–87, 102
    synaptic vesicles in, 83, 85, 86
    termination of, and cul-de-sac formation, 124
Pia mater, 281
Pial septa, 282–283
Pigment epithelium
    of ciliary body, 68, 226, 229, 239, 240, 241, 242
    foveomacular, 68–69
    of iris, 68, 198, 209, 210–214
    of retina, 61–70, 226
        actin filaments in, 64
        adhesion to sensory retina, 124
        basement membrane of, 61, 63–64, 219, 220, 225
        elastic lamina of, 61, 64
        endoplasmic reticulum in, 65, 67, 68
        gap junctions in, 65, 66, 67
        Golgi complex in, 70, 71
        lamina vitrea of, 61, 64
        lipofuscin granules in, 68–69
        macula communicans in, 65
        melanin granules in, 68, 71
        microperoxisomes in, 70
        myeloid bodies in, 70
        obstruction of intercellular passage from chorio-
            capillaris, 65, 67
        phagosomes in, 70
        relation to photoreceptors, 76, 80, 118
        residual bodies in, 68, 70
        ribosomes in, 68
        terminal bar region of, 63, 64, 65, 66
        villi of, 64, 68, 76, 80
Pigment granules, 26–27
Pigment seam or ruff, in iris, 209, 210
Pigmentation
    of iris, 197, 198, 199, 200, 212–213
        alterations in, 202
    of lids, 298
    of pars plana, 226
    and scleral spots, 187, 191
    suprachoroidal, 215, 216, 217
Pingueculum, 310
Pinocytotic vesicles, in canal of Schlemm, 258
Planes, of eye, 56
Plaques
    on cytoplasmic surface of plasmalemma, 33
    glial, of optic cup, 274
Plasma cells
    in connective tissue, 55
    in lacrimal gland, 326
Plasmalemma, 19–20
    active transport mechanisms in, 20
    adjacent
        attachments of, 33–36
        and intercellular cement, 33
    apical, 53
    basilar, 53

Plasmalemma (*continued*)
   cell growth affecting configuration of, 54
   of choriocapillaris endothelial cells, 216
   extracellular surface of, 6
   fenestrated, 33
   and intercellular space, 33
   of lacrimal gland acini, 329
   lateral, 53
   of lens epithelial cells, 155
   of photoreceptors, 74
   protoplasmic surface of, 6
   of Schwann cells, 273
   separation from basement membranes, 42–43
   sodium pump in, 20
   trilaminar structure of, 19
Platelets, in connective tissue, 55
Plexiform layer, retinal
   inner, 87, 90
   outer, 72, 82–87
Plica
   ciliaris, of pars plicata, 226
   semilunaris, of conjunctiva, 310, 315
Polysaccharides, 41
Pores
   in Bowman's membrane, 169
   capillary, 107
   in cell membrane, 19
   in drainage angle structures, 259
   nuclear, 21
Posterior chamber of eye, 251, 252
Premelanosome, 68
Prickle cells, in epidermis of lids, 295, 296
Processes
   ciliary, 226, 236
   iris, 268
Procollagen, 39
Proptosis, in vascular tumors, 321
Protein
   in cell membrane, 19–20
   residual, of vitreous body, 132
Prussian blue reaction, 42
Pterygium, 310
Ptosis, eyelid, 293–294
Puncta
   adherentes, 36
     and astrocyte attachments, 274, 280, 281
     of ciliary body, 229
     of photoreceptor synapses, 86, 87, 88
   lacrimal, 293
Pupil
   constriction of, 205
   dilation of, 206

Ranvier nodes, 274, 334
Rectus muscles, 56–57, 319, 321, 322, 339
   blood supply of, 191
Red cells
   in canal of Schlemm, 252, 255, 258, 260, 268
   in conjunctival capillaries, 314
   in iris stromal vessels, 204
Reflex
   annular, 120

Reflex (*continued*)
   central foveal, 113, 116, 120
   macular ring, 120
Relucency zones, in corneal stroma, 171, 174
Residual bodies, 28
   in retinal pigment epithelium, 68, 70
Reticulin, 40
Reticulum
   endoplasmic, 20–23. *See also* Endoplasmic reticulum
   Heinrich-Müller, 239
   sarcoplasmic, 333, 335
Retina, 61–124
   area centralis of, 111
   avascular region of, 111, 112, 113
   capillaries of, 283
   embryology of, 61, 62
   fovea of, 111–113, 114, 115
   foveola of, 111, 113, 115, 116–118
   ganglion cell layer of, 72, 92, 93, 94
   glial system in, 70, 73
   Henle fibers of, 72
   limiting membrane of
     external, 72, 73, 74, 226, 229
     internal, 72, 73, 230
     middle, 72, 73
   macula lutea of, 118–124
   neovascularization of, 88
     at periphery, 220
     subretinal, 64
   nerve fiber layer of, 72
   neural (sensory), 70–124
     adhesion to pigment epithelium, 124
   neuronal system in, 70, 71–99
   nuclear layer of
     inner, 72
     outer, 72
   ora serrata of, 122, 124
   peripheral, 111
     cystoid degeneration of, 123, 124
   pigment epithelium of, 61–70
   plexiform layer of
     inner, 87, 90
     outer, 72
   receptor AMP in, 44
   separation from adjacent nerve fibers, 277, 278
   subretinal space, 124
     cul-de-sac of, 123, 124
   topographic variations in, 111
   vascular system in, 70, 73, 103–111
Retinal artery, central, 107, 278, 281–282, 283, 284, 285, 320, 321
Retinal layer, of optic nerve, 274–278, 280
Retinal vein, central, 278, 281–282, 283, 285
Retrolental space, of Berger, 140
Rhabdomyosarcoma, orbital, 320
Ribbon synapse
   bipolar, 90, 91, 92
   photoreceptor, 86, 87
Ribonucleoprotein, 22
Ribosomes, 21, 26
   in photoreceptors, 74
   in retinal pigment epithelium, 68
Ridge, synaptic, 87
Ring, Schwalbe, 183, 184
   anterior, 251, 268, 269
   posterior, 252
Riolan muscle, 293, 303

RNA
  messenger, 22
  ribosomal, 22
Rods and cones. *See* Photoreceptors
Roll, scleral, 252, 253
Root, of iris, 197
Rubeosis iridis, 198

Sac
  conjunctival, 320
  lacrimal, 307, 308
Saccharides, 41
Saccules, Golgi, 24
Sagittal plane of eye, 56
Sarcolemma, 327, 334, 335
Sarcomeres, 330, 335
Sarcoplasm, 330
Sarcoplasmic reticulum, 333, 335
Satellite cells, 327, 335, 336
Schiff reagent, 42
Schlemm canal, 185, 191, 252–261
  canaliculi from, 266, 268
  collector channels of, 260–261, 262
  drainage from, 246
  juxtacanalicular connective tissue, 257, 258, 260, 268
  red cells in, 252, 255, 258, 260, 268
Schmidt-Lantermann clefts, 324, 334, 338
Schultze fiber baskets, 99
Schwalbe ring or line, 183, 184
  anterior, 251, 268, 269
  posterior, 252
Schwann cells, 273, 334, 338
Sclera, 55, 186–192
  attachment to choroid, 215
  emissaria of, 187–191
  episclera, 191
  fetal, 189
  lamina fusca of, 192
  pigment spots of, 187, 191
  stroma of, 191–192
Scleral layer, of optic nerve, 278–281
Scleral roll, 183, 185, 191, 252, 253
  attachment to ciliary muscle, 215
Scleral spur, 259
Scleral sulcus or furrow
  inner, 251, 253
  outer, 251, 253
Sebaceous glands, of eyelids, 298
Sectioning of ocular tissue, 3–4
Septa
  of canal of Schlemm, 252
  orbital, 291, 321
  pial, 282–283
Shagreen, lens, 154
Sheaths, optic nerve, 281–282
Sheen, retinal, 97, 111
Sialoglycan, 74
Silver tetraphenylporphine sulfonate, for staining of elastin, 9
Sinus, angular, 251
Sjögren's syndrome, 319, 327
Skin, of eyelids, 294–298

Sodium pump, in cell membrane, 20
Sondermann canals, 266
Space
  intercellular, 33
  intertrabecular, 265–266
  subarachnoid, 281, 282
  subdural, 281
  suprachoroidal, 215–216
  transtrabecular, 265
Sphenoid bone, 317, 318
Sphenopalatine ganglion, 318
Spherule
  calcific, in corneal basement membrane, 178, 181
  rod, 83, 85, 86, 87
Sphincter muscle, of iris, 203–206
Spiral of Tillaux, 57, 319
Spot
  Bitot, 310
  cherry-red, 116
Spurs
  Fuchs, 204, 205
  Michel, 205, 206
  scleral, 259
Staining of tissue, for electron microscopy, 9
Stars, macular, 122
Stevens-Johnson syndrome, 319
Strabismus, 319–320
Striae, pigmented, of pars plana, 226
Stroma
  choroidal, 216–226
  corneal, 169–171
  of iris, 198, 202–203
  scleral, 191–192
Strut, optic, 317
Subretinal space, 124
  cul-de-sac of, 123, 124
Substantia propria
  conjunctival, 307, 308, 309
  of limbus, 186
Sulcus
  orbitopalpebral, 291, 293
  scleral
    inner, 251, 253
    outer, 251, 253
Suture lines, lens, 149
Sweat glands, of lids, 291, 298
Synapse
  chemical, 87
  electrical, 87
  ribbon
    bipolar, 90, 91, 92
    photoreceptor, 86, 87
Synaptic densities, 87
Synaptic expansions
  bipolar cell, 90
  photoreceptor, 83–87
    in fovea, 118
Synaptic ridge, 87
Synaptic vesicles, 83, 85, 86, 335
  halo of, 86, 87

Tarsal muscle. *See* Müller muscle
Tarsus of eyelid, 299, 304, 305, 320

Tear film, of cornea, 163
Tears, lysozyme in, 326, 327
Temporal artery, 107, 293
Temporal veins, 293
Tenon's capsule, 191, 318, 320, 321, 322
Terminal bar region, 33–34
    apical portion of, 34
    basilar portion of, 34
    of capillary endothelial cells, 105
    of ciliary body epithelial cells, 226
    of iris blood vessels, 202
    junctional complex in, 34
    of retinal limiting membrane, external, 81, 82, 83
    of retinal pigment epithelium, 63, 64, 65, 66
Thiosemicarbazide, for glycogen detection, 9
Thrombosis, cavernous sinus, 322
Tillaux spiral, 57, 319
Tissue preparation, for transmission electron micros-
        copy, 3–4
    for scanning electron microscopy, 7
Tonofibrils, 33
    in corneal epithelium, 164
Tonofilaments, 33
    in conjunctival epithelium, 310, 311
    in corneal epithelium, 164
    in lid epidermis, 296, 297, 298
    in meibomian glands, 306, 308
    in Moll gland cells, 299
Trabeculae, iris, 198, 200
Trabecular meshwork, 261–269
Tracers, for studies of transport mechanisms, 10
Transport mechanisms, intracellular, tracers for studies
        of, 10
Trigeminal nerve, sensory nucleus of, 324
Trochlear nerve, 322, 323
Tropocollagen, 39
Tubes, aqueous, 266
Tubules. See Microtubules
Tumors. See also Melanoma
    of lacrimal gland, 326–327
    orbital rhabdomyosarcoma, 320

Uveal tract, 55, 197–245
    choroid, 215–226
    ciliary body, 225, 226–245
    episcleral tissue, 187
    iris, 197–214
    melanin granules in, 26
    nevi in scleral canals, 187
    venous drainage from, 246
Uveitis, sympathetic, 187

Vacuoles
    digestive, 28
    lipid, in orbital fat cells, 341
    secretion, 29
Vasculature. See Blood supply
Veins
    aqueous, of Ascher, 191, 261, 263
    ciliary
        anterior, 246

Veins, ciliary (continued)
        passage in sclera, 191
    cilioretinal, 283
    facial, 293
    intrascleral plexus, 261, 262
    opthalmic, 293
    orbital, 322
    retinal, central, 278, 281–282, 283, 285
    temporal, 293
    vortex, 56, 216, 246
        passage in sclera, 191, 215
Venules, retinal, 104, 107, 110, 111
Vesicles
    agranular, flattened, 24
    coated, 24
    membrane-coating, in epidermis of lids, 298
    micropinocytotic
        of canal of Schlemm, 257, 258
        of capillary endothelial cells, 105, 107
    optic, 61
    synaptic, 83, 85, 86, 335
Villi
    of canal of Schlemm, 252, 257, 258
    of capillary endothelial cells, 105
    of corneal endothelial cells, 178, 179
    of lacrimal gland acini, 325, 329
    of lacrimal gland duct cells, 332
    of Müller cell, 99
    of retinal pigment epithelium, 64, 68, 76
Vitrein, 132
Vitreous body, 131–144
    acid mucopolysaccharide in, 232, 233
    anterior attachments of, 138–140
    base of, 138, 139, 230
    boundaries of, 134
    central or medullary zone of, 140
    cortical zone of, 134, 138, 140–141
    embryology of, 131
    face of
        anterior, 140, 153, 232
        posterior, 138, 139
    fibrous component of, 132
    filaments of, 132
        aggregation into fibers, 141
        anterior, 140
        posterior, 134, 135
    hyaloid of
        anterior, 140
        posterior, 136, 137
    lateral attachments of, 138
    modifications in, 141–144
    mucinous component of, 134
    posterior attachments of, 134–138
        retracted, 136–137
    zones of, 140–141
Vitreous compartment, 251, 252
Vitrosin, 132
Vogt palisades, 310
Vortex veins, 56, 216, 246
    passage in sclera, 191, 215

Walls, orbital, 317–318
Warts

Warts (*continued*)
    Hassall-Henle, 176, 179, 182
    of pars plicata, 226, 237
Wieger ligament, 140
Wing cell layer, of cornea, 164, 166
Wolfring gland, 291, 309, 319

Z-line, of myofibrils, 330, 335
Zeis gland, 163, 291, 298, 299, 300
Zinn annulus, 319, 321, 322
Zinn-Haller circle, 281, 283
Zinn zonule, 141
Zones
    limbal, 183
    vitreous body, 140–141
Zonula adherens, 34
    of canal of Schlemm, 252, 256
    of capillary endothelial cells, 105, 106
    of choriocapillaris endothelial cells, 219

Zonula adherens (*continued*)
    of ciliary epithelial cells, 227, 228
    of lacrimal gland acini, 325, 329
    of lacrimal gland duct cells, 332
    of retinal limiting membrane, external, 82, 83
    of retinal pigment epithelium, 63, 64, 65, 66, 67
Zonula occludens, 34
    of capillary endothelial cells, 105
    of choriocapillaris endothelial cells, 219
    of ciliary epithelial cells, 227, 228
    of lacrimal gland acini, 325, 329
    of lacrimal gland duct cells, 332
    of retinal pigment epithelium, 63, 64, 65, 66, 67
Zonular fibers
    cilioequatorial, 144
    of lens, 40, 153
    orbiculoanterior, 144
    orbiculoposterior, 144
    of vitreous body, 141–144
Zonules, lens, 153
Zygomatic bone, 317
Zygomatic nerve, 319
Zymogenic granules, in lacrimal gland acini, 352, 327